NEW FRONTIERS IN
MAMMARY PATHOLOGY

NEW FRONTIERS IN
MAMMARY PATHOLOGY

Edited by
K. H. Hollmann
Marie-Lannelongue Surgical Center
Le Plessis Robinson, France

J. de Brux
Institute of Pathology and Applied Cytology
Paris, France

and
J. M. Verley
Marie-Lannelongue Surgical Center
Le Plessis Robinson, France

PLENUM PRESS · NEW YORK AND LONDON

Library of Congress Cataloging in Publication Data

Main entry under title:

New frontiers in mammary pathology.

Bibliography: p.
Includes index.
1. Breast—Diseases. 2. Breast—Cancer. I. Hollmann, K. H. II. Brux, Jean de. III.
Verley, J. M. [DNLM: 1. Breast neoplasms—Pathology—Congresses. 2. Breast neo-
plasms—Therapy—Congresses. WP 870 N533 1979]
RG491.N48   618.1'9   81-1547
ISBN 978-1-4757-0021-3   ISBN 978-1-4757-0019-0 (eBook)   AACR2
DOI 10.1007/978-1-4757-0019-0

Proceedings of the first Symposium on Mammary Pathology,
organized by the International Society against Breast Cancer,
and held December 3—7, 1979, in Paris, France

© 1981 Plenum Press, New York
Softcover reprint of the hardcover 1st edition 1981

A Division of Plenum Publishing Corporation
233 Spring Street, New York, N.Y. 10013

PREFACE

The first Symposium on Mammary Pathology organized
by the International Society against Breast Cancer was
held in Paris on December 3-7, 1979.

The programme was divided into sections with morning
lectures on current topics in mammary pathology given
by invited speakers, followed by discussions, and, in
the afternoon, emphasis on practical work, such as slide
seminars, technical explanations of tissue and cell
preparations for histology, cytology, electron microscopy
and tissue culture work.

The morning sessions were held at the Racing Club
of France, 5 rue Eblé, 75007 Paris and the organizers
of the meeting wish to thank the RCF and its President,
Mr. R. Menard for their kindness and generous help in
the arrangement of the symposium.

The afternoon workshops took place at the Institut
de Pathologie et de Cytologie Appliquée (Director
Professor J. de Brux), rue des Belles Feuilles, Paris XVI,
with the help of staff members from this Institute.

The editors of the Proceedings of the Symposium wish
to thank the contributors for their help in providing
manuscripts for publication and for complying with the
instructions given by the editors and the Plenum Publishing Company. Financial supports provided by the Ligue
Nationale Française contre le Cancer and the FEGEFLUC
are gratefully acknowledged. It is hoped that the present
volume will provide stimuli for future work on clinical
and basic research in mammary pathology.

K. H. Hollmann

CONTENTS

MAMMARY GLAND DIFFERENTIATION AND HORMONAL INFLUENCES

K.H. Hollmann

Hopital Marie-Lannelongue
133 avenue de la Résistance
92350 Le Plessis Robinson, France

Phylogenetically, mammary glands appeared in the animal kingdom about 100 million years ago, when the era of the egg-laying dinosaurs declined. At this time milk secretion became vital for the nourishment of an immature offspring and has remained so until our times. For only a few decades has the modern technical world increasingly replaced suckling by artificial nutrition.

Mammary glands are paired organs. Their number is grossly related to the number of newborns and varies from species to species and even in the same species, e.g., in rodents from 2 (guinea pig) to 14 (hamster) (for details see Anderson, 1978).

The fundamental architecture of the gland consists of dichotomically branching ducts and terminal lobules. The main ducts or galactophores originate in the nipple. In some mammals, as in the cow, there is only one galactophore (opening) per teat, whereas in others, as in humans, there are 15 and more (up to 25).

Each galactophore in the mature animal arises embryologically from a primary sprout as represented in Fig. 1, redrawn from Anderson (1978).

Different developmental stages may be distinguished in the following sequence : Band - streak - line-crest-hillock-bud-early teat formation - primary sprout - secondary sprout - canalization of primary sprout (= formation of galactophore).

1

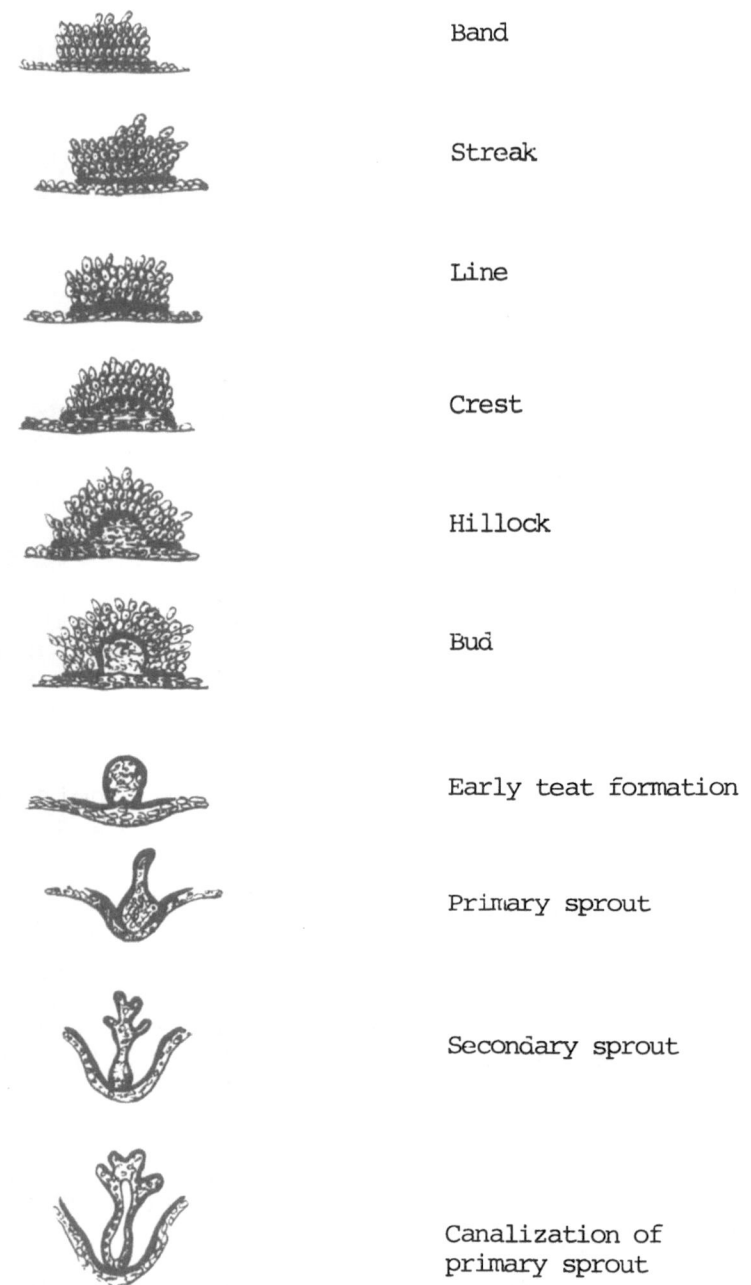

Band

Streak

Line

Crest

Hillock

Bud

Early teat formation

Primary sprout

Secondary sprout

Canalization of
primary sprout

Fig. 1. Sequential steps in mammary gland development. Schematic
representation from histologic cross sections.
(Redrawn from Anderson, 1978).

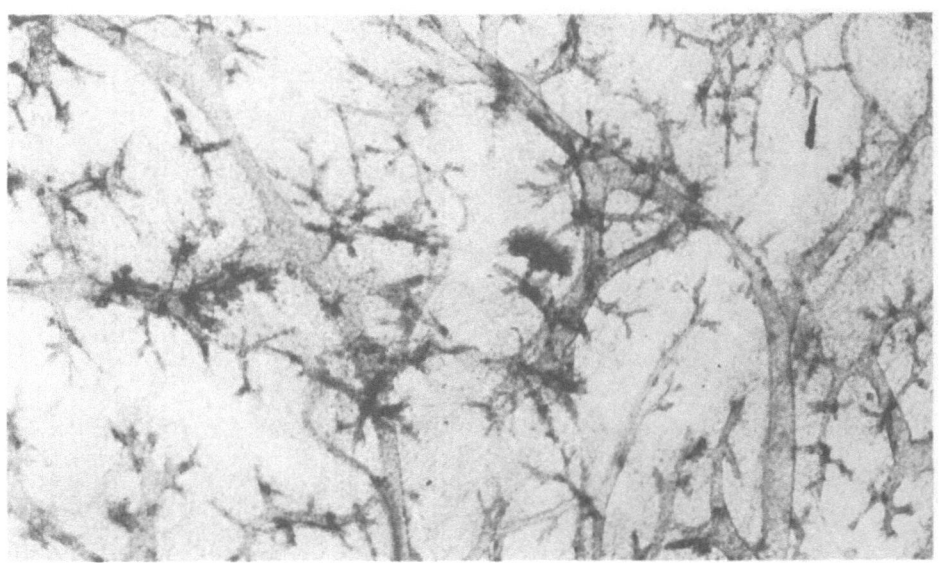

Fig. 2. Unstimulated mammary tree with branching ducts but almost no alveoli. (Whole mount, x 28).

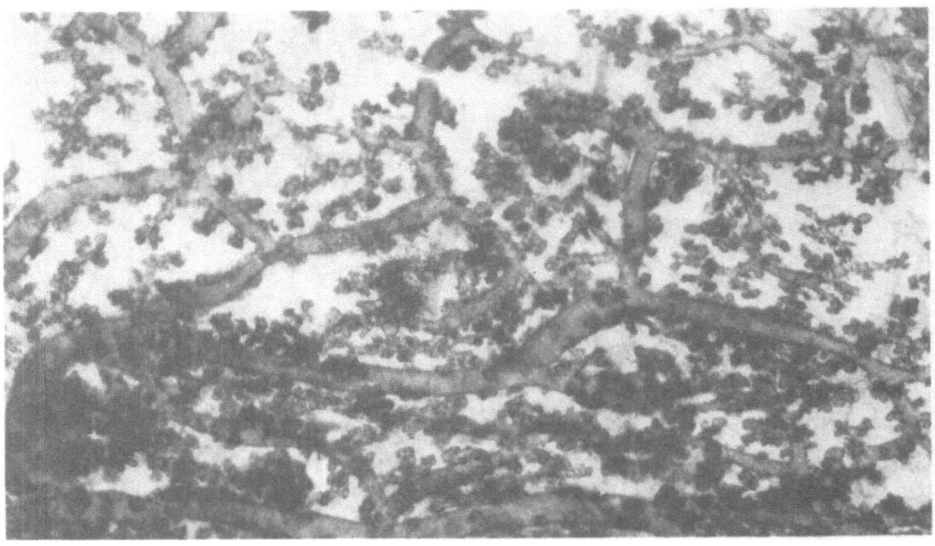

Fig. 3. Stimulated mammary tree with developing alveoli under the hormonal influence of beginning pregnancy. (Whole mount, x 16).

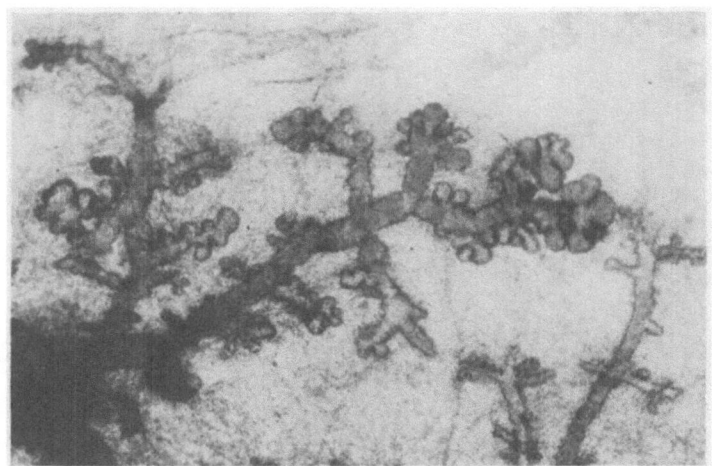

Fig. 4. Formation of terminal lobules in a hormonally stimulated
gland. (Whole mount, x 33).

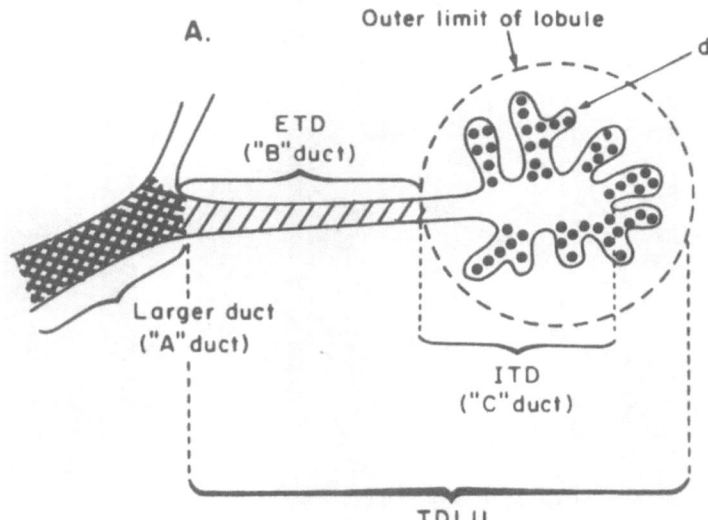

Fig. 5. Terminal ductal lobular unit (TDLU). (Slightly modified
from Wellings and Wolfe, 1978).
ETD = extralobular terminal duct
ITD = intralobular terminal duct
 d = ductule (or acinus / alveolus)
A, B, C, D indicate ducts of different (decreasing) size.

The branching ducts terminate in lobules, each of which being made up of numerous alveoli (Fig. 2 - 4). This basic organization is schematically represented in Fig. 5 (from Wellings and Wolfe, 1978).

The portion called "terminal ductal lobular unit" (TDLU) is particularly hormone-dependent and undergoes throughout life repeated modifications comprising differentiation and dedifferentiation. The continuous changes which take place in the TDLU during the different phases of mammary activity may account for a great deal of pathologic processes encountered at this site of the mammary tree (see Wellings et al., this vol.).

Ducts and alveoli are covered with glandular and myoepithelial cells. The larger ducts have a double-layered epithelium, the smaller ones and the alveoli a single layered covering. Gland cells in the distal portion of the mammary tree (alveoli) are more sensitive to hormonal stimulation than those in the proximal portion (larger ducts). If mammary gland cells become stimulated by adequate hormones they elaborate the different constituents of milk. The characteristic fine structure of mammary gland cells is very similar from one species to another although the composition of the different milks varies widely. As an example, horse or rhinoceros milk contains only traces of lipids, whereas the whale milk contains more than 50 %. Likewise, the protein content varies in different species from 1 to 20 % (it is low in primates and high in rabbits), as well as lactose levels (low in cetaceans, high in cows, etc).

As noted by Jenness (1979) the milk composition of only a few species is really well known, whereas it is totally unknown in about 4,000 species. This is also the case as far as the morphology of mammary glands is concerned and in particular their fine structure. Since the first description of the fine structure of the mammary epithelium of the rat by Bargmann and Knoop (1959) and of the mouse by Hollmann (1959) numerous investigations were devoted to the different aspects of functional activity and pathological modifications but only few other species such as the guinea pig, cow, goat, human were included.

Nevertheless, the knowledge accumulated in two decades has shown the intricate relationship between structure and function and has widened our insight in basic processes of mammary physiology, pathology and carcinogenesis.

Physiologic growth as well as pathological proliferations are under the influence of hormones. The relevant
hormones were studied in vitro and in vivo. In organ
culture studies, the respective role of insulin, corti-
costeroids and prolactin on growth and differentiation
of the mammary tree was studied and the following schematic representation was proposed (Fig. 6). Insulin alone
accelerates growth of the primary sprout but its action
is limited and it needs the presence of prolactin to
stimulate further growth and development. These two hormones combined with aldosterone promote ductal branching
and differentiation and the addition of progesterone
induces cell proliferation and secretion.

The hormonal action at the cellular level was followed
by Mills and Topper (1970) (Fig. 7). These authors studied
the effect of insulin, cortisol and prolactin on the fine
structure of mammary gland cells in vitro and found that
insulin alone for 96 h. had no effect at all. If administered together with cortisol for 96 h. it increased
slightly the amount of ergastoplasm. But only when prolactin is added to the two hormones does complete

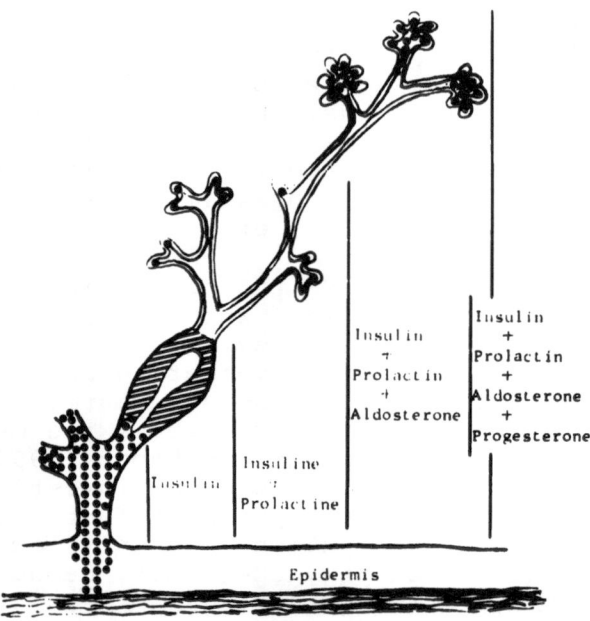

Fig. 6.   Diagram based on in vitro experiments indica-
          ting hormonal effects upon growth and diffe-
          rentiation of the mammary tree.
          (After Ceriani, 1970, taken from Anderson,
          1974).

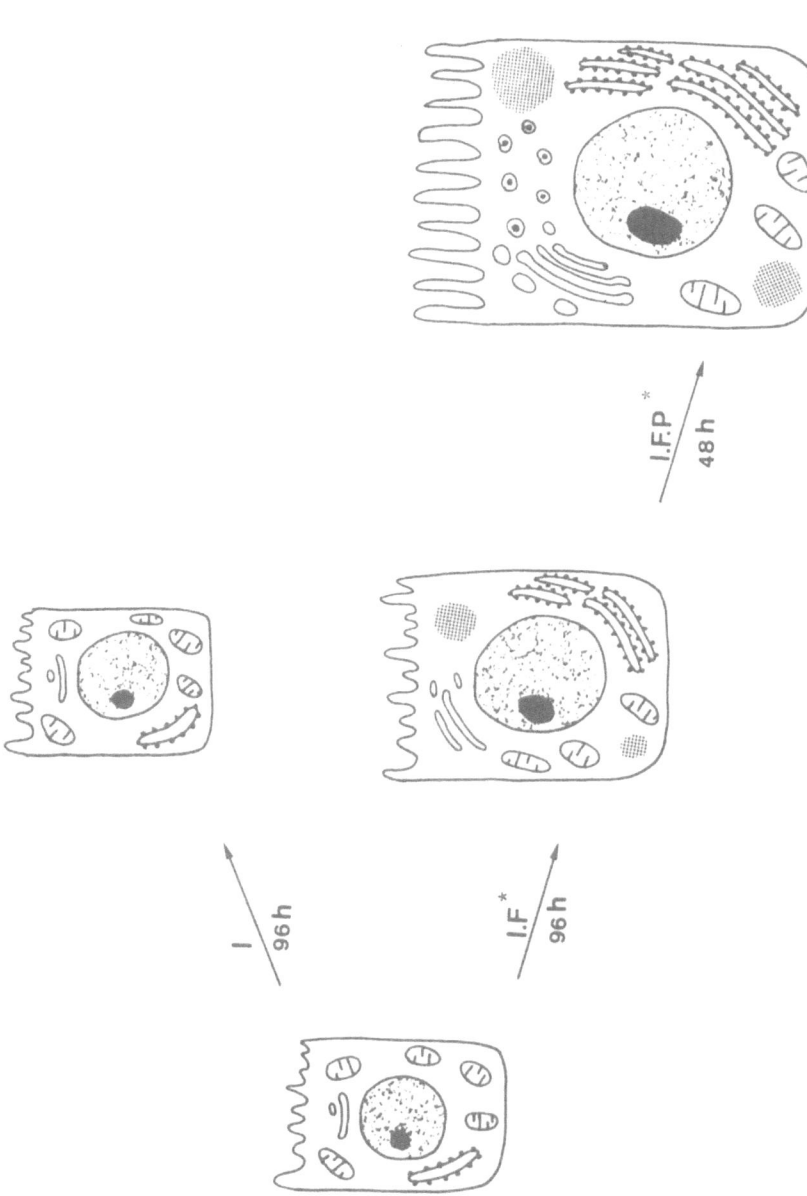

Fig. 7. Schematic representation of ultrastructural modifications in the glandular epithelium of explants of midpregnant mouse mammary tissues cultured in a synthetic medium with added hormones. I = Insulin, F = Hydrocortisone, P = Prolactin. (Modified after Mills and Topper, 1970).

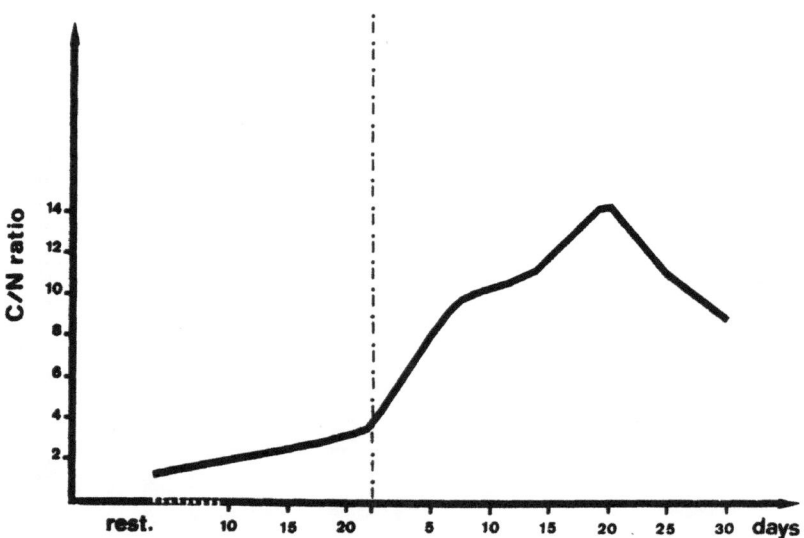

Fig. 8. Cytoplasmic-nuclear ratio (C/N) in mouse mammary gland
cells during different stages of secretory activity. The
relative amount of cytoplasm progressively increases from
pregnancy until the second half of lactation.

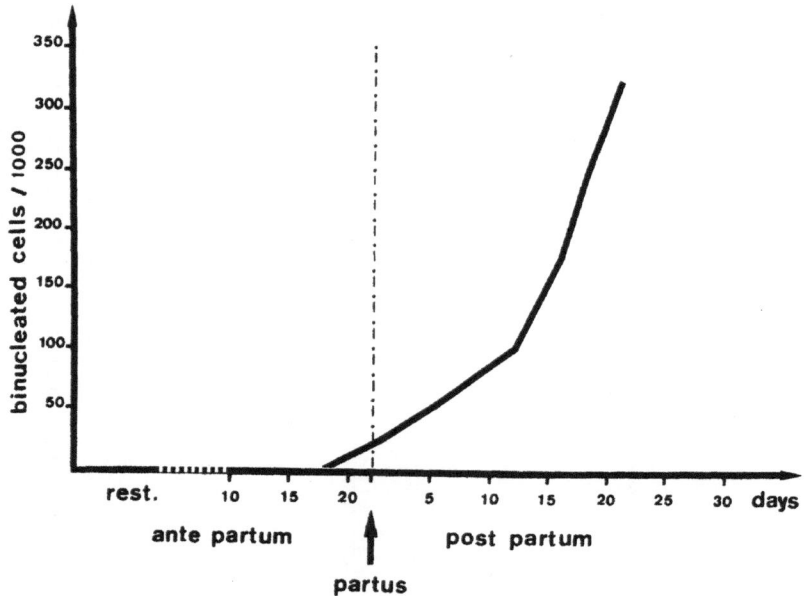

Fig. 9. The appearance of binucleated cells goes hand in hand with
the increase of the C/N ratio, reflecting the high functional activity of the cells about the 20th day of lactation.
(data from Kriesten, 1965).

development of ergastoplasm and the appearance of secretory activity occur. In vivo experiments demonstrated a similar situation. Wellings and Nandi (1968) treated ovari- adrenal- hypophysectomized mice and showed that a combination of MH, STH and a glucocorticoid (hydrocortisone or cortisone) is necessary to induce lactogenesis, almost indistinguishable from lactogenesis in intact animals.

STRUCTURE OF MAMMARY CELLS

As the different parts of the mammary tree respond in a different manner to hormonal stimulation, the structure of the mammary epithelium also differs from the main ducts to the distal ductuli.

Primary and secondary ducts are lined by cells with scalloped nuclei and a small rim of cytoplasm. They contain few, rather small mitochondria, an inconspicuous Golgi apparatus, free ribosomes and some rare ergastoplasmic cisternae.

Cells of tertiary ducts have more ergastoplasm (RER) and undergo, like alveolar cells, differentiation during pregnancy and become truly secreting (Sehkri et al., 1967).

Alveolar secretory cells are rapidly changing structures depending on the hormonal milieu. At the resting stage they differ from duct cells insofar as their cytoplasm is richer, their mitochondria, their ergastoplasm and their Golgi apparatus more developed. The apical membrane bordering the small acinar lumen is covered with short microvilli.

Under appropriate hormonal stimulation as during pregnancy and lactation the resting cells undergo differentiation. The cells become larger and the nuclei bigger and rounder. The cytoplasm increases and the cytoplasmic-nuclear ratio shifts, slightly until parturition, then profoundly during lactation (Fig. 8). This modification is paralelled by the appearance of binucleated cells as represented in fig. 9, according to Kriesten (1965).

Kriesten believes that the binucleated cells originate from amitotic divisions and that they reflect an increased functional activity of the epithelium. According to Saake and Heald (1974) this condition indicates that lateral plasmalemmas may break down without interrupting cell function but the authors do not exclude the

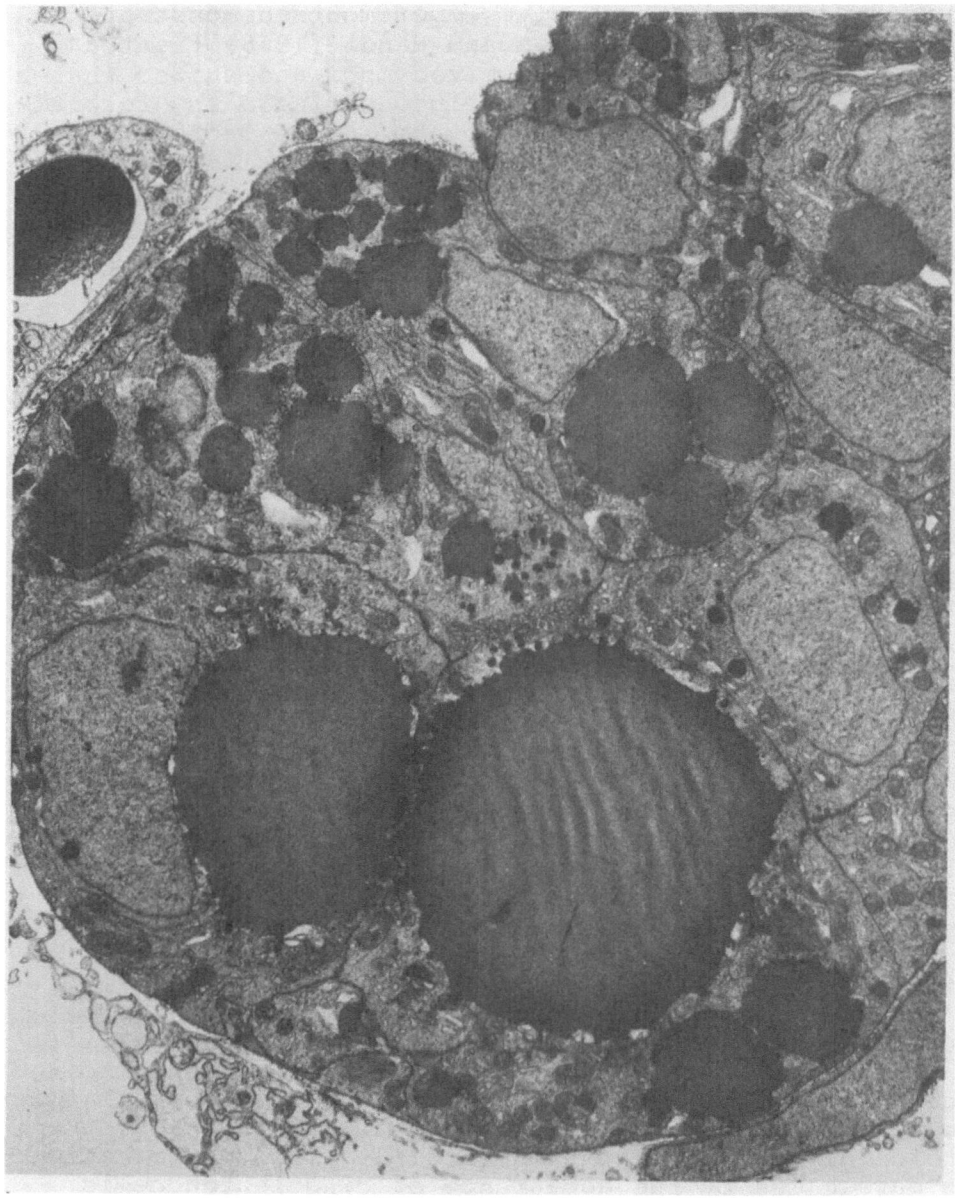

Fig. 10. Mouse mammary gland cells at the end of the
first half of pregnancy. The cells show a predominant elaboration and intracellular accumulation of lipid droplets, whereas others elaborate
and accumulate protein granules (Fig. 11).
(Electron micrograph, Lead citrate, x 7,500).

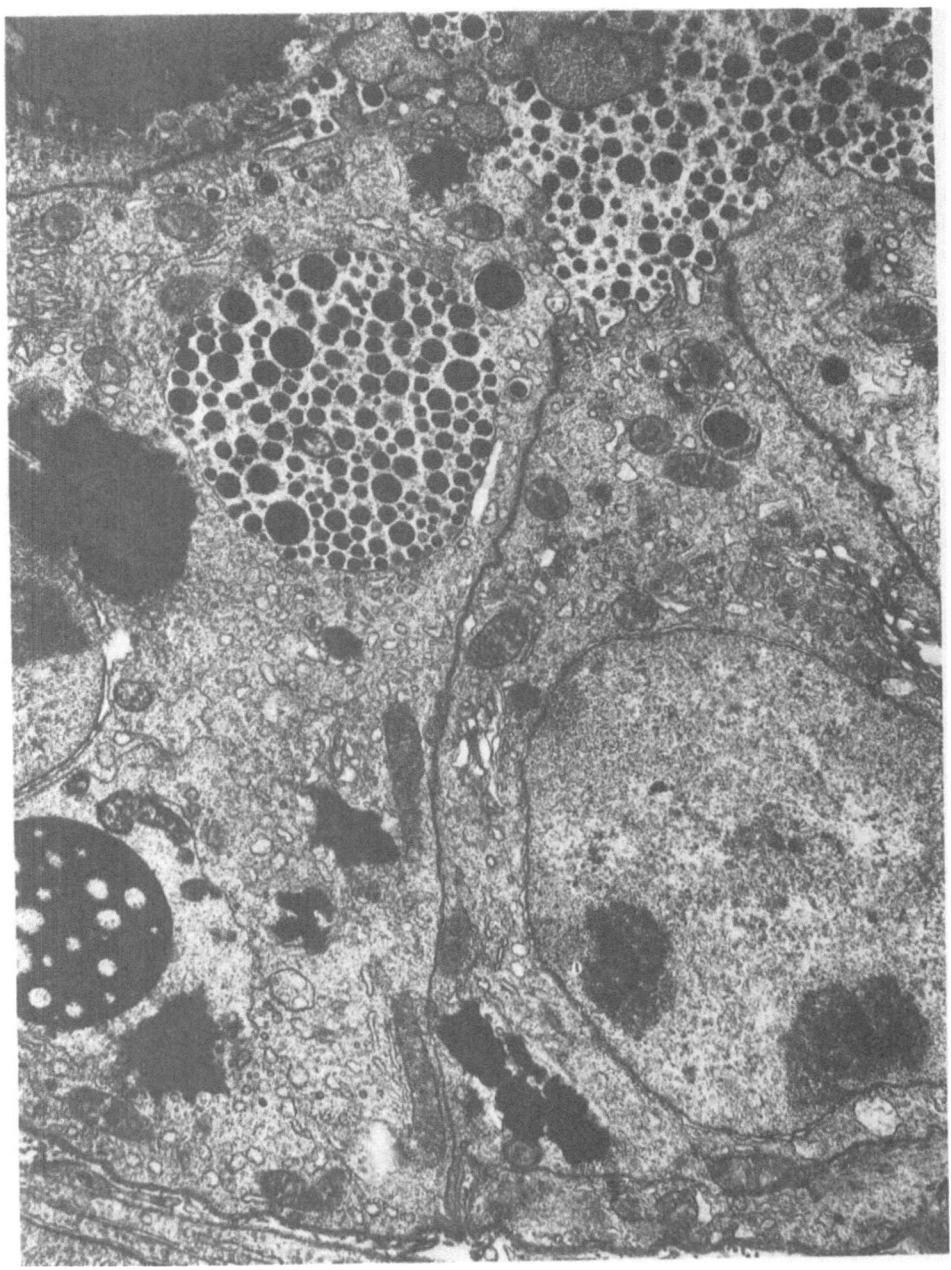

Fig. 11. Elaboration and stasis of protein granules at
the end of the first half of pregnancy. Compare
with fig. 10. (Electron micrograph, Lead citrate,
x 17,500).

possibility that such modifications may be an artefact
due to tissue preparation.

In any case the binucleated cells do not seem to
arise from mitosis, since mitotic divisions are frequent
during the growth of the mammary tree in the course of
pregnancy, but they are rare or almost absent during
lactation. In the rat mammary gland their number is less
than 0.1 % (Franke and Keenan, 1979).

The main cellular modification induced by the hormonal stimulus during pregnancy and lactation is the
development of the mitochondria, the ergastoplasm and the
Golgi elements.

At the same time, secretion phenomena appear. In the
mouse, at the end of the first half of pregnancy milk
fat droplets and casein granules appear in the cytoplasm
of the glandular cells which are ready for secretion
whereas others remain inactive (Figs. 10 and 11).

During the second half of pregnancy, the cellular
differentiation continues as can be clearly shown by
quantitative measurements. Ergastoplasm, mitochondria and
Golgi apparatus increase in surface and volume and the
secretory activity intensifies.

At the time of delivery, when most of the glandular
cells are ready for secretion, the complete cytoplasmic
differentiation is not yet accomplished, but will continue during the course of lactation, reflecting the increasing secretory activity of the epithelium. The
period preceding delivery is characterized by an increasing stasis of secretory material inside the cells as
shown by the measurement of fat droplet volume as a
percentage of cytoplasmic volume (Fig. 12). Immediately
before delivery the fat droplet volume attains up to
40 % of the cytoplasmic volume (Fig. 13). With parturition the stored secretory material is rapidly expelled
in the alveolar lumina and the intracellular fat droplet
volume falls sharply (Fig. 12). During lactation, when
the mammary gland is regularly emptied by suckling or by
milking (Fig. 14) the fat droplet volume inside the
cells amounts to about 10 % of the cytoplasmic volume.

The cell differentiation occurring physiologically
under the hormonal influences of pregnancy and lactation
can be followed by quantitative measurements (morphome-
try) of the ergastoplasm (RER), Golgi apparatus and
mitochondria.

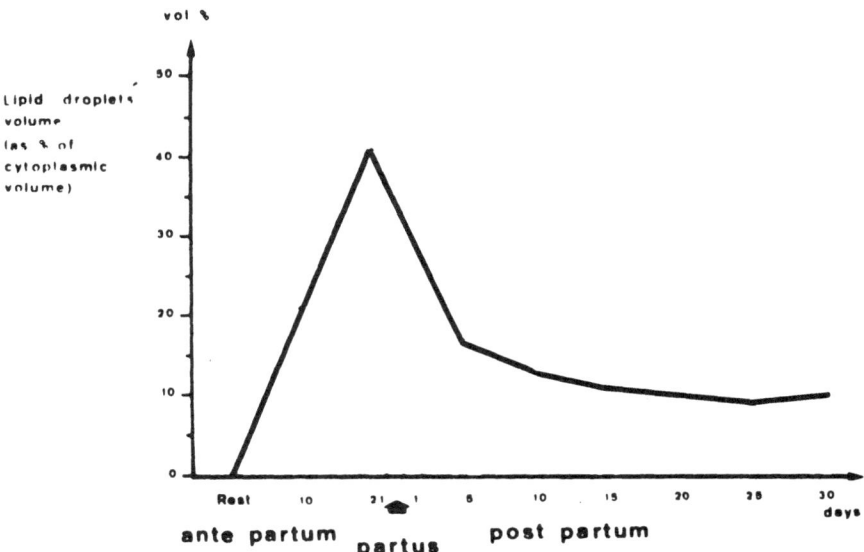

Fig. 12. Milk fat droplet volume in mouse mammary gland
          cells during pregnancy and lactation. The
          droplet volume is expressed as a percentage of
          the cytoplasmic volume (nucleus excluded). A
          peak of fat droplet accumulation is observed
          just before delivery (about 40 % of the cyto-
          plasmic volume). During lactation the milk
          fat droplets occupy about 10 % of the cyto-
          plasmic volume.

     The mitochondrial development comprising a large
increase in number, size and internal structure, is related to the increasing intensity in oxydative metabolism.
Epithelial cells from the mammary gland of virgin mice
contain few mitochondria of small size and poor organization. During pregnancy mitochondria increase in number
and become more complex in structure. Their matrix
darkens and the cristae increase in number and become
more closely arranged. This development continues during
the first days of lactation (Wellings et al., 1960)
(Figs 15 and 16). Incorporation of ^{3}H-Thymidine into mitochondrial DNA of mouse mammary gland cells was studied
by Sarma (1974) and shows the profile of fig. 17. From
morphology and marker studies Jones (1978) concluded
that the major mitochondrial replication phase is essentially coincident with cell proliferation. This is consistent with morphometric data (Hollmann, 1974) which
show an increase in mitochondrial volume during the
same period during which mitoses are frequent (Fig. 18).

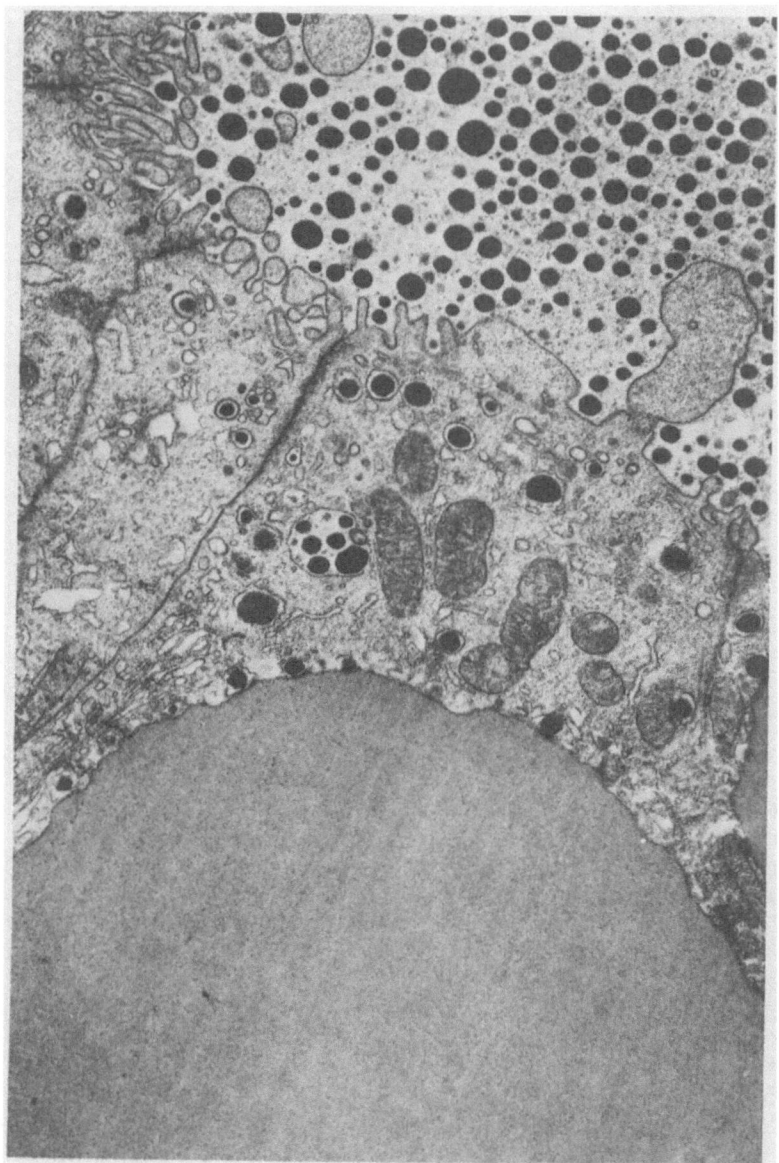

Fig. 13. Mouse mammary gland cells at the end of pregnancy.
Note large lipid droplet and casein granules
inside the cytoplasm. (Electron micrograph,
Lead citrate, x 17,500).

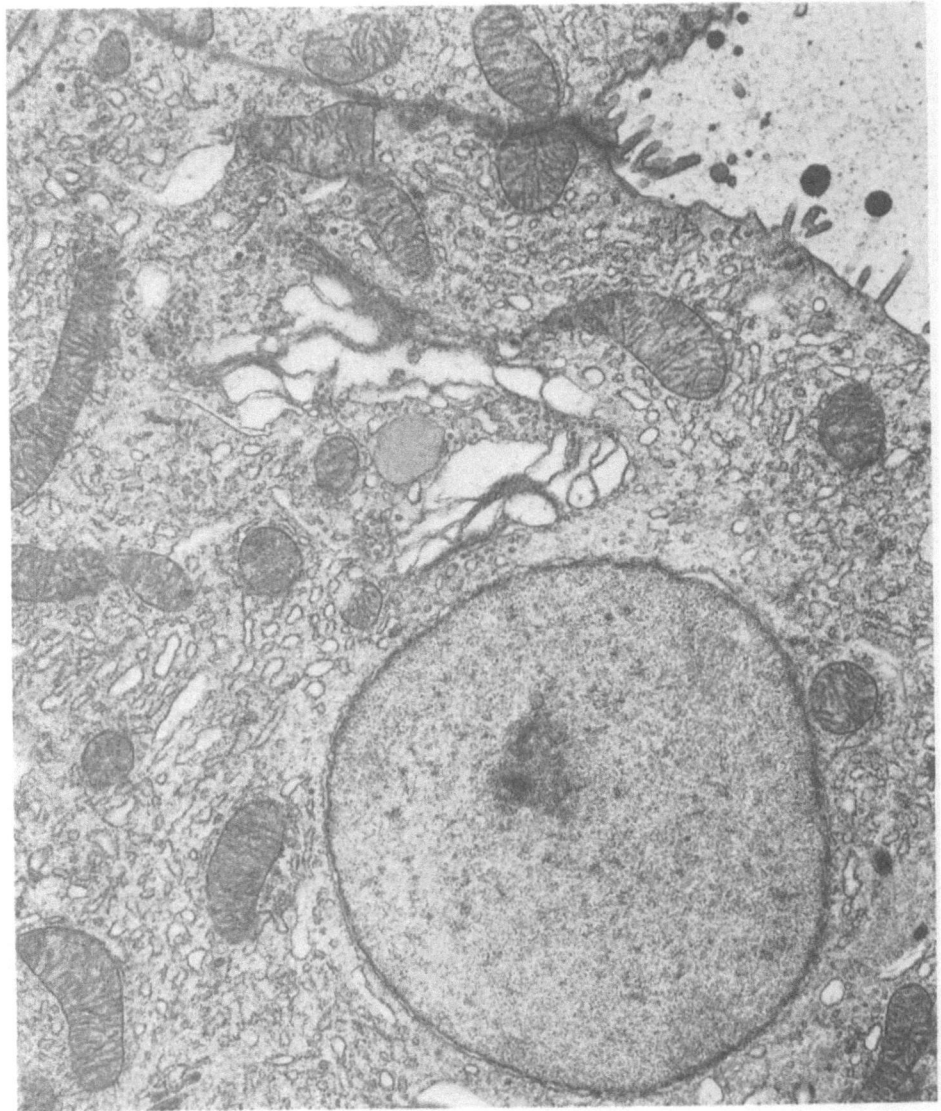

Fig. 14. Mammary gland cell at full lactation. As the gland is regularly emptied by suckling or milking, there is no stasis of secretory material inside the cytoplasm. (Electron micrograph, Lead citrate, x 18,000).

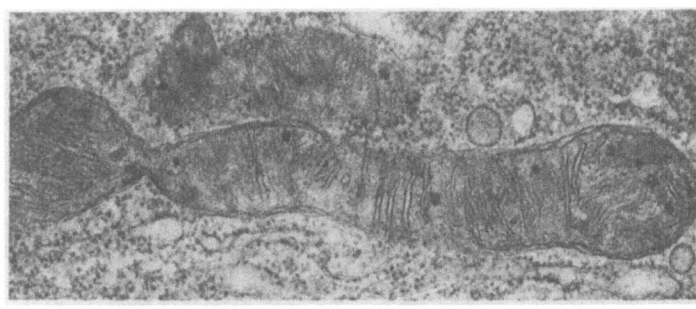

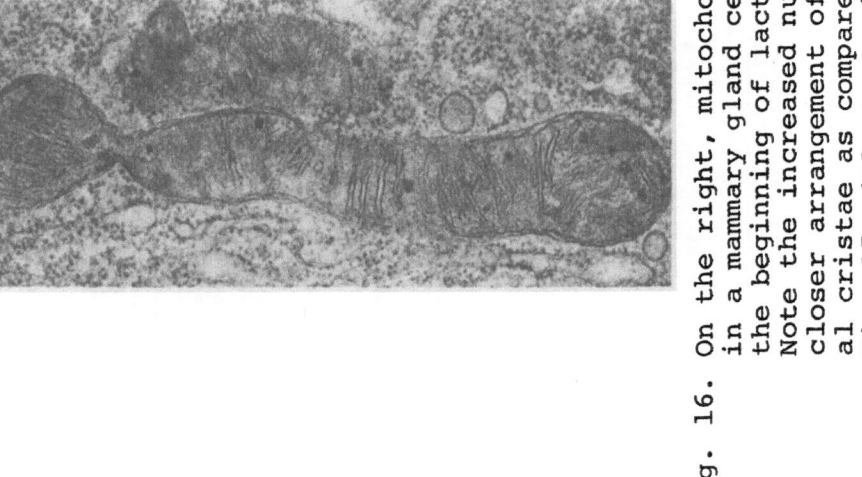

Fig. 16. On the right, mitochondrium in a mammary gland cell at the beginning of lactation. Note the increased number and closer arrangement of internal cristae as compared with Fig. 15. (Electron micrograph Lead citrate, x 72,000.

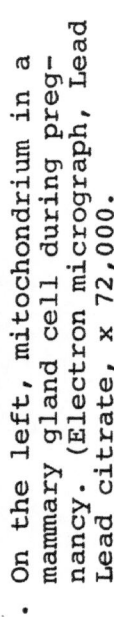

Fig. 15. On the left, mitochondrium in a mammary gland cell during pregnancy. (Electron micrograph, Lead Lead citrate, x 72,000.

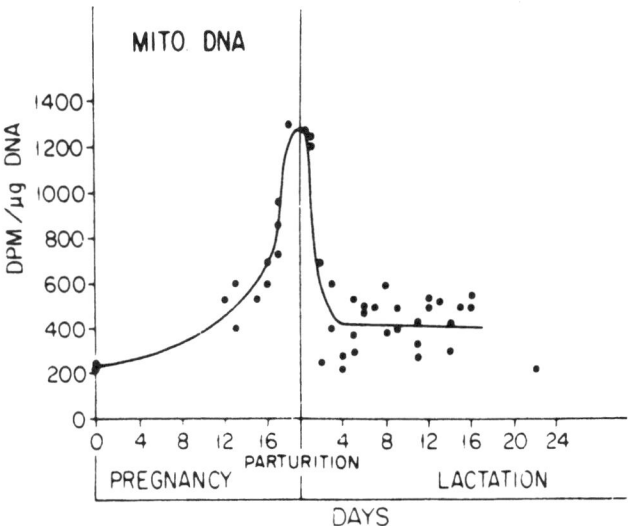

Fig. 17. The diagram indicates the rates of tritiated thymidine
         incorporation into mitochondrial DNA in the mouse mammary
         gland during pregnancy and lactation. (From Sarma, 1974,
         taken from Jones, 1978).

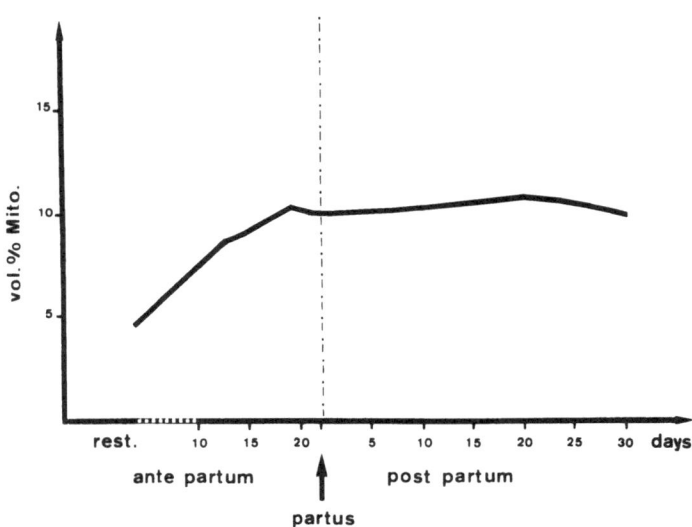

Fig. 18. The curve illustrates the increase of mitochondrial
         volume (as a percentage of cytoplasmic volume, nucleus
         excluded) during the same period in the mouse. (From
         Hollmann, 1974).

The half life of mitochondrial DNA as measured by labeling with ^{3}H-Thymidine was found to be seven days (Sarma,
1974) and was thus considerably shorter than that of
total cellular DNA, indicating that the mitochondria have
a more dynamic turnover than the epithelial cell proliferation (Jones, 1978).

Morphometric measurements have shown that the relative mitochondrial volume (as a percentage of the cytoplasmic volume, nucleus excluded, and not as a percentage
of the cellular volume as quoted by Jones, 1978) rises
from 4 % at the resting stage to about 8 % during mid-
pregnancy and approximately 10 % at the end of pregnancy,
remaining constant at this level until the end of lactation. During the same time the cytoplasmic-nuclear ratio
increases up to 12-fold. This means that the cytoplasmic
volume would increase 12-fold if the nuclear volume remained unchanged during the same period. But since the
latter also increases, the absolute volume of the cytoplasm is higher than 12-times that of the resting cell.
This should be considered if an attempt is made to evaluate the real increase of the mitochondrial population.
The curve in fig. 18 is only a measure of the mitochondrial volume as a percentage of the cytoplasmic volume
and does not take in account the number, the size and
the shape of the mitochondria. Changes in the latter
parameters during the different phases of mammary gland
activity have already been thoroughly described in the
rat fifty years ago (Weatherford, 1929). In the gland
of the virgin rat the mitochondria are mostly spherical.
During pregnancy, they increase in number and become
elongated and during lactation more and more filamentous
forms appear and become the predominant form during full
lactation. During this time the mitochondria have more
cristae and more electron dense matrix than in the prelactating state (Figs. 15 and 16) (Rosano et al., 1976).
These modifications of the internal structure are probably responsable for the increase in mitochondrial density on sucrose gradients, which rises from 1.18 to
1.20 gm/cm^3 from late pregnancy to day 8 of lactation in
the mouse (Rosano and Jones, 1976).

The ergastoplasmic development is the most spectacular change occurring during pregnancy and lactation.
Its surface can be measured (in μm^2 per μm^3 of cytoplasm) and rises from about 1.2 $\mu m^2/\mu m^3$ of cytoplasm at
the resting stage to 2.4 $\mu m^2/\mu m^3$ at mid-pregnancy, and
up to 5.3 $\mu m^2/\mu m^3$ at full lactation (5th day). This seems
to be the highest density per unit volume of cytoplasm

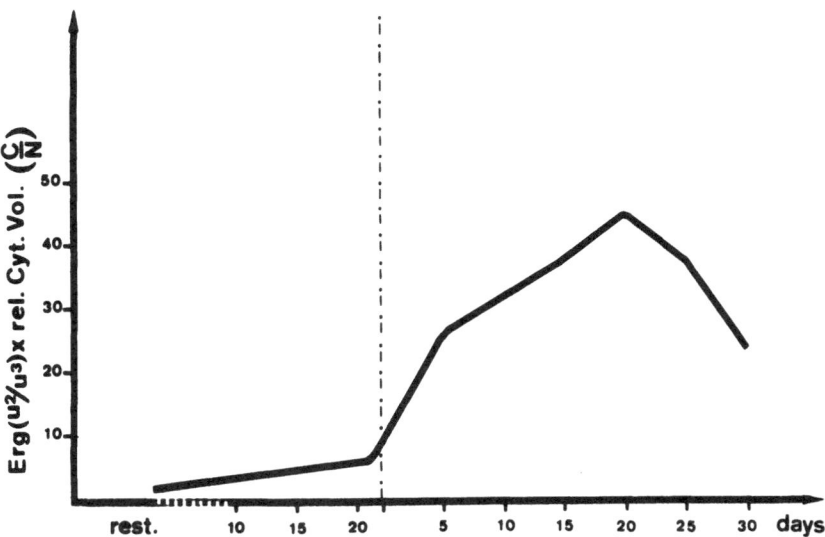

Fig. 19. The curve is an approximate expression of the
increase of total ergastoplasm in mouse mammary
cells, taking into account the value of μm^2 erg/
μm^3 cyto and the C/N ratio. There is a continuous increase until the 20th day of lactation.

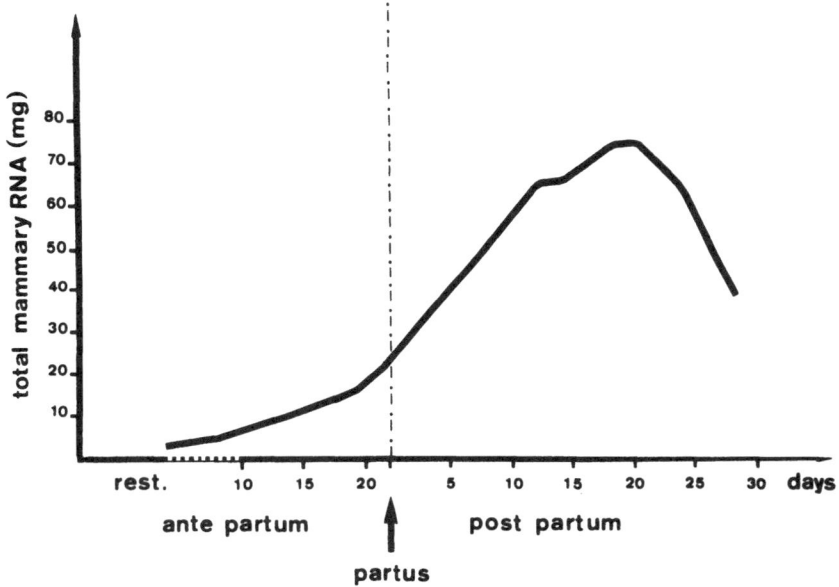

Fig. 20. This curve, illustrating the biochemically determined RNA content in mammary glands of rats
during the same period, parallels the curve of
fig. 19. (From Tucker, 1974).

but the absolute amount per cell will be attained later,
at about the 20th day (Figs 19 and 20), since as already
discussed the cytoplasmic nuclear ratio does not attain
its highest level, about 12:1, until that time.

Very grossly, it can be approximated that on the
peak of lactation, a single mammary cell contains about
18-20,000 μm^2 of ergastoplasm, which means, again very
grossly, 4.5-5 μm^2 per gram of lactating cells.

The development of Golgi membranes (in μm^2 per μm^3
of cytoplasm) and of Golgi vacuoles (in volume % of cytoplasm) closely follows the profile of ergastoplasmic development, but its absolute values remain lower. The
highest development attains about 1.5 $\mu m^2/\mu m^3$ of cytoplasm which corresponds to about 5-6,000 μm^2 in a single
fully lactating cell. Per gram of lactating cells, this
means a further 1.5 μm^2 to be added to the 4.5-5 m^2 of
ergastoplasm (RER).

The sequential steps of protein and fat synthesis in
the mammary gland cells have been followed by high resolution autoradiography (Wellings and Philp, 1964 ;
Verley and Hollmann, 1966 ; Stein and Stein, 1966, 1967 ;
Rohr et al., 1968 and others). From these studies it
emerges that the ergastoplasm is the primary site of protein synthesis while the Golgi apparatus plays a part
in the further elaboration and in the transport of the
proteinaceous secretory material. The following time
sequence was established : 20 minutes after i.v. injection
of tritiated leucine most of the radioactivity is localized over the ergastoplasm. 30 minutes after injection
the Golgi apparatus is heavily labeled and 60 minutes
after injection the tracer is found both over the Golgi
vacuoles and the alveolar lumen.

The different steps of lipid synthesis were studied
by Stein and Stein (1966, 1967). One minute after i.v.
injection of tritiated palmitate or oleate, 90 % of the
tracer was esterified into triglycerides and the radioactivity was observed over the ergastoplasmic cisternae
and over intracellular fat droplets. The labeled droplets
were of all sizes and situated at the base as well as at
the apex of the cell. At 30 and 60 minutes following
injection, radioactivity was found in the droplets near
the cell apex and in those extruded in the alveolar lumen.
No tracer was found over the Golgi apparatus and the se-

cretion vacuoles. It was therefore concluded that these
organelles are not involved in fat droplet synthesis.

The release mechanism of the secretory material has
been elucidated by electron microscopy. Bargmann and
Knoop (1959) suggested that the extruded milk fat droplet
is surrounded by a membrane which derives from the apical
plasmalemma of the mammary cell. The authors described
a process of umbilication during which the protruding fat
droplet becomes progressively enveloped by the plasmalemma and finally pinched off into the alveolar lumen.
According to this description the entire envelope of the
fat droplet is supplied by the apical plasmalemma. Later,
Wooding et al.(1970) and Wooding (1971) suggested that
part of the envelope originates from Golgi vacuoles.
Indeed, Golgi derived vacuoles are frequently observed in
the periphery of apically located fat droplets and discharge their content concomittantly with the expulsion
of the fat droplet. Thus, it is likely that in this way
they contribute to the fat droplet membrane which therefore has a dual origin : one part deriving from the
plasmalemma and the other from vacuole membranes.

Apart from their participation in the formation of
the fat droplet membrane, the transport vacuoles loaded
with casein granules and other milk constituents such
as lactose release their contents by reverse pinocytosis
or exopinocytosis. This implies that the vacuole membrane
fuses with the plasmalemma whereby the vacuole opens and
frees its contents. In that way, the membrane of the
vacuole becomes a part of the plasmalemma. This mechanism
is a source of resplenishment for plasma-membranes lost
during the extrusion and umbilication of the fat droplets.
Millions of fat droplets with a diameter of 1 to 10 μm
are discharged in every milliliter of milk and a number
of square meters of milk fat droplet membranes are contained in every liter. This tremendous loss must conti-
nually be replaced and the Golgi derived secretory vacuoles play an important role in this process. It appears
that there is a continuous membrane flow in the mammary
cell which involves the different compartments of the
endomembrane system (Keenan et al., 1974) : the nuclear
envelope, the rough endoplasmic reticulum (or ergastoplasm), the smooth endoplasmic reticulum (endoplasmic
reticulum devoid of ribosomes), the Golgi apparatus, the
secretory vacuoles derived from the Golgi apparatus and
carrying secretory material, and finally the plasma
membrane. The endomembrane system is schematically represented in fig. 21.

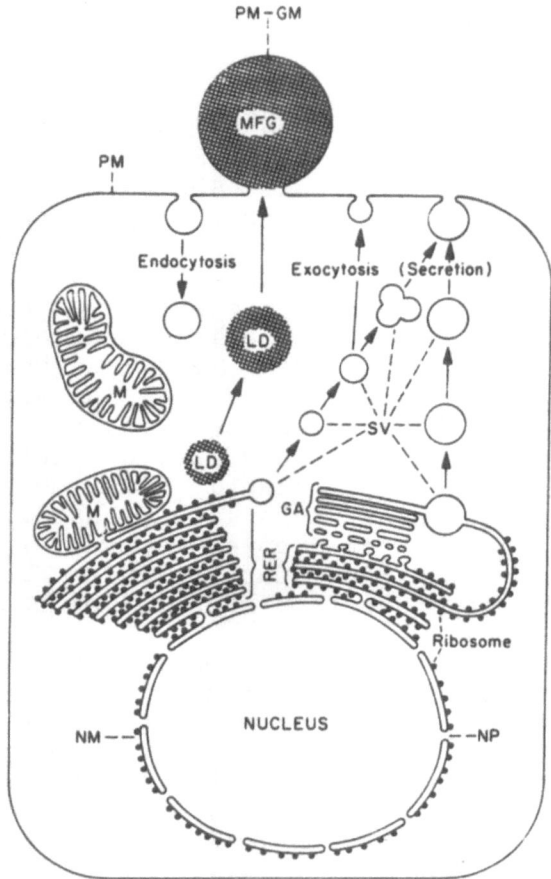

Fig. 21. Diagram illustrating the different components of
the functionally continuous endomembrane system
in the mammary gland cell. This system is the
morphological substratum for the membrane flow
hypothesis.
NM = nuclear membrane
NP = nuclear pore
RER = rough endoplasmic reticulum (ergastoplasm)
GA = Golgi apparatus
SV = secretory vacuole
M = mitochondria
PM = plasma membrane
PM-GM = plasma membrane enveloping a milk fat
globule (MFG)
LD = lipid droplets synthesized in the cytoplasm
grow in size as they rise toward the cell apex.
The droplets inside the cytoplasm are devoided
of a membrane. (From Keenan et al., 1974).

REFERENCES

Anderson, R.R., 1978, Embryonic and fetal development of
        the mammary apparatus. In : Lactation, vol. 4,
        Larson, B.L. (ed), Academic Press, New York and
        London, pp 3-40.
Bargmann, W., and Knoop, A., 1959, Über die Morphologie
        des Milchsekretion. Licht und elektronmikroskopi-
        sche Studien an der Milchdrüse des Ratte. Z. Zell-
        forsch., 49, 344-388.
Ceriani, R.L., quoted by Anderson, R.R., 1974, Endocrino-
        logical control. In : Lactation vol.1, Larson, B.L.
        and Smith, V.R. (eds), Academic Press, New York
        and London, pp 97-140.
Franke, W.W., Keenan, T.W., 1979, Mitosis in milk secre-
        ting epithelial cells of mammary gland : an ultra-
        structural study. Differentiation, 13, 81-88.
Hollmann, K.H., 1959, L'ultrastructure de la glande
        mammaire normale de la souris en lactation. J.
        Ultrastruct. Res., 2, 423-443.
Hollmann, K.H., 1969, Quantitative electron microscopy
        of sub-cellular organization in mammary gland
        cells before and after parturition. In : Lacto-
        genesis : the initiation of milk secretion at
        parturition. Reynolds, M. and Folley, S.J. (eds),
        University of Pennsylvania Press, Philadelphia,
        pp 27-42.
Hollmann, K.H., 1974, Cytology and fine structure of the
        mammary gland. In : Lactation, vol.1, Larson, B.L.
        and Smith, V.R. (eds), Academic Press, New York
        and London, pp 3-95.
Hollmann, K.H., and Verley, J.M., 1971, Morphology of
        secretion in mammary gland cells. In : Lactation,
        Falconer, I.R. (ed), Butterworth, London, 31-45.
Jennes, R., 1974, The composition of milk, In : Lactation,
        vol. 3, Larson, B.L. and Smith, V.R. (eds), Aca-
        demic Press, New York and London, pp 3- 107.
Jones, D.H., 1978, The mitochondria of the mammary pa-
        renchymal cell in relation to the pregnancy-
        lactation cycle. In : Lactation, vol. 4, Larson,
        B.L. (ed), Academic Press, New York and London,
        pp 503-512.
Keenan, T.W., Morre, D.J., and Huang, C.M., 1974, Mem-
        branes of the mammary gland. In : Lactation,
        vol.2, Larson, B.L., and Smith, V.R. (eds),
        Academic Press, New York and London, pp 191-233.
Kriesten, K., 1965, Über den Funktionswandel des Milchdrü-
        senepithels bei der weissen Maus. Inaugural-
        Dissertation (Dr. Rer. nat.) Köln, 27 p.

Mills, E.S., and Topper, Y.J., 1970, Some ultrastructural
    effects of insulin , hydrocortisone, and prolactin
    on mammary gland explants. J. Cell Biol., 44,
    310-328.
Rohr, H., Seitter, U., and Schmalbeck, J., 1968, Vorausset
    zungen und derzeitige Grenzen der quantitativen
    elektronenmikroskopischen Autoradiographie bei
    Kinetikstudien an Drüsenzellen. Z. Zellforsch.,
    85, 376-397.
Rosano, T.G., and Jones, D.H., 1976, Developmental changes
    in mitochondria during the transition into lacta-
    tion in the mouse mammary gland. I. Behavior on
    isopycnic gradient centrifugation. J. Cell Biol.,
    69, 573-580.
Rosano, T.G., Lee, S.K., and Jones, D.H., 1976, Develop-
    mental changes in mitochondria during the tran-
    sition into lactation in the mouse mammary gland.
    II. Membrane marker enzymes and membrane ultras-
    tructure. J. Cell Biol., 69, 581-588.
Saake, R.G., and Heald, C.W., 1974, Cytological aspects
    of milk formation and secretion. In : Lactation,
    vol. 2, Larson, B.L., and Smith, V.R. (eds), Aca-
    demic Press, New York and London, pp 147-189.
Sarma, M.H., 1974, Ph. D. Dissertation, Albany Medical
    College of Union University, Albany, New York.
Sekhri, K.K., Pitelka, D.R., and DeOme, K.B., 1967,
    Studies of mouse mammary glands. I. Cytomorphology
    of the normal mammary glands. J. Nat. Cancer Inst.,
    39, 459-490.
Stein, O., and Stein, Y., 1966, Formation of milk glyce-
    rides in lactating mice, studied by electron-
    microscopic autoradiography. Israel J. Med. Sci.
    6, 773-778.
Stein, O., and Stein, Y., 1967, Lipid synthesis, intra-
    cellular transport and secretion. II. Electron
    microscopic radioautographic study of the mouse
    lactating mammary gland. J. Cell Biol., 34,
    251-263.
Tucker, H.A., 1974, General endocrinological control of
    lactation. In : Lactation, vol.1, Larson, B.L.
    and Smith, V.R. (eds), Academic Press, New York
    and London, pp 277-327.
Verley, J.M., and Hollmann, K.H., 1966, Synthèse et
    réabsorption des protéines dans la glande mammaire
    en stase. Etude autoradiographique au microscope
    électronique. Z. Zellforsch., 75, 605-610.
Weatherford, H.L., 1929, A cytological study of the
    mammary gland ; Golgi apparatus, trophospongium
    and other cytoplasmic canaliculi, mitochondria.
    Am. J. Anat., 44, 199-281.

Wellings, S.R., DeVault, M., Jenfoft, V., Richards, J., Yang, J., Nandi, S., Guzman, R., and Faulkin, L.J., Early lesions of the human mammary gland and their relationship to precancerous lesions of other species, this volume.

Wellings, S.R., and Nandi, S., 1968, Electron microscopy of induced secretion in mammary epithelial cells of hypophysectomized-ovariectomized-adrenalectomized BALB/cCrgl mice. J. Nat. Cancer Inst., 40, 1245-1258.

Wellings, S.R., and Philp, J.R., 1964, The function of the Golgi apparatus in lactating cells of the BALB/cCrgl mouse. Z. Zellforsch., 61, 871-882.

Wellings, S.R., and Wolfe, J.N., 1978, Correlative studies of the histological and radiographic appearance of the breast parenchyma. Radiology, 129, 299-306.

Wellings, S.R., DeOme, K.B., and Pitelka, D.R., 1960, Electron microscopy of milk secretion in the mammary gland of the C3H/Crgl mouse. I. Cytomorphology of the prelactating and the lactating gland. J. Nat. Cancer Inst., 25, 393-421.

Wooding, F.B.P., 1971, The mechanism of secretion of the milk fat globule. J. Cell Sci., 9, 805-821.

Wooding, F.B.P., Peaker, M., and Linzell, J.L., 1970, Theories of milk secretion : Evidence from the electron microscope examination of milk. Nature, 226, 762-764.

EARLY LESIONS OF THE HUMAN MAMMARY GLAND AND THEIR RELATIONSHIP TO PRECANCEROUS LESIONS OF OTHER SPECIES

S.R. Wellings[1], M. DeVault[1], Virginia Jenfoft[1],
J. Richards[2], J. Yang[2], S. Nandi[2], R. Guzman[2],
and L.J. Faulkin[3]

1. Department of Pathology, School of Medicine,
   University of California, Davis, California,
   95616.
2. Cancer Research Laboratory, University of
   California, Davis, California, 95616.
3. Department of Anatomy, School of Veterinary
   Medicine, University of California, Davis,
   California, 95616

Preneoplastic pathological lesions are tissue formations possessing an increased probability of developing neoplasia in comparison to the probability that the corresponding type of neoplasm will develop in adjacent morphologically normal tissue. Lesions with presumed preneoplastic potential have been described in the mammary glands of mice, rats, dogs, subhuman primates, and humans. In every instance the lesions stand out from the normal background as focal, multicentric, and hyperplastic. The epithelial cells of preneoplastic lesions have variable degrees of so-called premalignant atypia (anaplasia), and on this basis can be arranged in an arbitrary morphological continuum linking normal to pre-invasive carcinoma. In mice there is direct experimental proof that more cancers arise from precancerous mammary tissue than from normal tissue. In the human, however, techniques for such direct observation are not as yet perfected and the assignment of risk to particular focal lesions of the human breast is based on morphological and statistical inference.

Table 1. Average numbers of lesions per breast

Lesion	185 Random autopsy breasts	107 Cancer associated breasts (cancer containing or controlateral)	Probability that the 2 samples are drawn from different populations (t test)	Standard abbreviation for lesion
A. Fibrocystic complex				
1. epithelial cyst	0.85	1.44	0.853	EP cyst
2. stromal cysts	0.08	0.25	0.853	S cyst
3. apocrine cysts	4.47	14.88	> 0.999	APO cyst
4. sclerosing adenosis	1.83	1.82	0.015	SA
5. hyperplastic duct (larger than terminal)	0.12	0.62	0.938	HD
6. hyperplastic terminal duct, all grades	0.08	1.82	> 0.999	HTD
7. hyperplastic terminal duct, with papilloma	0.22	5.78	0.964	HTD-PAP
8. atypical lobules, type A, all grades (1–4) (proposed precancerous to ductal carcinoma)	10.31	44.50	> 0.999	ALA
9. atypical lobules, type B, all grades (1–4) (proposed precancerous to lobular carcinoma)	0.03	0.80	0.999	ALB

Table 1 (continued)

B. Carcinoma in situ				
1. ductal carcinoma in situ	0.08	5.47	0.996	DCIS
2. lobular carcinoma in situ	0.00	0.75	0.950	LCIS
C. Other tumors				
1. fibroadenoma	0.40	1.11	>0.999	FA
2. duct papilloma	0.23	1.70	0.999	D-PAP
D. Other lesions				
1. persistant lobule (remaining after menopause in otherwise atrophic breast)	8.31	24.77	>0.999	PL
2. large lobule (exceeding average lobule size by 3x or more)				LL
E. Average number all lesions/ breast	27.01	105.41		

PRESUMPTIVE PRENEOPLASTIC LESIONS OF HUMAN BREAST

     While there is difference of opinion, it is the
majority view that certain of the epithelial proliferations of hyperplastic fibrocystic disease (HFCD) (mammary
dysplasia complex) are preneoplastic. This assumption
is based largely on imperfect statistical and morphological correlations linking the presence of HFCD to past,
present, and future development of breast carcinoma
(Foote and Stewart, 1945 ; Geschicter, 1945 ; Ingleby
and Gershon-Cohen, 1960 ; Gallagher and Martin, 1969 ;
Wellings et al., 1975). Morphological intermediates are
observed between normal and pre-invasive carcinoma in
ordinary histology slides. Black and Chabon (1969) and
others have devised methods for semiquantitative grading
of preneoplastic atypia, and these methods appear to
have validity (Black and Chabon, 1969 ; Wellings et al.,
1975 ; Wellings and Wolfe, 1978). However, there is no
direct proof of the preneoplastic nature of any human
mammary epithelial lesions and the attendant difficulties
have been discussed by McDivitt et al. (1968).

     Our own studies (Wellings et al., 1975 ; Wellings
and Rice, 1978) give clear representations of the terminal ductal lobular units (TDLU) (Fig. 1a,b) which
appear to give origin to most kinds of human mammary
pathology. Two hundred and ninety-two whole human breasts
were studied by us using a subgross method with histological confirmation permitting the identification, classification, and enumeration of all pathological lesions
large enough to be observed with the dissecting microscope (Table 1). Of these breasts, 185 were from random
autopsies, and 107 were breasts which either contained
a cancer or were controlateral to one. A statistical
comparison reveals that HFCD is more frequent in women
with breast cancer than in those without. HFCD with
marked epithelial atypia is especially likely to be
present in breast cancer patients. Included among the
hyperplastic lesions observed with increased frequency
are apocrine cystic formations of the TDLU (Fig. 2a,b)
and a group of lesions of the TDLU which we interpret
as atypical lobules (AL) (Fig. 3). The commonest of AL,
which we have termed atypical lobule, Type A (ALA)
(Fig. 3) has epithelial populations with easily recognized morphological transitions between normal epithelial cells and the cells of carcinoma-in-situ of the
classical ductal type. ALA are hyperplastic lobule-like
formations composed of blindly ending, enlarged termina+
ting tubular structures which may be regarded as either
ductules or duct end buds. In spite of their terminal,

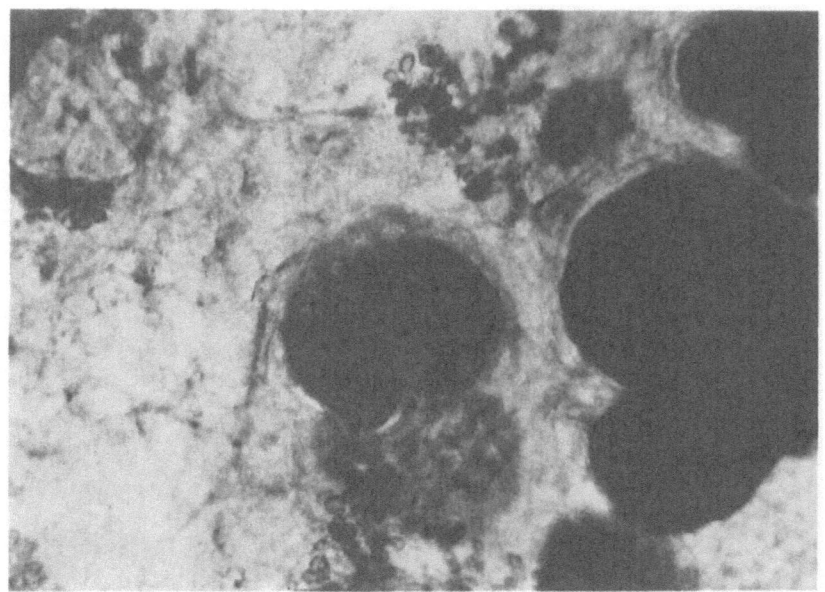

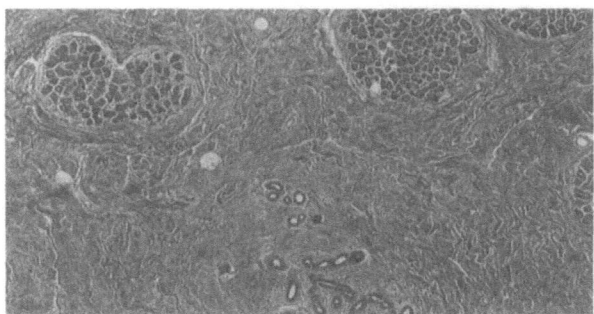

Fig. 1a. Subgross photograph of breast of a 22 year
          old woman. Note mixture of relatively well
          developed dense ovoid lobules (right) with
          smaller lobules (left). Hematoxylin stain,
          28x.

Fig. 1b. Corresponding histology of well developed
          and smaller lobules. Hematoxylin and eosin,
          30x.

lobule-like structure, there have been objections to
referring to this lesion (ALA) as of lobular nature,
inasmuch as it appears to be related to classical pre-
invasive and invasive "ductal" carcinoma, rather than

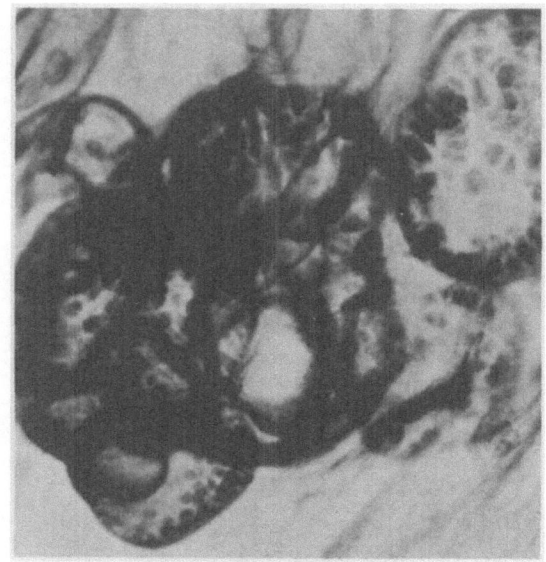

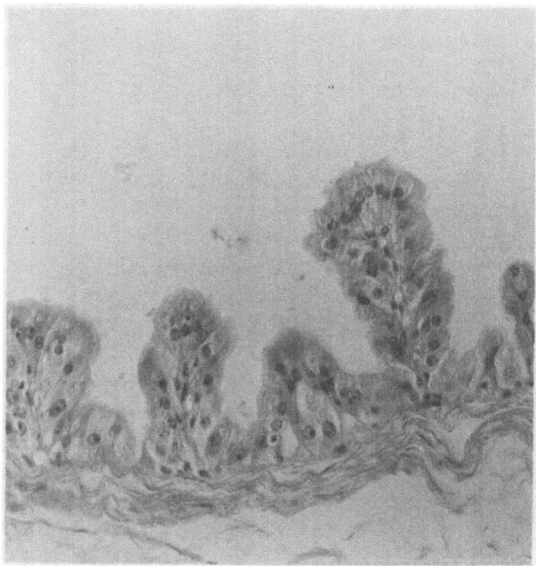

Fig. 2a.   Subgross photograph of a lobule with papillary
           cystic apocrine (pink cell) change. Hematoxylin
           stain, 28x.
Fig. 2b.   Corresponding histology with apocrine (pink
           cell) change. Hematoxylin and eosin, 252x.
           H & E.

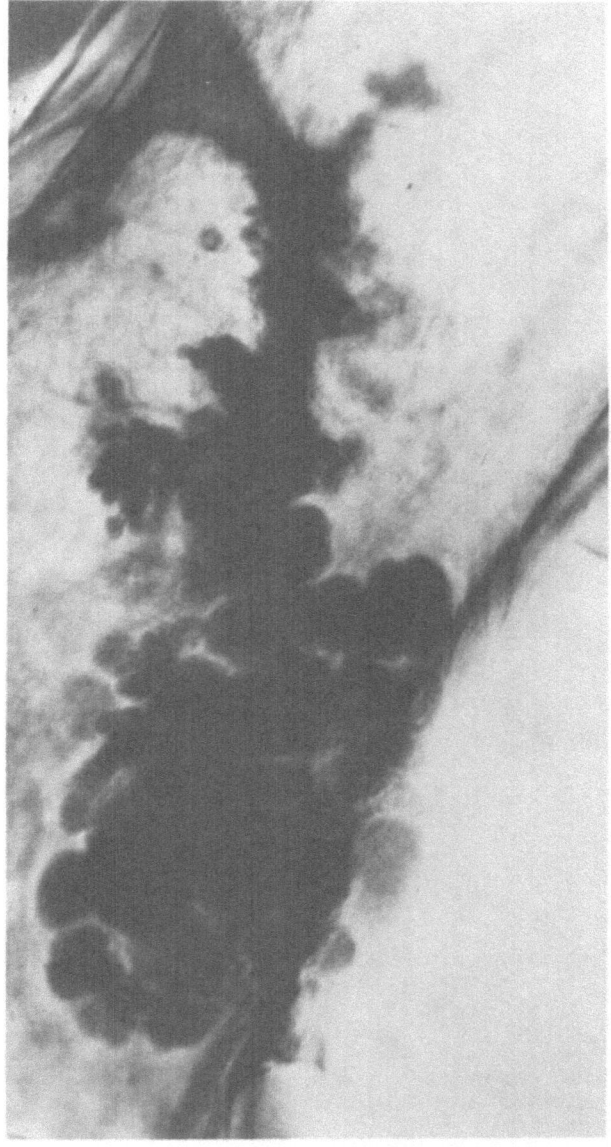

Fig. 3a. Subgross preparation of an atypical lobule,
type A (ALA). This ALA is essentially a giant
lobule with greatly enlarged ductules (acini).
Hematoxylin stain, 43x.

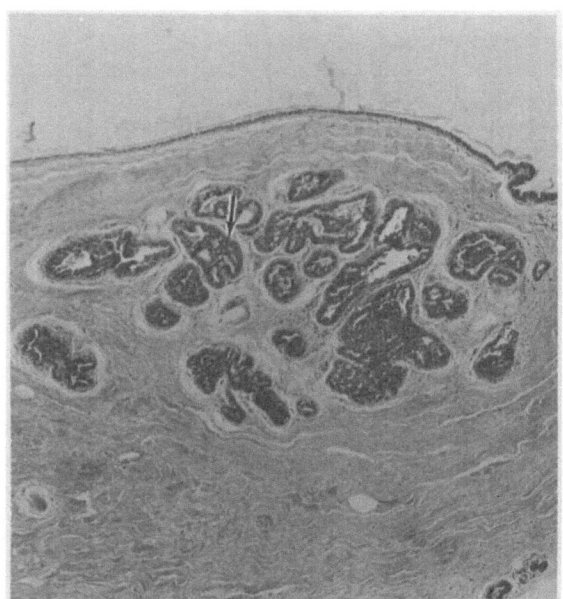

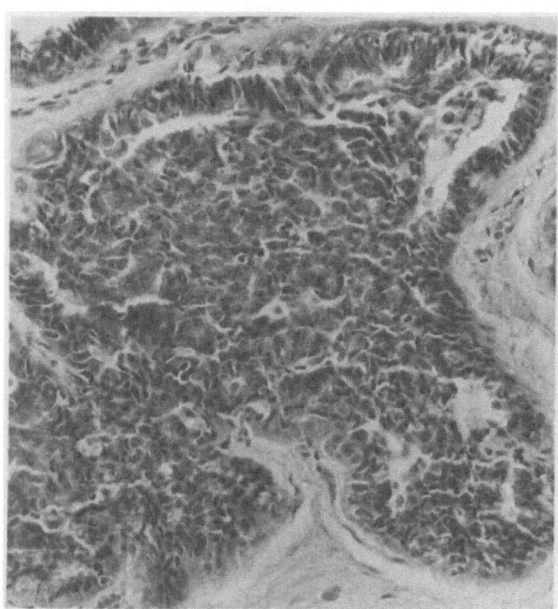

Fig. 3b, c. Corresponding histology of Fig. 3a. Note
            hyperplastic epithelium (arrow). Hemato-
            xylin and eosin, 44x and 262x, respecti-
            vely.

"lobular" carcinoma. Moreover, ALA closely resemble
lesions referred to by some pathologists as "blunt duct
adenosis". Dr. W. Coulson (personal communication) has
suggested that the term "hyperplastic adenosis" be used
for this and related lesions. This term alleviates somewhat the above conflict in terminology which is so dis-
turbing to the surgical pathologist in America. In order
to avoid the issue as to whether the structures are
lobules or hyperplastic abnormally grouped duct end buds,
we have at times referred to ALA as "hyperplastic terminal groupings of ducts and/or ductules", abbreviated
HTG. For our present purposes we will continue to use
the term ALA for the form of hyperplastic adenosis, illustrated below, for which the evidence for precancerous
potential is especially convincing. It needs to be borne
in mind that the exact cell types giving rise to human
mammary carcinomas are at this time unknown.

Typical ALA are illustrated in Figures 3 and 4. It
is to be emphasized that ALA are focal, lobule-like formations which stand out from the background of more
normal appearing TDLU. Further, ALA have hyperplastic
epithelial populations identifiable in ordinary histological slides. In our preparations, hyperplastic epithelial lesions of ducts larger than those found in the
TDLU are exceedingly rare and logic would indicate that
so-called ductal carcinoma does not arise in larger ducts,
but rather in the terminal ducts and ductules of the
TDLU.

We are transplanting normal lobules, ALA, and cancer
into the host gland free mammary fat pad (DeOme et al.,
1959) of the nude athymic mouse. As noted in Figure 5a,
b,c, human mammary epithelium derived from normal lobules
and ALA forms hyperplastic outgrowths in nude mice. The
human tissue grows usually by expansion, sometimes by
infiltration, and may have numerous mitotic figures. No
transplants of normal lobule or ALA have as yet given
rise to carcinoma. Transplants of carcinomatous tissue
invariably grow as expanding spherical or ovoid masses
with marginal infiltration and numerous mitoses (Fig. 6a,
b). The histo-pathology of the growing cancer xenografts
closely duplicates the appearance on control microslides
fixed at the time of transplantation. Further studies of
this kind may provide direct evidence of preneoplastic
potential for certain human breast lesions.

The most recent preliminary results indicate that
purified normal, hyperplastic and carcinomatous human
mammary epithelial cells can be grown in primary cell

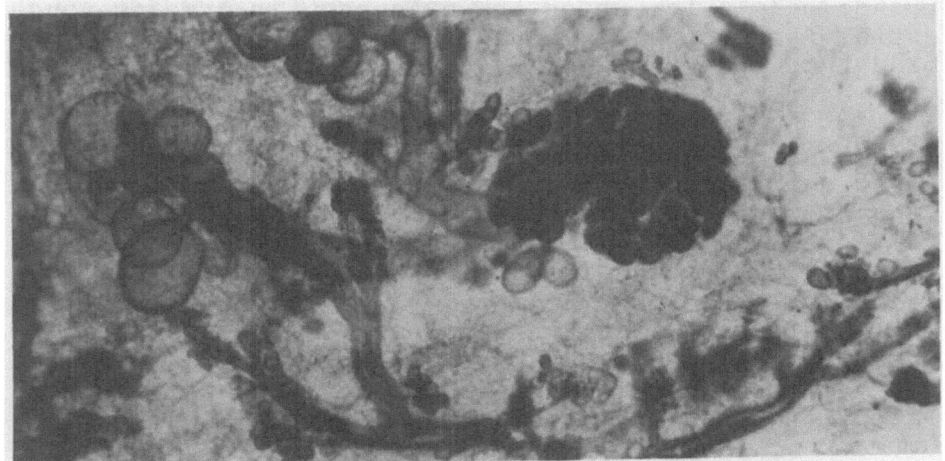

Fig. 4a.   Subgross of another ALA. Hematoxylin stain,
           34x.

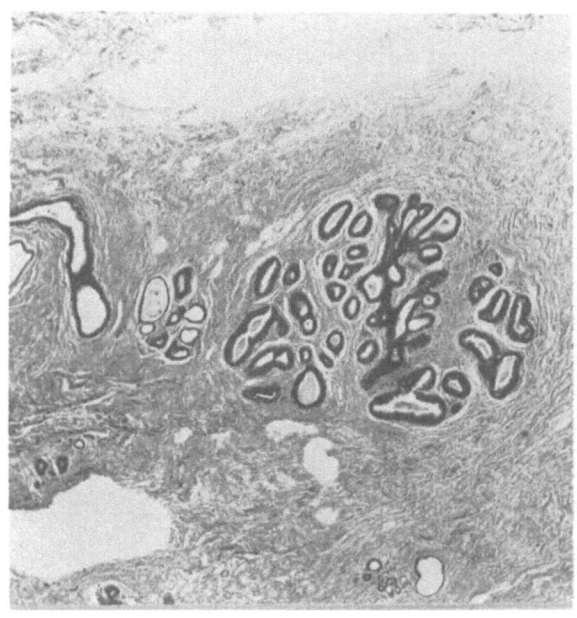

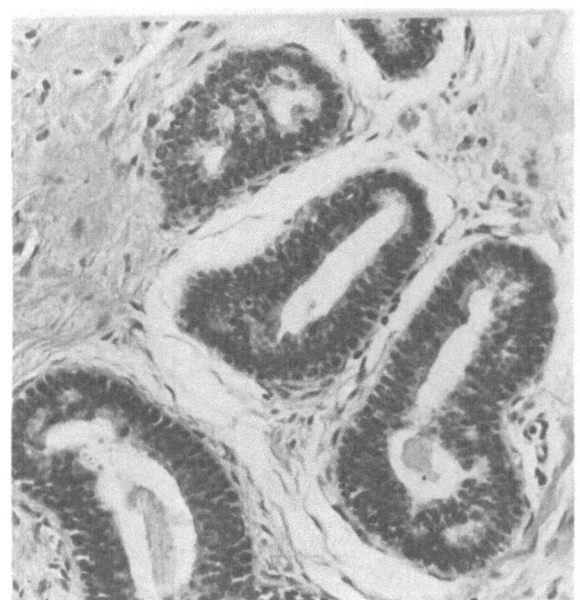

Fig. 4b,c.Corresponding histology. Hematoxylin and
        eosin, 44x and 262x, respectively.

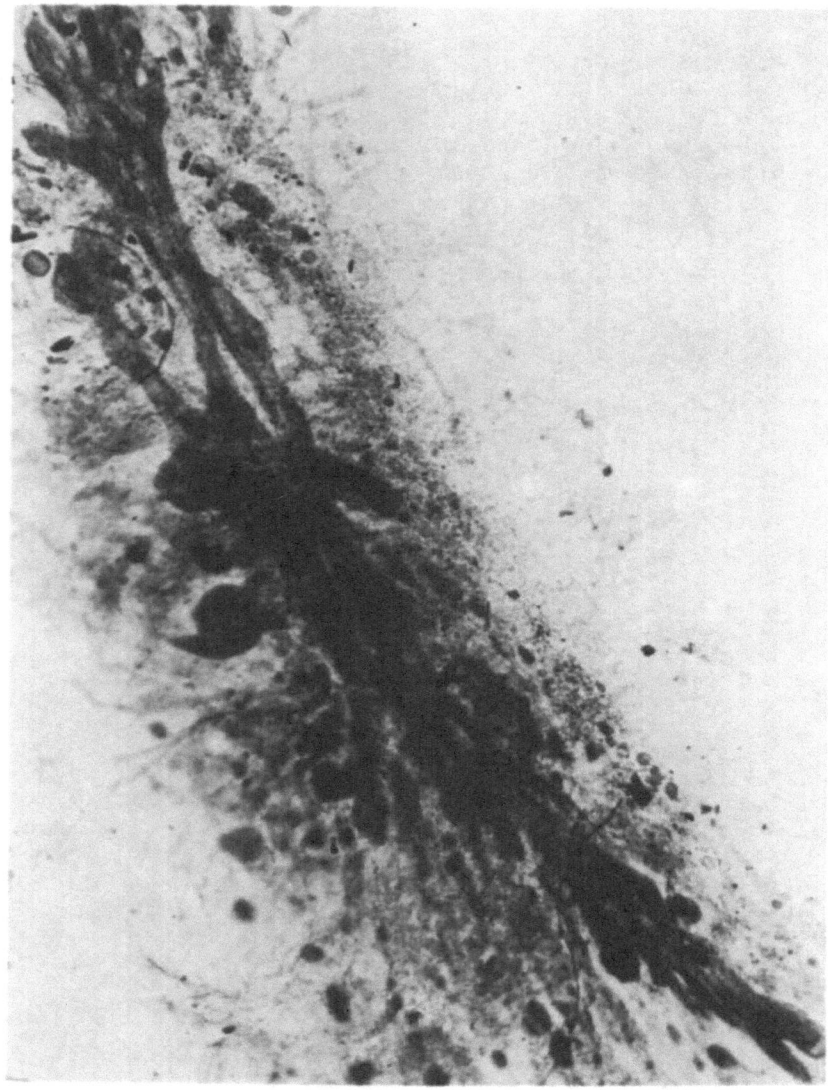

Fig. 5a. Subgross preparation of a proliferation of
         normal and "fibrocystic" human mammary epi-
         thelial cells in the host gland free mammary
         fat pad of a "nude" athymic mouse. Note tubular
         structures and buds. Hematoxylin stain, 32x.

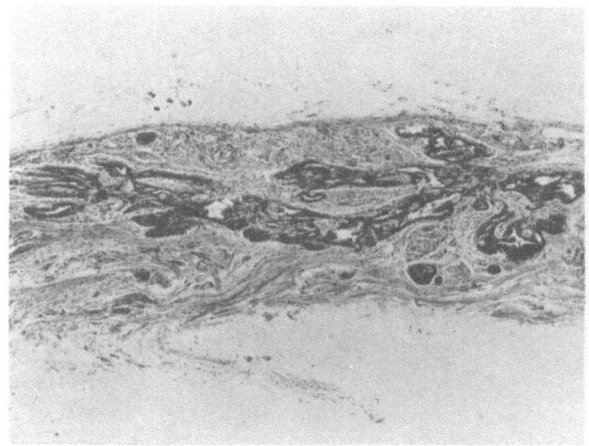

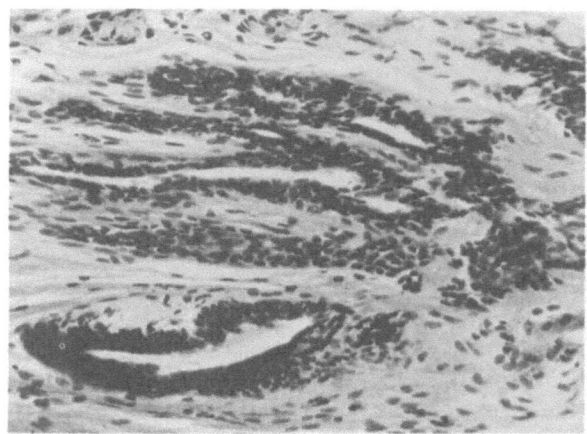

Fig. 5b, c. Corresponding histology of Fig. 5a. Hema-
        toxylin and eosin, 31x and 197x, respec-
        tively.

cultures without fibroblasts (Yang et al., 1979). This
is accomplished by a combination of tissue digestion,
epithelial cell purification in density gradients, and
growth in collagen gel cultures with special media.
Figure 7a,b illustrates a pure epithelial culture derived
from tissue composed of a mixture of normal ducts and
lobules with focal mild, nonproliferative fibrocystic
changes.

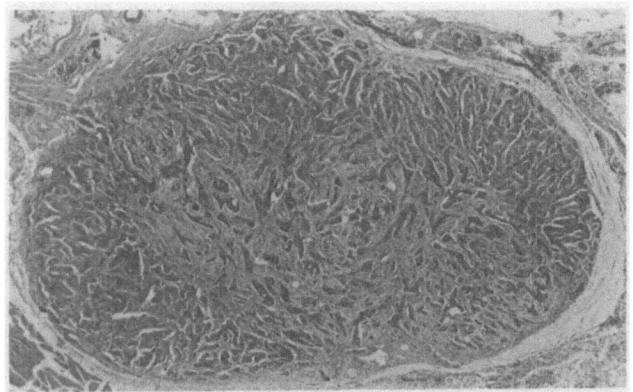

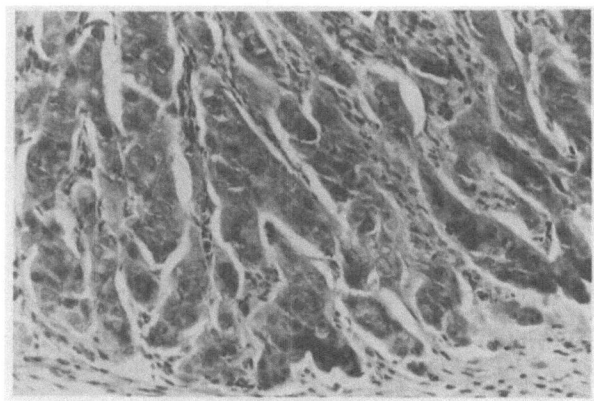

Fig. 6a. Histology of human mammary carcinoma ("infil-
          trating duct carcinoma") growing in host gland
          free mammary fat pad of nude athymic mouse.
          Hematoxylin and eosin, 27x.
Fig. 6b. Same at higher magnification. Hematoxylin and
          eosine, 171x.

RELATIONSHIP OF HUMAN LESIONS TO PRECANCEROUS MAMMARY
LESIONS OF OTHER SPECIES

Mouse

     Inbred mouse strains have been used for decades for
experimental mammary studies. High and low mammary tumor
strains were created by selective breeding practices. The
degree of inbreeding within strains is sufficient to
allow tissue transplantation without rejection. Multiple
factors are involved in mouse mammary tumorigenesis and

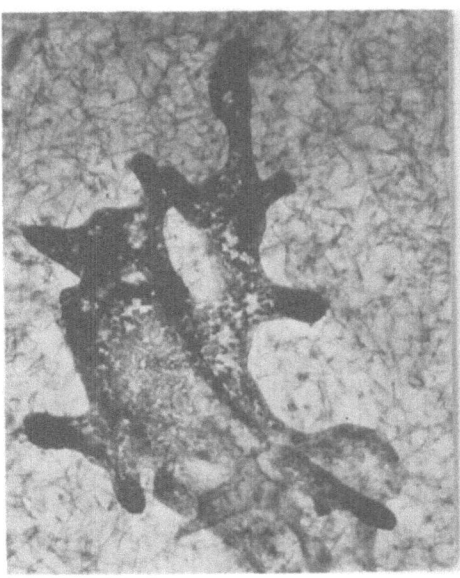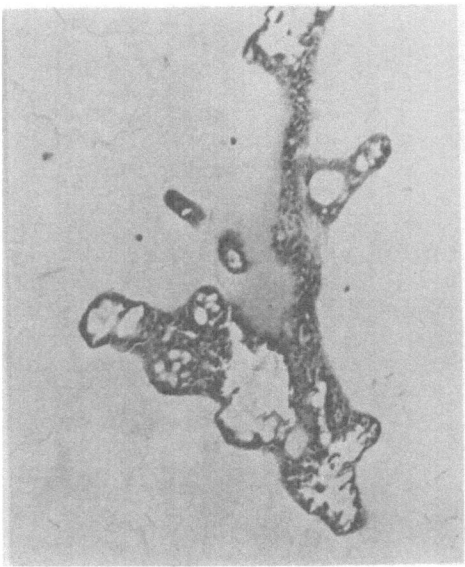

Fig. 7a. Colony of human mammary epithelial cells growing in collagen gel cultures for 4 weeks. Note branching pattern of hollow tubes. Unstained, 44x.

Fig. 7b. Corresponding histology. Note formations of epithelial cells with central lumens. There are no fibroblasts. Hematoxylin and eosin, 68x.

these have been extensively reviewed by several authors (Bentvelzen, 1974 ; Bern and Nandi, 1961 ; Heston and Parks, 1975 ; Medina, 1973 ; Nandi and McGrath, 1973). The multiple factors involved can be classified chiefly as genetic, hormonal, and viral ; tumor incidence is the result of interaction of these factors.

The mammary tumors of mice are generally adenocarcinomas which grow slowly by expansion and may develop increasing tissue and cellular pleomorphism as they enlarge. Those attaining large size frequently have pulmonary and lymph nodal metastases. The tumors are relatively hormonally independent and deprivation of mammogenic hormones by endocrine organ ablation gives little or no effect on tumor growth.

At least one common preneoplastic lesion has been extensively investigated since first recognized at the

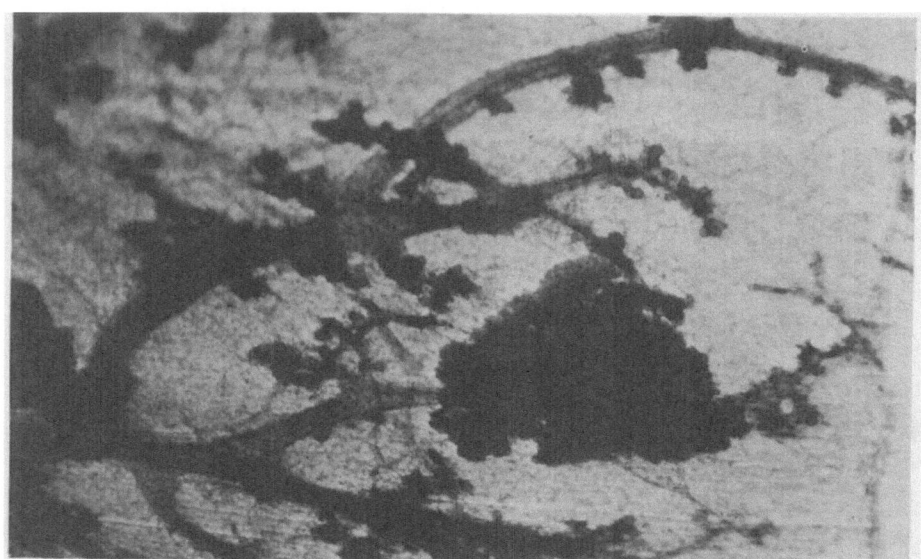

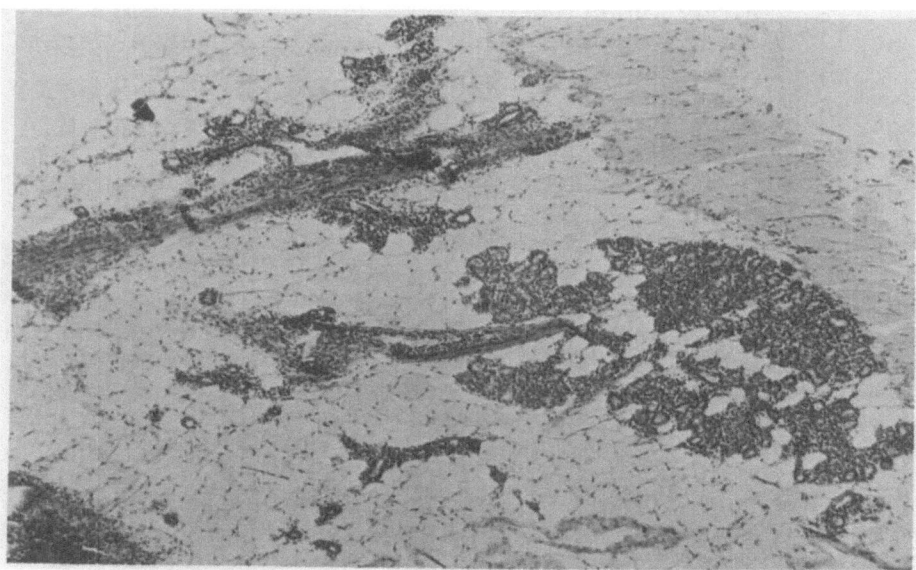

Fig. 8a.   Subgross preparation of hyperplastic alveolar
           nodule (HAN) of female high mammary tumor
           strain C3H mouse. Note lobuloalveolar charac-
           ter of HAN. Hematoxylin stain, 32x.
Fig. 8b.   Corresponding histology. Hematoxylin and
           eosin, 71x.

turn of the century. This lesion, the hyperplastic alveolar nodule (HAN) was first observed by Apolant (1906)
and Haaland (1911). Heston and Vlahakis (1971) describe
the variations in morphology and frequency of HAN within
different strains. DeOme, Faulkin and co-workers (1959)
clearly demonstrate a preneoplastic potential for HAN
by direct experimental means. This is accomplished by
demonstrating that more adenocarcinomas arise from HANs
than from normal gland when these are transplanted into
host gland free mammary fat pads of isologous mice.

HAN are individually lobuloalveolar in design
(Fig. 8), and are geographically multicentric throughout
the mammary glands. They increase in number with time,
and appear several months prior to the appearance of the
mammary adenocarcinomas to which they give rise. HAN
have clear alterations in hormonal sensitivity, since
they exist in the resting mammary gland of the non-
pregnant animal under hormonal circumstances not suppor-
ting the maintenance of normal lobuloalveolar structure.
Thus, HAN persists in the hormone milieu of the nonpre-
gnant animal. In serial transplantation studies HAN
produce hyperplastic epithelial outgrowths with life
spans of indefinite duration.

Induction of HAN occurs by various experimental
maneuvers involving hormones, mammary tumor virus,
chemical carcinogens and x-radiation.

DeOme and Medina (1969) propose a two-step model
for mammary tumorigenesis in mice : 1. normal to preneoplasia, and 2. preneoplasia to neoplasia. The reaction is driven toward neoplasia by experimental treatments with certain hormones, mammary tumor virus, and
chemical carcinogens. Much experimental data is also
consistent with a multistep hypothesis, and both models
are compatible with the human system in which the
commonest preneoplastic lesions (ALA) appear also to be
of lobuloalveolar nature and to include aberrant epithelial cell populations in the terminal ducts and
lobules.

Rat

Mammary tumorigenesis in the rat has not been
studied as extensively as in the mouse. It is clear
that certain strains of rats have very high incidence
of spontaneous mammary tumors, usually appearing late
in life. Most of the tumors are fibroadenomata. Whole

mount subgross preparations of rat mammary gland reveal
lobuloalveolar lesions similar to the HAN of mice. These
lesions are more frequent in mammary glands of strains
with a high incidence of spontaneous mammary tumors,
and increase in number with age. Beuving et al. (1967a)
transplanted spontaneous HAN from inbred Fischer rats
to the host gland free mammary fat pads of the same
strain. Normal outgrowths appear, but no tumors are
observed, suggesting that the HAN of the Fischer rat
is not clearly preneoplastic, and has a very low tumor
producing potential.

HAN-like lesions and ductal proliferations are
observed in Sprague-Dawley and Fischer rats following
treatment by DMBA (Beuving et al., 1967b). Similar lesions are produced by x-radiation of Sprague-Dawley
rats (Faulkin et al., 1967). Using Lewis rats, Beuving
(1968) gives evidence for preneoplastic nature of rat
HAN in an experiment in which 8 of 37 nodules produced
tumors following transplantation.

Cat

Mammary tumorigenesis from hyperplastic lesions
has not been extensively studied in the house cat,
Felis domesticus. Dorn et al. (1968) found that mammary
tumors were the third most frequent neoplasm of cats,
with an incidence of 156/100,000 in Alameda and Contra
Costa Counties, California. Age incidence data (Weijer
et al., 1972) give average age of onset at 10.8 years,
with a range of 2.5 to 19 years. Feline mammary tumors
are usually adenocarcinomas and over 80 % have metastases at autopsy (Weijer et al., 1972). Hyperplastic
alveolar lesions, suggestive of the HAN of mice, were
recently observed in 2 cats (Wellings, 1978, unpublished
data). There is no direct evidence bearing on the preneoplastic nature of any focal lesion in the cat mammary
gland.

Dog

Mammary cancer in dogs has been studied extensively
and several classification schemes proposed (Fowler et
al., 1974 ; Misdorp et al., 1971, 1972, 1973). Schneider
et al. (1969) classified 93 mammary tumors as follows :
carcinoma, 61 cases ; malignant mixed tumors, 22 cases ;

benign mixed tumors, 2 cases ; and unknown, 3 cases.
Mixed tumor is a designation used for mammary tumors
containing both epithelial elements and osseous or
cartilagenous tissue as part of the tumorous proliferation.

Cameron and Faulkin (1971) report studies based
on examination of whole mount subgross preparations of
canine mammary gland. These workers observe a variety of
focal lesions, the most frequent of which is a hyperplastic alveolar nodule (HAN), closely resembling that
observed in mice. The lesions increase in number with age
from a very few at 3 or 4 years to several hundred at
12 years. Morphological intermediates forming an arbitrary continuum between HAN and neoplastic lesions are
observed. Evidence for preneoplastic potential of the
dog HAN is circumstantial since direct experimentation
such as that done with mouse mammary gland is not possible due to the lack of sufficiently inbred strains of
dogs. Normal, hyperplastic and neoplastic tissue transplanted to the host gland free mammary fat pad of nude
athymic mice produces no growth after 60-70 days.
However, if the mice are given estrogen and progesterone,
normal and hyperplastic tissue grow to several times
the original size in 70 days (Faulkin et al., unpublished
data).

Subhuman Primates

Literature dealing with mammary tumors of subhuman
primates is sparse. Appleby et al. (1974) present three
cases and review a total of thirteen. These occur in
seven different genera, and four different families of
primates. Six of the cases are in rhesus monkeys (Maccaca
mulatta). Four of these six are adenocarcinomas, one is
designated simply carcinoma, and one is squamous cell
carcinoma with local invasion. Metastases are not observed. The general lack of age information and reproductive history in most instances of reported primate tumors
weaken natural historical analysis which might bear on
the development of mammary tumors in primates. Virus
has been isolated in some rhesus tumors (Chopra and
Mason, 1970) without any direct evidence that virus is
tumorigenic. Hyperplastic lesions, some of which resemble
hyperplastic alveolar nodules (HAN) of mice of high mammary tumor strains are observed by some workers (Speert,
1940 ; Nelson and Shott, 1973 ; Cameron and Faulkin,
1974).

DISCUSSION AND SUMMARY

Precancerous lesions are observed in the mammary glands of several species. Only in the instance of inbred strains of mice and the Lewis rat is there direct experimental proof of precancerous nature of these lesions. In other species, including the human, the evidence for precancerous potential is circumstantial, and based on imperfect statistics and arbitrary morphological sequencing.

In humans the indirect evidence is strong ; the commonest presumptive preneoplastic lesions appear to arise as abnormal terminal ductal lobular units (TDLU) and usually consist of ductules (acini) together with intralobular and extralobular terminal ducts. These lesions, termed atypical lobules, type A (ALA) for convenience, contain atypical epithelial cell populations which grade into carcinoma-in-situ of the classical intra-ductal type (DCIS). ALA are readily distinguished from another type of easily recognizable formation, called atypical lobule, type B (ALB) for which the evidence suggests a relationship to so-called lobular carcinoma-in-situ (LCIS). ALB and LCIS are not illustrated in this paper but the reader is referred to Wellings et al. (1975) and Wellings and Rice (1978).

ALA are somewhat similar to the hyperplastic alveolar nodules of mice ; they increase in number with age until the menopause, after which new ones probably do not form. ALA are significantly more frequent in the breasts of women judged to be at high risk on the basis of clinical history, in the breasts of women with coincident breast cancer (Wellings et al., 1975) and in women whose breasts fall into xeromammographic risk categories P2 and DY, as determined by the method of Dr. John Wolfe (Wellings and Wolfe, 1978).

Normal human TDLU, ALA, and mammary cancer can be successfully grown in "nude" athymic mice which lack T-cell lymphocyte capabilities. Moreover, preliminary studies show that human mammary epithelial cells from these structures can now be grown in relatively pure culture without fibroblasts. In view of these new methodological developments, the way is open for detailed analysis of growth requirements, and sensitivity to hormones and chemotherapeutic agents. The basic biology of the various types of human mammary cells, and the mechanisms of neoplastic transformation can now be explored.

ACKNOWLEDGEMENTS

This work was supported by Grants CA 21366, CA 21523, CA 05388, and CA 09041 from the National Cancer Institute, U.S. Public Health Service, DHEW.

REFERENCES

Apolant, H., 1906, Die epithelialen Geschwülste der Maus. Arb. Kgl. Inst. Expt. Therapie, Frankfurt, pp. 11-62.

Appleby, E.C., Keymer, I.F., and Hime, J.M., 1974, Three cases of suspected mammary neoplasia in non-human primates. J. Comp. Pathol., 84, 351-364.

Bentvelzen, P., 1974, Host-virus interactions in murine mammary carcinogenesis. Biochem. Biophys. Acta, 355, 236-259.

Bern, H.A., and Nandi, S., 1961, Recent studies of the hormonal influence in mouse mammary tumorigenesis. Prog. Exp. Tumor Res., 2, 90-144.

Beuving, L.J., Bern, H.A., and DeOme, K.B., 1967a, Occurence and transplantation of carcinogen-induced hyperplastic nodules in Fischer rats. J. Natl. Cancer Inst., 39, 431-447.

Beuving, L.J., Faulkin, L.G., DeOme, K.B., and Bergs, V.V., 1967b, Hyperplastic lesions in the mammary glands of Sprague-Dawley rats after 7,12 dimethylbenz(a)anthracene treatment. J. Natl. Cancer Inst., 39, 423-429.

Beuving, L.J., 1968, Mammary tumor formation within outgrowths of transplanted hyperplastic nodules from carcinogen-treated rats. J. Natl. Cancer Inst., 40, 1287-1291.

Black, M.M., and Chabon, A.B., 1969, In situ carcinoma of the breast. In : Pathology Annual, S.C. Sommers ed., Appleton-Century-Crofts, New York, pp. 185-210.

Cameron, A.M., and Faulkin, L.J. Jr., 1971, Hyperplastic and inflammatory nodules in the canine mammary gland. J. Natl. Cancer Inst., 47, 1277-1287.

Cameron, A.M., and Faulkin, L.J., 1974, Subgross evaluation of the nonhuman primate mammary glands : Method and initial observations. J. Med. Primatol., 3, 298-310.

Chopra, H.C., and Mason, M.M., 1970, A new virus in a spontaneous mammary tumor of a rhesus monkey. Cancer Res., 30, 2081-2086.

DeOme, K.B., Faulkin, L.J., Bern, H.A., and Blair, P.B., 1959, Development of mammary tumors from

hyperplastic alveolar nodules transplanted_in the
gland-free mammary fat pads of female C3H mice.
Cancer Res., 19, 515-520.
DeOme, K.B., and Medina, D., 1969, A new approach to
mammary tumorigenesis in rodents. Cancer, 24,
1255-1258.
Dorn, C.R., Taylor, D.O.N., Frye, F.L., and Hibbard, H.H.,
1968, Survey of animal neoplasms in Alameda and
Contra Costa Counties, California. II. Cancer
morbidity in dogs and cats from Alameda County.
J. Natl. Cancer Inst., 40, 307-318.
Faulkin, L.J., Shellabarger, C.J., and DeOme, K.B., 1967,
Hyperplastic lesions of Sprague-Dawley rat mammary
glands after x-irradiation. J. Natl. Cancer Inst.,
39, 449-458.
Foote, F.W., and Stewart, F.W.,1945, Comparative studies
of cancerous versus noncancerous breasts. Ann.
Surg., 121, 6-53, 197-222.
Fowler, E.H., Wilson, G.P., and Koestner, A., 1974,
Biologic behavior of canine mammary neoplasms
based on a histogenetic classification. Vet.
Pathol., 11, 212-229.
Gallagher, H.S., and Martin, J.E., 1969, Early phases
in the development of breast cancer. Cancer,
24, 1170-1178.
Geschickter, C.F., 1945, Diseases of the breast : Diag-
nosis, Pathology and Treatment, Lippincott,
Philadelphia, p. 413.
Haaland, M., 1911, Spontaneous tumors in mice, Imperial
Cancer Research Fund, Great Britain, Fourth
Scientific Report, Her Majesty's Stat. Off.,
London, pp. 1-113.
Heston, W., and Parks, W., 1975, Mouse mammary tumor
virus and host genome in the transmission and
causation of mammary tumors in mice. Can. J.
Genet. Cytol., 17, 493.
Heston, W.E., and Vlahakis, G., 1971, Mammary tumors,
plaques and hyperplastic alveolar nodules in
various combinations of mouse inbred·strains and
the different lines of the mammary tumor virus.
Int. J. Cancer, 7, 141-148.
Ingleby, H., and Gershon-Cohen, J., 1960, Comparative
Anatomy, Pathology and Roentgenology of the
Breast, Univ. Pennsylvania Press, Philadelphia,
pp. 291-309.
McDivitt, R.W., Stewart, F.W., and Berg, J.W., 1968,
Tumors of the breast, in : Atlas of Tumor Patho-
logy, Second Series, Fascicle 2, A.F.I.P.,
Washington, D.C.

Medina, D., 1973, Preneoplastic lesions in mouse mammary
        tumorigenesis. In : Methods in Cancer Research,
        Vol. 7, H. Busch, ed., Academic Press, New York,
        pp. 1-53.
Misdorp, W., Cotchin, E., Hampe, J.F., Jabara, A.G.,
        and von Sandersleben, J., 1971, Canine malignant
        mammary tumors. I. Sarcomas. Vet. Pathol., 8,
        99-117.
Misdorp, W., Cotchin, E., Hampe, J.F., Jabara, A.G.,
        and von Sandersleben, J., 1972, Canine malignant
        mammary tumors. II. Adenocarcinomas, solid car-
        cinomas and spindle cell carcinomas. Vet. Pathol.,
        9, 447-470.
Misdorp, W., Cotchin, E., Hampe, J.F., Jabara, A.G.,
        and von Sandersleben, J., 1973, Canine malignant
        mammary tumors. III. Special types of carcinomas,
        malignant mixed tumors. Vet. Pathol.,10, 241-256.
Nandi, S., and McGrath, C.M., 1973, Mammary neoplasia
        in mice. Adv. Cancer Res., 17, 353-414.
Nelson, L.W., and Shott, L.D., 1973, Mammary nodular
        hyperplasia in intact rhesus monkeys. Vet. Pathol.
        10, 130-134.
Schneider, R., Dorn, C.R., and Taylor, D.O.N., 1969,
        Factors influencing canine mammary cancer deve-
        lopment and postsurgical survival. J. Natl.
        Cancer Inst., 43, 1249-1261.
Speert, H., 1940, Hyperplastic mammary nodules in the
        castrate female rhesus monkey. Bull. Johns
        Hopkins Hosp., 67, 414-426.
Weijer, K., Head, K.W., Misdorp, W.,and Hampe, J.F.,
        1972, Feline malignant mammary tumors. I. Mor-
        phology and biology : some comparisons with
        human and canine mammary carcinomas. J. Natl.
        Cancer Inst., 49, 1697-1704.
Wellings, S.R., Jensen, H.M., and Marcum, R.G., 1975,
        An atlas of subgross pathology of the human breast
        with special reference to precancerous lesions.
        J. Natl. Cancer Inst., 55, 231-273.
Wellings, S.R., and Rice, J.D., 1978, Preneoplastic
        lesions in the human breast. Cancer Campaign,
        Vol. 1,Gustav Fischer Verlag, Stuttgart, New
        York, pp. 91-106.
Wellings, S.R., and Wolfe, J.N., 1978, Correlative
        studies of the histological and radiographic
        appearance of the breast parenchyma. Radiology,
        129, 299-306.
Yang, J., Richards, J., Bowman, P., Guzman, R., Enami,
        J., McCormick, K., Hamamoto, S., Pitelka, D.,
        and Nandi, S., 1979, Sustained growth and

3-dimensional organization of primary mammary
tumor epithelial cells embedded in collagen
gels. Proc. Natl. Acad. Sci., $\underline{76}$(7), 3401-3405.

NATURAL HISTORY OF BENIGN BREAST TUMORS

J. de BRUX

Institut de Pathologie
53 rue des Belles Feuilles
75116 Paris, France

Benign breast tumors are lesions of various sizes and morphology. Although the vast majority of them have a good prognosis, women with benign tumors should be considered more apt than others to develop subsequent carcinoma : they should therefore have regular check-ups for the rest of their lives.

The histological aspect of benign mammary tumors is related to the embryology of the gland. Mammary glands have, similar to salivary or sudoriparous glands, an ectodermic origin. They derive from epidermic thickenings which penetrate the underlying tissue and form buds. Towards the 20th week of embryonic development the branches develop lumina, thus creating the main galactophores and the ducts. As in the other ectodermic glands, the ductal system is outlined by two layers of cells : glandular and myoepithelial cells, both surrounded by a distinct basal membrane.

Hamperl (1970) and Bässler (1970) showed that the myoepithelium plays a complex part in mammary pathology. Physiologically, it is contractile and allows the transfer of metabolic substances and hormones between the surrounding connective tissue and the secretory cells. It probably takes part in the resorption of substances remaining in the ductal and acinar lumina. Myoepithelial cells may, in certain cases, secrete glycoaminoglycans and are capable of reconstituting the vanishing basal membrane of the regressing lobules at the end of lactation.

   Moreover, the outer cell layer comprising the myo-
epithelia is the cell layer which regenerates glandular
cells, thus explaining the morphology of some tumors :
mixed tumors, cylindroma, adeno-myoepithelioma and car-
cino-sarcoma. This pathology is much more frequent in
female dogs than in women.

   In a study of mastosis, Vogler (1947) was the first
to describe the presence of argyrophilic granules in ductal cells of a case of fibrocystic disease. More recently
Cubilla and Woodruff (1977) reported a case of a primary
carcinoid tumor of the breast without a clinical carcinoid syndrome. Another case in a man was observed by
Kaneko et al. (1978). This tumor was hormonally active
and associated with a slightly increased level of epi-
nephrin. Finally Azzopardi et al. (1979) observed argy-
rophil granules in the clear cytoplasm of hyperplastic
myoepithelial cells in a fibroadenoma. These cases
illustrate the extraordinary differentiation potential
of mammary cells, as related to their embryonic potentials

   The intralobular connective tissue (mantel tissue),
which is thin and edematous, with a fine reticular network, develops during puberty, changes under hormonal
action, and transmits the metabolites necessary for
secretory activity of the gland cells. The two tissues,
mesenchymal and glandular, are physiologically intimately
connected.

   At female puberty, the ducts develop and penetrate
into the connective tissue, forming lobes separated by
a fibro-vascular network.

   Benign breast tumors develop from any component of
the gland and may show two major gross morphologies :
unitissular tumors, localized and generally well delimited
and tumors with mixed mammary components, poorly delimited
They may originate in two locations : lobules, or ducts
and galactophores.

TUMORS OF LOBULAR ORIGIN

   These tumors originate in lobules, consisting of
intralobular terminal ducts and acini surrounded by the
intralobular connective tissue, and the extralobular
terminal ducts. They are classified according to the
predominating component :

- tumors consisting mainly of gland cell proliferation, with little participation of myoepithelial cells and connective tissue : adenomas,
- tumors in which participation of the myoepithelial cells is clearly predominant : sclerosing adenosis and adenomyoepithelioma,
- tumors in which intralobular mesenchymal tissue exceeds epithelial tissue : fibroadenoma.

Adenomas

The entity of a "pure breast adenoma" has only recently been accepted (Persaud et al., 1968 ; Hertel et al., 1976). These adenomas are of two sorts : tubular and lactating.

Tubular adenoma is clinically a hard and well delimited tumor and resembles fibroadenoma radiologically. Although it is without a true capsule, retraction of the neighboring connective tissue makes its excision easy. Histologically (Fig. 1), this lesion is characterized by a considerable development of the lobules, practically no longer separated by a stromal tissue. The acini, increased in number and size, have small lumina lined with regular epithelial cells and some myoepithelial cells visible at irregular intervals. Sometimes, the epithelial cells have prominent nucleoli and a few secretion vacuoles in the cytoplasm. The lumina often contain an eosinophilic substance. Mitoses are scarce and without atypia. The neoformed ducts and ductules are surrounded by a fine network of reticulin. They are separated by sclerosis of variable thickness, sometimes hyaline, so that in certain cases the small ducts tend to separate from one another and their lumina collapse.

Electron microscope study of tubular adenoma shows cells identical to those found in normal ductules : glandular cells, myoepithelial cells in an uninterrupted layer, and an intact epithelium to stroma interface with fibroblasts.

These tumors should not be confused with fibroadenoma, which shows hyperplasia of the intralobular connective tissue without multiplication of the ductules. In certain cases, Hertel et al. (1976) were able to show coexistence of a tubular adenoma and a fibroadenoma side by side without any transition zone. But the histological differences suggest that they are two separate entities, without transition from one to the other. Tubular adenoma

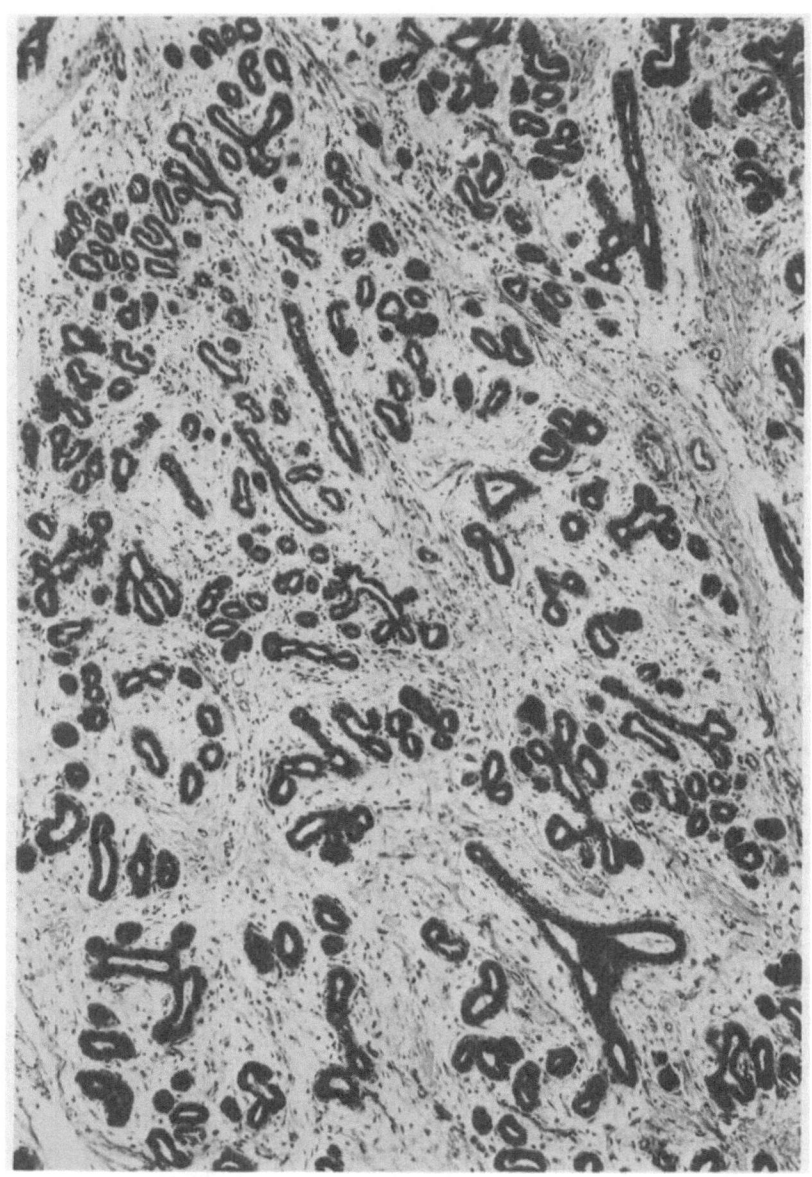

Fig. 1.   Tubular adenoma in a young girl at puberty.
H & E, x 125.

should neither be mistaken for sclerosing adenosis, which is distinguishable by the absence of delimitation with the rest of the mammary gland and considerable multiplication of myoepithelial cells, nor for well differentiated ductal carcinoma, even if ductule density is considerable.

The etiology of tubular adenomas remains unclear. Pregnancy, contraception or estrogen therapy do not seem to play a decisive part in their formation.

Lactating adenoma is the histological expression of induced secretory activity in an adenoma or fibroadenoma either preexisting or most likely formed during pregnancy. It is characterized by hyperplasia and signs of secretion. Such focal hyperplasia appears in areas with an increased hormonal sensitivity.

Grossly these tumors are well delimited from neighboring tissue and have a softer consistency than tubular adenomas. Upon section, the tumor is yellowish, 1-4 cm in diameter, without hemorrhage or necrosis.

Histologically, the lactating adenoma is rather well lobulated by fibrous septa, but is not surrounded by a true capsule.

At low magnification, it shows a network of large alveoli separated by fine fibro-vascular sheets. The alveolar lumen, filled with foamy material, is lined with epithelial cells with an abundant cytoplasm and small nuclei. The substance contained in the alveolar lumina has the histochemical characteristic of milk. Sometimes, mitoses are observed, but without cellular atypia. Myoepithelial cells are poorly distinguishable.

A somewhat special form has been observed by Hertel et al. (1976) in women pregnant for less than six months. The adenoma consists not of dilated alveoli, but of more or less oval-shaped and irregular gland structures, covered with a single-layered epithelium rich in vacuoles and in fat droplets. Mitoses are frequent. The remaining part of the breast shows the modifications corresponding to the stage of pregnancy. This lesion could be a form of transition between true tubular adenoma and lactation adenoma, since small-sized or slow-growing benign tumors begin to grow rapidly with the onset of pregnancy and even more rapidly during lactation.

Generally, adenoma evolution is strictly benign. However, an exceptional case was reported by Hill and Miller (1954) who observed a carcinoma in situ becoming invasive seven months after the removal of lactation adenoma without any atypia.

Sclerosing adenosis

Sclerosing adenosis is a lesion that can be localized and unnoticed in the midst of other lobular and ductal lesions, but which, in certain cases, may evoke carcinoma both clinically and histologically. It appears as a hard, round, nodular and multicentric lesion, resembling cancer in certain aspects, particularly scirrhous cancer and cancers with central sclerosis or elastic hyalinosis.

Morphologically, this swirling and multinodular lesion is highly cellular. Two different forms can be distinguished : the flourishing form and the regressive form.

In the flourishing form, the terminal ducts and acini multiply and become surrounded by hyperplastic myoepithelial cells, which in accumulating progressively compress the glandular lumina. The lesion is therefore of lobular origin, but the extra- and intralobular ducts may participate in the process (Tanako and Oota, 1970). In addition, the lumina may be filled with calcifications, which, upon mammography, can be mistaken for lobular carcinoma in situ (McErlean and Nathan, 1972).

The regressive form is the result of glycoaminoglycan secretion by the myoepithelial cells which constitute a ground substance in which the myoepithelial cells become modified and transformed into fibroblasts, thus provoking a dense sclerosis. The ground substance may be hyaline and contains elastic fibers. The epithelial constituents disperse in the modified sclerosing adenosis mass leading to mistaken diagnosis of invasive cancer, particularly since Norris and Taylor (1967), Gould et al. (1975), Eusebi and Azzopardi (1976) and more recently Fisher et al. (1979) all stressed the fact that infiltration in the peri-vascular and peri-neural lymph vessels can be found in 10 % of sclerosing adenosis cases. Caution should therefore be the rule before affirming benignity, and the lesion should be examined in step sections after embedding in paraffin. Comprehension on the part of the surgeon, the patient and his family is of great importance

Adeno-myoepithelioma

Adeno-myoepithelioma is an extremely rare disease, first described by Hamperl (1939). We observed one case, which differed from that of Finck et al. (1968) who described a clear cell hidradenoma ; it was similar to that of Toth (1977) who considered it a pure myoepithelioma resembling a multifocal leiomyoma. The tumor consisted

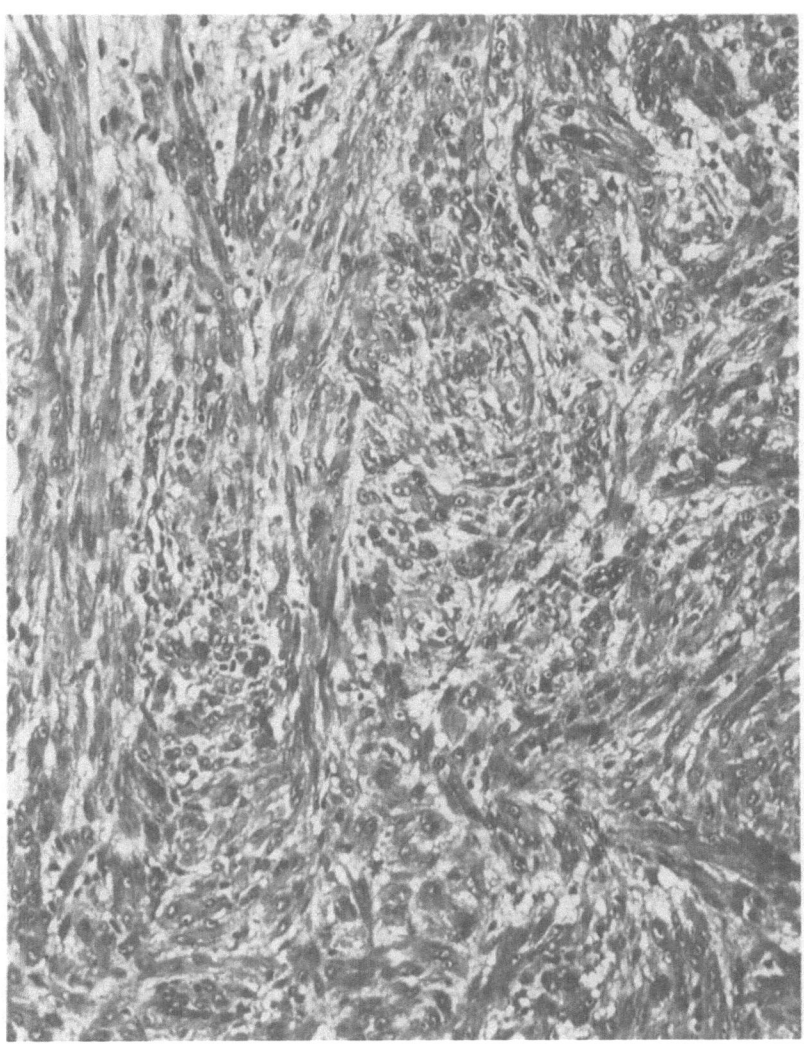

Fig. 2.   Adeno-myoepithelioma, made up by hyperplastic myoepithelial cells. H & E, x 200.

of large bundles of cells lying either in parallel fasci-
cles or in swirls, sometimes with a few remaining ducts
bordered by epithelial cells (Fig. 2 and 3).

The investigation of Van Bogaert and Maldague (1977)
revealed the presence of acid polysaccharides secreted
by the myoepithelial cells, thus explaining the existence
of some interstitial sclerosis.

In the rare instances of malignant transformation,
the myoepithelial cells account for the development of
mixed, salivary type tumors (Hamperl, 1970), with or
without cartilaginous and osseous metaplasia, similar
to mammary tumors in the dog, carcinosarcomas (Harris
and Persaud, 1974 ; Kahn et al., 1978), or even the rare
leiomyosarcomas or rhabdomyosarcomas which can be associated with carcinosarcomas (Govan, 1945).

Fibroadenoma

Fibroadenomas are the most frequent benign tumor
of the breast. They are characterized by the proliferation of the intralobular connective tissue and, depending
on the mode of proliferation, can be divided into two
types : intra- and pericanalicular fibroadenomas.

The intracanalicular form is the most frequent. The
hyperplastic intralobular connective tissue proliferates
between and into the glandular structures, stretching
them lengthwise and compressing the lumina so that the
apical poles of the bordering cells come into contact with
one another. The compression may attain such a degree
that the epithelium vanishes and the ducts appear as a
mere line of flattened cells.

Pericanalicular fibroadenomas are less frequent.
The intralobular connective tissue proliferation does
not modify lobular topography. Intralobular ducts are
isolated one from the other by a pericentric increase
in intralobular connective tissue. In both types of
fibroadenoma, the extralobular ducts are either compressed
or distended and cystic.

Fibroadenomas are devoid of a true capsule. Excision
can easily be performed, however, due to the compression
of the neighboring connective tissue. But the delimitation may sometimes be imprecise, because in the early
stages small fibroadenomas develop either contiguous to
or outside of the main tumor.

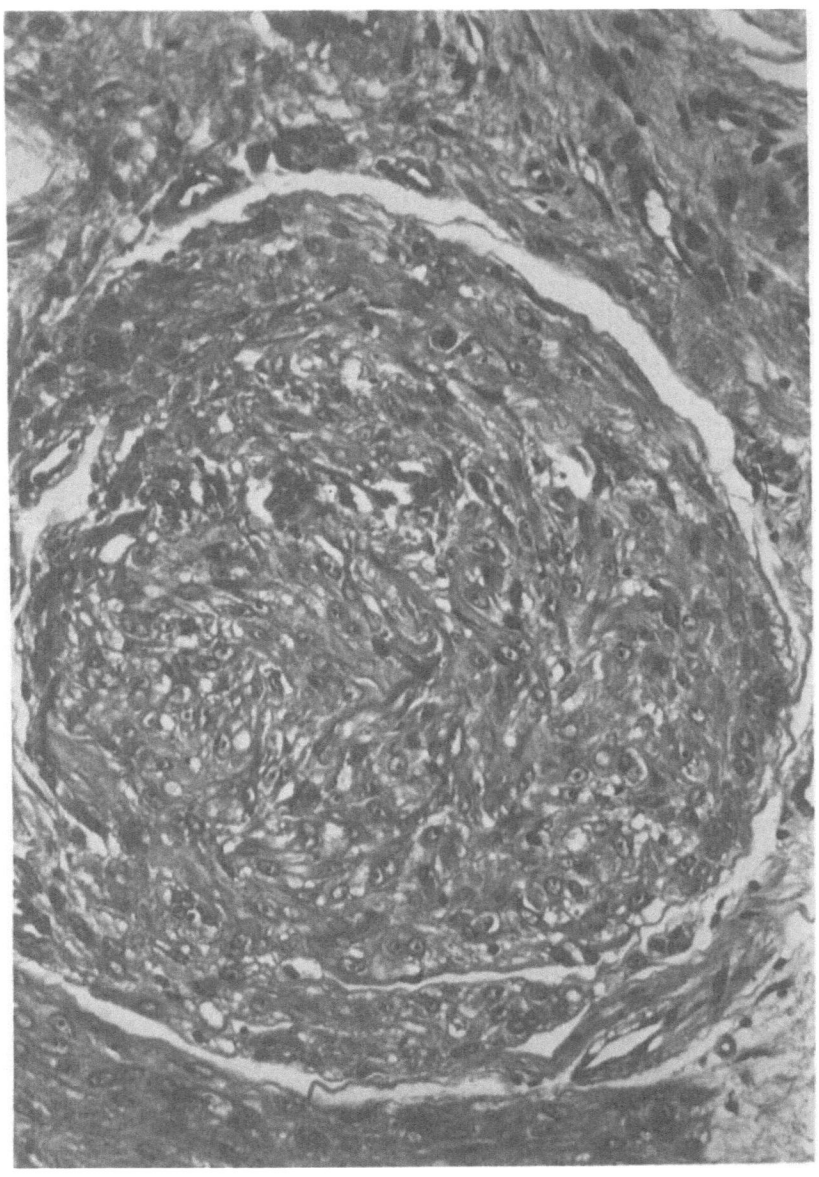

Fig. 3. Same tumor as fig. 2, showing intermingled
hyperplastic myoepithelial cells.
H & E, x 315.

Epithelial hyperplasia is fairly uncommon but may exist and mitoses may occur. Sometimes, particularly in young girls, small clusters of cells resembling those found in gynecomasty are observed, but benignity is the rule.

The rare cases of adenocarcinoma which develop in fibroadenoma (1/1000) are easy to distinguish due to their lobular or, less frequently, ductal morphology. They are usually carcinoma in situ, but sometimes they may invade neighboring mammary tissue (McDivitt et al., 1967).

Idrosadenoid metaplasia infrequently occurs in the more or less compressed glandular structures. More frequently these changes are found in the cysts in the periphery of the tumor, which represent the extralobular ducts either of the fibroadenoma itself or of the neighboring lobules.

Very rarely, multiplying myoepithelial cells may show argyrophilic granulations, as demonstrated by Hamperl (1970). Such granules also occur in the salivary and sudoriparous glands, and in their malignant tumor, cylindroma. Another rare aspect is the epidermoid metaplasia, as described by Salm (1957). According to Azzopardi et al. (1979), this change occurs more frequently in cystadenoma phyllodes.

Infarction of fibroadenoma was described by Delarue and Redon (1949), and in three of their cases a carcinoma was present. Other authors have drawn attention to this complication (Wilkinson and Green, 1964 ; Haagensen, 1971 ; Newman and Kahn, 1973 ; Majmudar and Rosales-Quintana, 1975). The lesion resembles an hemorrhagic infarction surrounded by a sclerous zone. Probably, such an event is related to circulatory trouble or thrombosis can be assimilated to similar changes found in leiomyoma.

Modifications in intralobular connective tissue are not well understood. Fibroblast density may vary and the mantel tissue become hyalin and at times calcified. Azzopardi et al. (1979) reported transformation into smooth muscle fibers, a lesion considered by certain authors as an hamartoma (Riddell and Davies, 1973). Calcifications occurring at the junction of the intralobular connective tissue and the myoepithelial cells are rather voluminous rounded or polygonal, and differ from those observed in carcinoma in situ.

<u>Giant fibroadenomas</u> appear mainly in Negro and Asian
women, and in caucasian women at puberty (Wulsin, 1960).
They consist of very pronounced hyperplasia of the epithelial and mesenchymal structures (Fig. 4) and may
evoke phyllode tumors. But neither cell density abnormalities nor mitoses are found.

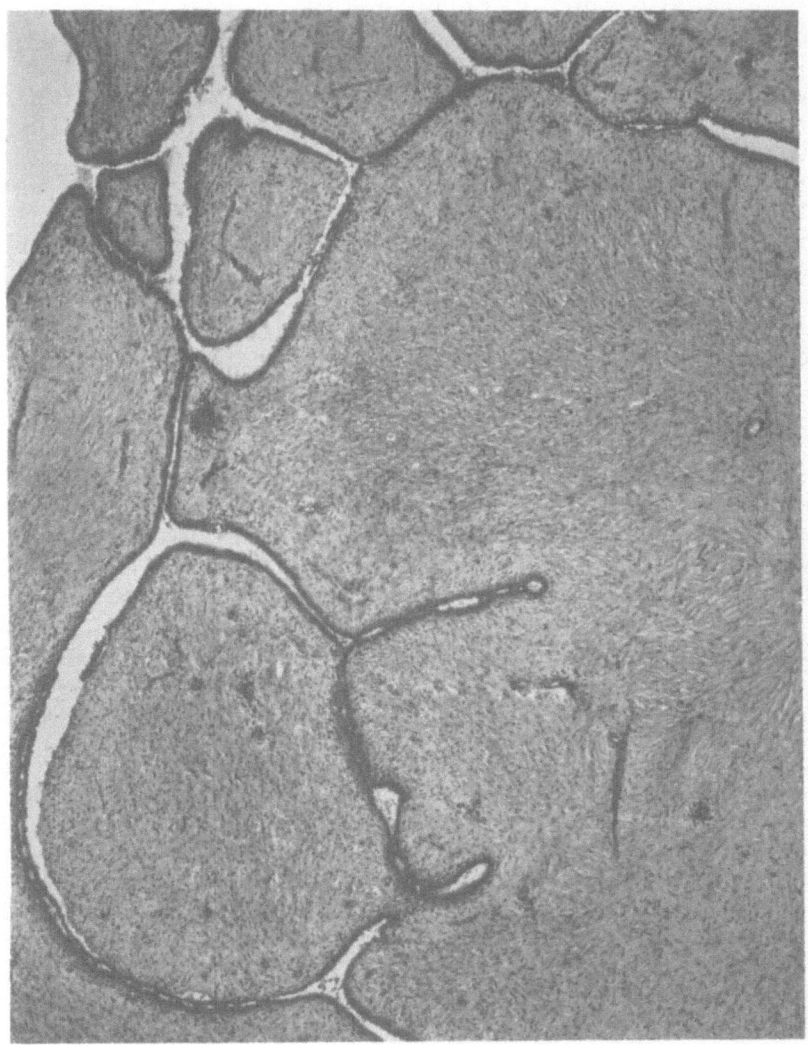

Fig. 4.   Giant fibroadenoma
H & E, x 160.

Phyllode tumor

    Phyllode tumors were first described by Chelius
(1828) and by Muller (1838). These rare tumors have a
well known histological aspect but their prognosis is
difficult to evaluate. Their terminology is therefore
particularly abundant, depending upon whether they are
considered benign with possible local recurrence or on
the contrary malignant, sarcoma-like. McDonald and
Harrington (1950) thus call this lesion the "27-name
tumor".

    The basic structure of the tumor is mainly that of
a fibroadenoma, and both lesions have a mesenchymal
origin with epithelial participation. But whereas in the
ordinary or the giant type of fibroadenoma there exists
an equilibrium between mesenchymal and epithelial cell
proliferation, in phyllode tumors the mesenchymal structures generally predominate and show considerable cell
density associated with abnormal mitoses. Zones of
epithelial proliferation of various intensity may be
observed and may then evoke a carcinoma in situ. Cyto-
sarcoma phyllodes can thus be classified between fibroadenoma and sarcoma.

    The clinical examination does not allow to differen-
ciate between giant fibroadenoma and tumor phyllodes.
The usual form evokes sarcoma because its development is
very rapid. The tumor is polylobulated, movable, painless
and hard. The skin may be edematous with a visible venous
network but without adherence to the deeper structures.
Axillary lymph nodes are generally not involved, except
in the observations of Treeves and Sunderland (1951).
The tumor may attain a volume of 10-15 cm in diameter and
exceptionally a bilateral tumor may occur. Phyllode tumor
can be distinguished from fibroadenoma by the presence of
several small knobby adjacent tumors which are more voluminous than an ordinary fibroadenoma. Furthermore, it
is deeply situated in the parenchyma and apparently
attached to the gland, in contrast with the perfectly
movable and encapsulated fibroadenoma. The evolution of
these tumors varies from a few weeks to several decades.
At later stages, invasion of the neighboring mammary
tissue may occur, but fascias and the skin are respected,
and ulcerations are of purely mechanical origin.

    From the etiological point of view, the role of
hormones has been suggested but not yet proven. Phyllode
tumors occur at the two extremities of sexual life.

Pregnancy and lactation do not appear to influence this
type of tumor.

At macroscopic examination the tumor appears encapsulated, but a small peduncular zone always exists,
attaching the tumor to the gland. Upon section, the tumor
is more fragile than fibroadenoma, white, myxoid-like,
and with pseudo-cystic formations filled with a gelati-
nous substance.

On sectioning, the tumor shows multiple lobulated or
finger-like formations which protrude and evoke the
aspect of a puzzle or a leaf ("phyllode" meaning "leaf-
like").

Histologically, tumor phyllodes consist, as fibroadenoma, of a proliferation of mensenchymal and epithelial
cells (Fig. 5).

The mesenchymal component predominates, accounting
for the particularity of the tumor and its subsequent
evolution. The ground substance varies in appearance.
Sometimes it appears edematous containing fibroblasts
and a fibrillar reticulum that reticulin staining
clearly reveals. At times, it is hyaline and contains
collagen fibers, thus representing the oldest part of
the tumor. The cellular elements of the stroma also have
different aspects : star-shaped cells and fibroblasts
of normal shape and size, and low cell density, evoking
giant fibroadenoma ; or more cellular hyperplastic stroma
and cellular abnormalities such as voluminous chromatic
nuclei, numerous mitoses or anaplastic pattern, giving
the tumor a sarcomatous appearance. The dense cellular
zones are sometimes located in the periphery of large
edematous digitations which either project, like polyps,
into the distended cystic lumina of the ducts, or
compress their lumina, thus producing a mosaic-like
effect. The glandular structures are usually compressed
and the central lumina reduced and occasionally completely absent, showing mere T or Y-shaped slits lined by
a flattened epithelium. In some tumors, the mesenchymal
cells undergo metaplasia and induce cartilaginous or
osseous transformation of the ground substance. In other
areas, the ducts are dilated, some of which are cystic
and show a polypoid proliferation of mesenchymal buds.
Haagensen (1971) describes five types of epithelial
proliferation which may be associated :

1. small areas of epithelial polypoid hyperplasia
filling the ducts,

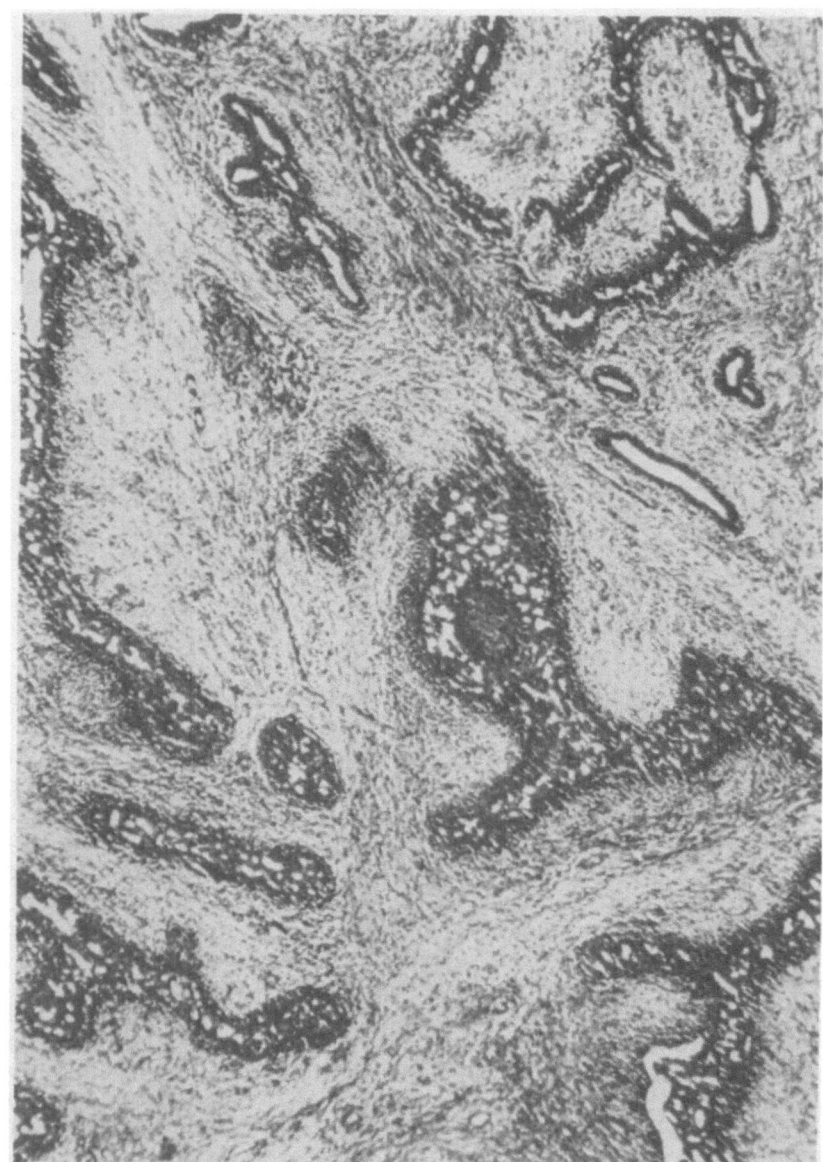

Fig. 5.   Cystadenosarcoma phyllodes. High cellular
          density of the intralobular connective tissue
          and hyperplasia of the ductal cells.
          H & E, x 125.

2. areas of adenosis,
3. areas of epidermoid metaplasia filling the lumina (Norris and Taylor, 1967),
4. areas of intraductal lobular neoplasia (cancer in situ),
5. invasive carcinoma.

Criteria for malignancy are difficult to establish, due to the inconsistency of both the clinical and histological signs.

Neither size nor growth rate are features of malignancy. The classification of a cystosarcoma as benign or malignant is based solely on changes observed in the stromal portion of the tumor, i.e. the degree of cellular pleomorphism of the stromal cells. However, a certain number of such histologically malignant tumors have proven benign in evolution, although the opposite case has also been observed. Lester and Stout (1954), studying 58 cases, discovered 5 metastases. In reviewing the primary tumor sections, they found that only two had been classified as malignant. Lester and Stout's criteria for malignancy are the infiltration on the margin of the mammary gland, the degree of atypia in the stromal cells and the number of mitoses. For Treeves and Sunderland (1951), however, the presence of bizarre or giant cells is not necessarily an indication of malignancy.

Complexity of lobular lesions

Most lesions described under the name of mastosis, mastopathy or mammary dystrophy, are composed of multiple, closely intricated, poorly delimited foci resembling different types of benign tumors. Areas of adenosis are frequently associated with sclerosing adenosis and/or small fibroadenomas. The epithelial structures of sclerosing adenosis may break up within hyaline or fibrinoid layers and then evoke a beginning carcinoma. Similarly some lobules with clear cell proliferation may be found in small fibroadenomas and be mistaken for in situ lobular carcinoma. The intermingling of these various lesions is associated with small cyst formation, with metaplastic alterations of the lining epithelium, and, frequently, with hyperplasia of the epithelium of the intra- and extralobular ducts. At these critical regions carcinoma in situ takes origin.

TUMORS OF DUCTS AND GALACTOPHORES

We shall set aside cysts and consider benign tumors
originating in the walls of large or medium sized ducts
and galactophores. Such tumors are papillomas which
develop from the ductal wall, forming finger-like projections in the lumen, and consist of a central, generally ramified, gradually thickening peduncle, bearing
a central capillary. The covering epithelium consists of
myoepithelial and glandular cells. The former tend to
vary in aspect. Sometimes they are hyperplastic and
myxoid, sometimes flattened, and it seems that they secrete acid mucopolysaccharides and account for progressive growth of the central axis. Touching of the distal
extremities of the papillary projections may evoke
pseudoacini, whence the misleading name "dendritic
adenoma".

The surface cells are cuboidal with a rather voluminous, generally pale, nucleus. Mitoses are rare. The
epithelium frequently undergoes various types of metaplasia, the most frequent being the apocrine type with
the presence of ceroid pigments which are found in the
mammary discharge, the first clinical symptom of the
tumor.

Two varieties of intraductal papilloma can be
distinguished :

- Solitary papilloma, rather large-sized, attaining
3 cm in diameter, is usually situated in a cystic dila-
tion or in the large galactophores ;
- Multiple papillomas of smaller size, occuring in
one or both breats, are much more frequently associated
with carcinoma than solitary papilloma, either by
transformation of the preexisting tumor or by subsequent
development of another papillary and primary malignant
tumor.

The diagnostic difficulty of the two lesions is
generally due to the fact that they are either underes-
timated or overestimated. The presence, amid the
papillae, of a connectivovascular axis, an uninterrupted
layer of myoepithelial cells and an unchanged nucleo-
cytoplasmic ratio plead for benignity.

Intraductal papilloma may be associated with other
dystrophies, the most common of which is ductal ectasia.
Although coexistence with ductal carcinoma in situ exists,

differential diagnosis is easy on mammary discharge
cytology.

Several cytological criteria should be considered :
variation in cell size and shape; nuclear volume and hyperchromatism; mitoses, although certain highly differentiated carcinomas have practically none; piling of
several layers of only one cell type with loss of pola-
rity in carcinoma, whereas in intraductal papilloma the
two types of ductal cells can be recognized; eosinophilic apocrine metaplasia, which, according to Kraus and
Neubecker (1962), is absent in papillary carcinoma,
whereas for Haagensen (1971) it may occasionally be found.

Histologically, the following criteria can be
applied : the connective axes, which are thick in benign
papilloma, are thin or absent in carcinoma ; the papillae
are organized in a regular glandular aspect in adenoma,
whereas they are much more irregular in cancer, where
pseudoglands penetrate the stroma.

Other criteria are : in benign papilloma, dilated
ductal walls are thickened, sclerotic, dotted with spots
of pigmented histiocytes ; in carcinoma, this aspect is
usually associated with invasion of the neighboring
stroma ; in papilloma, dystrophy and dysplasia of the
mammary tissue are frequently associated, in particular
sclerosing adenosis ; in cancer this association is
practically nonexistent.

CONCLUDING REMARKS

The natural history of benign breast tumors can be
interpreted on embryological and microanatomical grounds.

The vast majority of benign breast tumors originate
in the lobules and only a minority in the epithelium of
the ducts.

In tumors of lobular origin the predominance of one
cell component determines the structural pattern without
eliminating the participation of other structural components.

In fibroadenoma, predominance of intralobular connective tissue proliferation does not exclude hyperplasia
of the epithelium. In adenoma, hyperplasia of glandular
structures prevails, but the myoepithelial cells and
the intralobular connective tissue are also hyperplastic.

In sclerosing adenosis, there is a predominance of the myoepithelial cells. Multiple metaplastic lesions then appear and induce sclerotic regression of the lesion. Multiplying myoepithelial cells push away the glandular elements, thus creating adeno-myoepithelioma. In other cases, the myoepithelial cells secrete hydroxylase-type substances, inducing tissular degeneration with secondary elastosis, giving some benign lesions the aspect of malignant tumors.

In breast cancer patients, 2.5 % have case histories of benign breast lesions (Black and Leis, 1973 ; Monson et al., 1976). Although the relationship between breast cancer and previous existence of benign breast tumor has not yet been established, this fact may be explained by various factors, such as race and family history, cocan-cerogenous factors, mammary cell receptivity to hormones and immunological deficiency. Finally, Fisher and Paulson (1978) demonstrated by karyotype studies that chromosomal abnormalities exist in benign breast tumors similar to those found in invasive carcinomas.

REFERENCES

Azzopardi, J.G., Ahmed, A., and Millis, R.M., 1979, In :
    Problems in Breast Pathology, Vol. II in the
    Series "Major Problems in Pathology", W.B. Saunders
    London, Philadelphia, Toronto.
    "Infarction of fibroadenoma" p. 43, "Argyrophilic
    cells in Fibroadenomas" p. 52, "Eccrine spiradenoma-
    like tumour" p. 340.
Bässler, R., 1970, The morphology of hormone induced
    structural changes in the female breast. In :
    Current Topics in Pathology, pp 1-89, Springer,
    Berlin.
Black, M.M., and Leis, H.P. Jr., 1973, Cellular responses
    to autologous breast cancer tissue. Sequential
    observations. Cancer, 32, 384.
Chelius, 1828, Talanziektasie, Heidelb. Klin. Ann.,
    4, 449.
Cubilla, A.L., and Woodruff, J.M., 1977, Primary carci-
    noid tumor of the breast. A report of eight pa-
    tients. Am. J. Surg. Path., 4, 283-292.
Delarue, J., and Redon, H., 1949, Les infarctus des
    fibroadénomes mammaires, problème clinique et
    pathogénique. Sem. Hôp. Paris, 25, 2991-2996.
Eusebi, V., and Azzopardi, J.G., 1976, Vascular infil-
    tration in benign breast disease. J. Pathology,
    118, 9-16.

Finck, F.M., Schwinn, C.P., and Keasbey, L.E., 1968,
    Clear cell hidradenoma of the breast. Cancer,
    22, 125-135.
Fisher, E.R., Palekar, A.S., Kotwal, N., and Lipana, N.,
    1979, A nonencapsulated sclerosing lesion of the
    breast. Am. J. Clin. Path., 71, 3 240-246.
Fisher, E.R., and Paulson, J.D., 1978, Karyotypic abnor-
    malities in precursor lesions of human cancer of
    the breast. Am. J. Clin. Path., 69, 284-288.
Gould, V.E., Miller, J., and Jao, W., 1975, Ultrastruc-
    ture of medullary, intraductal, tubular and
    adenocystic breast carcinomas. Comparative patterns
    of myoepithelial differentiation and basal lamina
    deposition. Am. J. Path., 78, 401-407.
Govan, A.D.T., 1945, Two cases of mixed malignant tumour
    of the breast. J. Path. Bact., 56, 397-404.
Haagensen, C.D., 1971, Diseases of the breast. 2nd ed.
    W.B. Saunders, Philadelphia, London, Toronto.
Hamperl, H., 1939, Uber die Myothelien (myo-epithelialen
    elements) der Brustdrüse. Wirchow Arch. Path.
    Anat., 305, 171-215.
Hamperl, H., 1970, The myothelia (myoepithelial cell).
    in : Currents Topics in Pathology, Springer,
    Berlin, pp. 161-220.
Harris, M., and Persaud, V., 1974, Carcinoma of the
    breast. J. Pathology, 112, 99-105.
Hertel, B.F., Zaloudek, C., and Kempson, R.L., 1976,
    Breast adenomas, Cancer, 37, 2891-2905.
Hill, R.P., and Miller, F.N. Jr., 1954, Adenomas of breast
    with case report of carcinomatous transformation
    in adenomas. Cancer, 7, 318-324.
Kahn, L.B., Uys, C.D., Dale, J., and Rutherfoord, F.,
    1978, Carcinoma of the breast with metaplasia to
    chondrosarcoma : a light and electron microscopic
    study. Histopathology, 2, 93-106.
Kaneko, H., Hojo, H., Ishikawa, S., Yamanouchi, H.,
    Sumida, T., and Saito, R., 1978, Norepinephrine
    producing tumors of bilateral breast. A case
    report. Cancer, 41, 2002-2007.
Kraus, F.T., and Neubecker, R.D., 1962, The differential
    diagnosis of papillary tumors of the breast.
    Cancer, 15, 444-455.
Lester, J., and Stout, A.P., 1954, Cystosarcoma phyllodes.
    Cancer, 7, 335-353.
McDivitt, R.W., Stewart, F.W., and Farrow, J.H., 1967,
    Breast carcinoma arising in solitary fibroadenomas.
    Surg. Gynecol. Obstet., 125, 572-576.
McErlean, D.P., and Nathan, B.E., 1972, Calcification in
    sclerosing adenosis simulating malignant breast

calcification. Brit. J. Radiology, 45, 944-945.

McDonald, J.R., and Harrington, S.W., 1950, Giant fibroadenoma of the breast "cysto-sarcoma phyllodes".
Ann. Surgery, 131, 243-251.

Majmudar, B., and Rosales-Quintana, S., 1975, Infarction
of the breast fibroadenomas during pregnancy.
JAMA, 231, 963-964.

Monson, R.R., Yen, S., and McMahon, B., 1976, Chronic
mastitis and carcinoma of the breast. Lancet,
224-226.

Müller, J., Ueber dem feinern Bau und die Formen der
krankhaften Geschwülste. Berlin, G. Reimer, 1838.

Newman, J., and Kahn, L.B., 1973, Infarction of fibroadenoma of the breast. Brit. J. Surg., 60, 738-
740.

Norris, H.J., and Taylor, H.B., 1967, Relationship of
histologic features to behavior of cystosarcoma
phyllodes. Analysis of ninety-four cases.
Cancer, 20, 2090-2099.

Persaud, V., Talerman, A., and Jordan, R., 1968, Pure
adenoma of the breast. Arch. Pathology, 86,
481-483.

Riddell, R.H., and Davies, J.D., 1973, Muscular hamar-
tomas of the breast. J. Path., 111, 209-211.

Salm, R., 1957, Epidermoid metaplasia in mammary fibroadenoma with formation of keratin cysts. J. Path.
Bact., 74, 221-222.

Tanaka, Y. and Oota, K., 1970, A stereomicroscopic study
of the mastopathic human breast. I. Three dimensional structures of abnormal duct evolution and
their histologic entity. Virchows Arch. A. Pathology, 349, 195-214.

Toth, J., 1977, Benign human mammary myoepithelioma.
Virchows Arch. A, Pathology, 374, 263-269.

Treeves, N., and Sunderland, D.A., 1951, Cystosarcoma
phyllodes of the breast : a malignant and a
benign tumor ; a clinico-pathological study of
77 cases. Cancer, 4, 1286-1332.

Van Bogaert, L.J., and Maldague, P., 1977, Histologic
variants of lipid secreting carcinoma of the
breast. Virchows Arch. A. Pathology, 375, 345-353.

Vogler, E., 1947, Über das basilare Helle-Zellen-Organ
der menschlichen Brustdrüse. Klinische Medizin,
2, 159-168.

Wellings, S.R., and Roberts, P., 1963, Electron microscopy of sclerosing adenosis and infiltrating duct
carcinoma of the human mammary gland. J. Natl.
Cancer Inst., 30, 269-287.

Wilkinson, L., and Green, W.O., Jr., 1964, Infarction of
       the breast lesions during pregnancy and lactation.
       Cancer, 17, 1567-1572.
Wulsin, J.H., 1960, Large breast tumors in adolescent
       females. Ann. Surgery, 152, 151-159.

CYSTOCARCOMA PHYLLODES

F. Cabanne

Centre Georges-François Leclerc
1 rue du Professeur Marion
21034 Dijon Cedex, France

Since the first description of cystosarcoma phyllodes, more than 150 years ago, the question concerning the true nature of the growth has not yet been answered. Its etiology is still unknown. Its incidence is about 1 to 3 % of all mammary tumors and it occurs almost exclusively in females and may be found from puberty until senescence (Table 1).

From the practical point of view the diagnosis of the lesion and the histoprognostic evaluation should be the object of particular attention.

The following remarks are based on 11 personal observations. The diagnosis of the tumor may present some difficulties. Cystosarcoma phyllodes is, like fibroadenoma and particularly like giant fibroadenoma, an fibro-epithelial growth. However, several microscopic features, sometimes difficult to elucidate, distinguish it from fibroadenoma. The most characteristic feature concerns the connective portion of the tumor : predominance of the latter compared to the epithelial component ; formation of voluminous digitations protruding in the lumina of the ducts and pushing ahead the lining epithelium ; edematous, myxoid or partially hyalinized aspect occasionally with areas of osteo-cartilagenous metaplasia ; star-like cells anastomosing together, or fibroblastic spindle cells either ramdomly scattered or grouped in bundles and in dense clusters ; finally cell abnormalities.

TABLE 1

Cystosarcoma phyllodes. Age incidence.

AUTHORS	Number of cases	Age range
Lester and Stout (1954)	58	13 - 88
Barbeau et al. (1956)	11	22 - 62
Norris and Taylor (1967)	94	15 - 86
West et al. (1971)	15	13 - 77
Centre Georges-François Leclerc (Dijon)	11	12 - 71

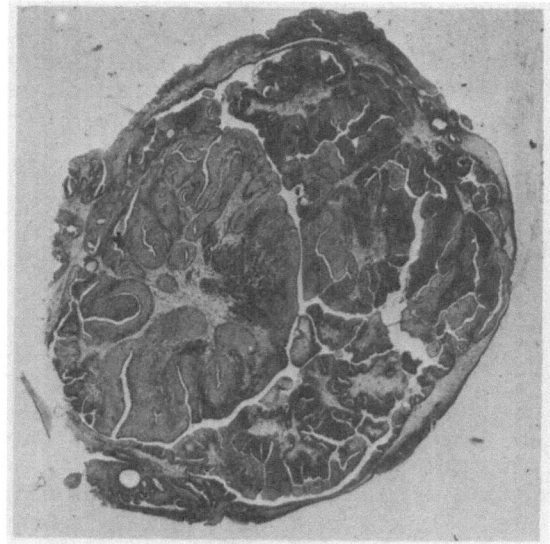

Fig. 1. Low power of cystosarcoma phyllodes, type 1,
        showing the digitations of the connective tissue
        and the resulting clefts of the compressed
        ducts. The lesion in well circumscribed.

TABLE 2

Histological classification of cystosarcoma phyllodes, after Contesso et al., 1978.

Type	Epithelial component	Connective tissue component	
		Cells	Intercellular tissue
I benign		abundant loosely arranged sometimes atypical	edematous
II benign	more or less hyperplastic stratified papillary	very abundant arranged in dense bundles sometimes atypical	myxoid cystic necrotic
III benign		very abundant randomly arranged atypical normal mitoses	cartilaginous or osteoid metaplasia
IV malignant	persistent tubular formations	irregular atypical abnormal mitoses	dense irregular

The ducts are either dilated and cystic, or compressed to small clefts. The ductal epithelium is rarely
cubic or flattened. It usually participates in the proliferative process and shows hyperplastic protrusions in
the lumina.

The observation of the above-described alterations,
which are more or less intricate from one tumor field to
another, leads to the diagnosis (Fig. 1).

The evolutivity of the growth varies from case to
case. In about 85 % of the cases the evolution resembles
that of a benign tumor or of a locally invading and
recurring tumor which ultimately is cured surgically.
About 15 % of the cases progress as a true cancer giving
rise to loco-regional and distant metastases and resembling a sarcoma or less frequently, a carcinosarcoma or
even a carcinoma.

The prognosis is even more difficult to establish
than the diagnosis. The density of the spindle cells,
the high number of mitoses per microscopic field, the
infiltration of the mammary gland at the borderline of
the tumor, the disappearance of the epithelial component,
are strong arguments in favor of a malignant growth. On
the other hand, the presence of polymorphous cell atypias
should not give rise to excessive pessimism.

Aside from the cases which are clearly malignant,
it is always difficult to predict the evolution of the
tumor from a histological point of view and to distinguish
the cystosarcoma which remains benign from that which
reccurs or which becomes cancer. Table 2 shows the histological classification proposed by Contesso et al.
(1978) in an attempt to distinguish between different
degrees of evolutivity. Reccurence is rare in type I,
except incomplete resection, less rare in types II and III,
and the rule in type IV, which is further characterized
by metastases.

REFERENCES

Barbeau, A., Lefebvre, R., Cholette, C., 1956, Le cysto-
        sarcome phyllode. Union médicale du Canada, 85,
        653-663.
Contesso, G., Genin, J., Lasser, Ph., 1978, Tumeurs
        phyllodes du sein. Revue du praticien, 28,
        1031-1037.

Lester, J., Stout, A.P., 1954, Cystosarcoma phyllodes.
        Cancer, 7, 335-353.
Norris, H.J., Taylor, H.B., 1967, Relationship of histo-
        logic features to behavior of cystosarcoma phyllo-
        des. Analysis of ninety-four cases. Cancer, 20,
        2090-2099.
West, T.L., Weiland, L.H., Clagett, O.T., 1971, Cystosar-
        coma phyllodes. Annals of surgery, 173, 520-528.

ASPIRATION CYTOLOGY AND CYTO-PROGNOSIS OF BREAST LESIONS

A. Zajdela and M.A. de MAUBLANC

Department of Cytopathology
Institut Curie, 26 rue d'Ulm
75005 Paris, France

INTRODUCTION

The cytological analysis of tumors by puncture aspiration with a fine needle is not a new method : it has been used for half a century, since Martin and Ellis (1930, 1934) showed its usefulness and effectiveness.

In the last twenty years, the literature has been much enriched, especially in the field of breast lesions, by numerous publications (Cornillot and Verhaeghe, 1955 ; Godwin, 1956 ; Zajdela, 1963 ; Franzen and Zajicek, 1968 ; Kreuzer and Zajicek, 1972 ; Hajdu and Melamed, 1973 ; Zajicek, 1974 ; Lopez Cardozo, 1976). Some of these studies were based on a very large number of cases (Franzen and Zajicek, 1968 ; Cornillot et al., 1971 ; Zajdela et al., 1975), and it was shown that needle biopsy is a very safe examination. Robbins et al. (1954), in a major clinical report and Burn et al.(1968), in an experimental study on rats bearing Walker's adenocarcinoma showed that this type of sampling did not influence survival in any way.

Without expounding on the aspiration technique already described by different authors (Cornillot and Verhaeghe, 1955 ; Godwin, 1956 ; Franzen and Zajicek, 1968 ; Zajdela, 1963 ; Zajdela et al., 1975), we will stress that the success of the method depends mostly on mastering the technique. It is carried out with a 20 or 30 ml syringe and a 7 to 8/10th mm needle. The puncture is practically painless and requires no local anaesthesia.

The aspirates are stained according to the May-Grunwald-Giemsa technique, which allows examination of the preparations 20 minutes after the puncture.

At the Institut Curie, in Paris, we have carried out aspiration cytology on breast lesions since 1954, associated systematically with the other usual breast examinations.

In 1974, our data included 3,583 breast tumors cytologically studied on aspiration smears and histologically proved. All the tumors with uncertain histological diagnoses were excluded from the study.

We propose to discuss here the validity of aspiration cytology in diagnosis of breast tumors (including postradiotherapy residual lesions) and the determination of its value in the prognosis of breast cancers, by measurement of the diameter of the nuclei and by the application of Scarff, Bloom and Richardson's histological parameters to smear cytology.

VALIDITY OF ASPIRATION CYTOLOGY IN THE DIAGNOSIS OF BREAST CANCER

Patients not treated by radiotherapy

The cytology and histology of 3,583 breast tumors, 2,071 of which histologically malignant and 1,512 histologically benign, were compared (Zajdela et al., 1975).

Out of the 2,071 malignant tumors (Table 1), the histological and cytological results agreed, in 87.4 % of the cases (1,810 cases) and disagreed in 12.6 % (261 cases). Out of the latter cases, 3.7 % (77 cases) were considered cytologically suspect, 3.8 % wrongly benign (79 "false benign" reports) and 5.1 % insufficient in aspiration (105 cases).

Out of the 1,512 benign tumors (Table II), the histological and cytological results were consistent in 89.7 % (1,357 cases) and inconsistent in 10.3 % (155 cases). The latter cases were broken down as follows : 52 cases (3.5 %) were considered cytologically suspicious ; 4 cases (0.3 %) were mistakenly considered to be malignant (false malignant reports) ; and in 99 cases (6.5 %), aspiration was insufficient.

TABLE I

VALUE OF ASPIRATION CYTOLOGY IN DIAGNOSIS OF MALIGNANT BREAST

TUMORS

HISTOLOGIC DIAGNOSIS	N°	CYTOLOGIC DIAGNOSIS			
		concordant	suspicious	false benign	insufficient cell material
Carcinoma	2,055*	1,795*	76	79	105
Melanoma	2	2			
Malignant lymphoma	11	11			
Fibrosarcoma	3	2	1		
TOTAL	2,071	1,810	77	79	105
PERCENTAGE		87.4 %	3.7 %	3.8%	5.1 %

*Including 45 cases of colloid carcinoma, 3 of adenoid cystic carcinoma, 7 medullary carcinoma, 2 apocrine carcinoma and 3 carcinoma with squamous metaplasia. All diagnosed by aspiration cytology.

TABLE II

VALUE OF ASPIRATION CYTOLOGY IN DIAGNOSIS OF BENIGN BREAST TUMORS

HISTOLOGIC DIAGNOSIS	N°	CYTOLOGIC DIAGNOSIS			
		concordant	suspicious	false malign.	insufficient cell material
Adenoma and fibro-cystic disease	893	786	38	4*	65
Benign cystic tumors	502	481	14		7
Inflammation	69	59			10
Lipoma	42	28			14
Tuberculosis	3	1			2
Granular cell myo-blastoma	2	2			
Actinomycosis	1				1
TOTAL	1,512	1,357	52	4	99
PERCENTAGE		89.7 %	3.5 %	0.3 %	6.5 %

*Three cases proved to be fibroadenoma and one fibrocystic disease.

An analysis of these results shows that the consistency between the histological and cytological diagnoses is good, both in the malignant (87.4 %) and in the benign tumors (89.7 %). Nevertheless, the diagnostic value of aspiration cytology varies, depending on whether the tumor is malignant or benign. In malignant tumors, the value is high because there were very few false malignant reports (0.3 %). Note also that among the 1,810 malignant tumors in which the histology and cytology concurred, 102 cases (5.6 %) had been considered to be benign upon clinical examination.

On the other hand, in benign tumors the value of cytological diagnosis cannot be considered to be definite, despite the good histological and cytological concordance, because there is a rather high level (3.8 %) of false benign reports (i.e. cancers which have not been recognized cytologically). These false benign reports are practically impossible to avoid, even by the most highly trained cytologist.

These errors can result from an aspiration outside the tumor area, from a carcinoma without morphological changes, especially some well differentiated adeno- or scirrhus carcinomas, and from a benign tumor lying next to a carcinoma, the latter having not been reached by the puncture needle. (We saw 5 such cases of cysts which we diagnosed as benign, although there was an adjacent carcinoma).

Finally, it is important to note that the percentages of malignant diagnoses, false malignant reports and false benign reports are nearly the same in the 3 largest statistical cyto-histological studies published to date, i.e. those by Franzen and Zajicek (1968) on 1,680 cases, the report by Cornillot et al. (1971) on 2,267 cases and our own study on 3,583 cases (Tables III and IV).

Patients previously submitted to radiotherapy

The postradiotherapy follow-up of breast cancer is often very difficult because neither the clinical nor the radiographical signs allow differentiation between postradiotherapy sclerosis and further evolution of the cancer, particularly since the two can be associated.

Between 1968 and 1975, 202 cases of breast cancer treated exclusively by irradiation (182 cases) or by lumpectomy and post-operative irradiation (20 cases) were investigated by fine needle cytology during the radio-

TABLE III

INCIDENCE OF FALSE BENIGN REPORTS IN HISTOLOGICALLY CHECKED BREAST TUMORS

AUTHORS	HISTOLOGY Malignant tumors TOTAL	CYTOLOGY Concord. %	CYTOLOGY False benign reports %
FRANZEN & ZAJICEK (1968)	873	89.2	4.8
CORNILLOT et al. (1971)	1,335	87.8	4.6
ZAJDELA et al. (1975)	2,071	87.3	3.8

TABLE IV

INCIDENCE OF FALSE MALIGNANT REPORTS IN HISTOLOGICALLY
CHECKED BREAST TUMORS

AUTHORS	HISTOLOGY Benign tumors TOTAL	CYTOLOGY False malignant reports %
FRANZEN & ZAJICEK (1968)	807	0.1
CORNILLOT et al. (1971)	932	0.4
ZAJDELA et al. (1975)	1,512	0.3

logical and clinical follow-up (Zajdela and de Maublanc, 1979). The histological diagnosis was confirmed by drill-biopsy before treatment (182 cases) or by histology after lumpectomy (20 cases).

The cytological aspirations were carried out either on a residual tumor, or in a suspicious area having appeared after a periòd of normalization. More than half of the aspirates were carried out in the first two years ; nearly all within 5 years after irradiation. The extremes were between 4 months and 23 years after treatment.

The following cytological findings were recorded : presence of viable carcinomatous cells, corresponding histologically to an evolutive carcinoma ; presence of suspicious cells, corresponding to a doubtful histological lesion ; and absence of carcinomatous cells, corresponding to the absence of an active carcinoma on histology.

The cytology results in these 202 cases were compared with those of histological examination of the surgical specimen. In 181 cases there was histologically active cancer, in 2 cases the lesion was suspicious and in 19 cases there was no active carcinoma on the histological slides.

Out of the 183 cases of evolutive or suspicious lesions, the cytological diagnosis concorded in 144 cases (79 %) and was in discordance with the histological diagnosis in 39 cases (21 %). The 144 concordant cases included the 2 cases of lesions which were only histologically suspicious. Out of the 39 cytologically discordant cases, the cytological examination was suspicious in 11 cases (6 %), benign (wrongly, i.e., a false benign report) in 4 cases (2 %) and there was insufficient cellular aspirate in 24 cases (13 %).

In the 19 cases in which there was no active cancer in the histological slides, the cytology results gave 15 concordant results (79 %), 2 smears were diagnosed as suspicious (10.5 %) and 2 others were given false malignant reports (10.5 %).

The results show that the diagnostic value of this cytological examination is good even after irradiation of the breast, because a high percentage of active breast cancers (79 %) were revealed by this method.

The proportion of false malignant reports (10.5 %) and false benign reports (2 %) is not negligible, but

it should be noted that : although the 2 cases of false
malignant reports were regrettable, they were somewhat
compensated for by the fact that a previous cancer of
the breast had already been treated and the cure was not
certain ; the 4 cases (2 %) of false benign reports were
not serious, as we consider that a negative cytology
report does not have a definite value and does not allow
the conclusion to be drawn that there is no active carcinoma ; and the high level of cases (24 cases, 13 %) in
which there was insufficient aspirate is due to the difficult conditions of drawing the sample in post-radiotherapy
tissue, mainly because of fibrosis.

Nevertheless, for this method to be valid, certain
basic technical conditions must be respected : 9/10 mm
needles sould be used so that cells can easily be aspirated from a tissue which has often been altered by
radiotherapy ; there should be a minimum time lapse of
4 months between the end of treatment and aspiration
cytology ; and sufficient cellular material should be
aspirated.

As for interpretation of the results, it should be
kept in mind that a good knowledge of the cytological
changes following irradiation is necessary ; that the
absence of carcinomatous cells or the presence of only
benign cells does not mean that there is no active carcinoma ; and that there are no "absolute" morphological
criteria for the viability of irradiated tumor cells.

EVALUATION OF FINE NEEDLE ASPIRATION CYTOLOGY IN THE
PROGNOSIS OF BREAST CANCER

As discussed above, this method is useful in the
diagnosis of breast cancer. But it is also useful in
establishing prognosis. In our work, we first measured
the diameter of the nuclei of neoplastic cells and then
applied the histoprognostic methods of Scarff, Bloom and
Richardson to cytology.

Measurement of the nuclei of neoplastic cells

Histological grading methods have already been used
for cancer of the breast in which the size of the nucleus
is taken into account. Black and Speer (1957) showed a
better survival rate in patients with breast cancer with
regular and small nuclei. Kister et al. (1969), as well
as Eichner et al. (1970), used a system of grading nuclei
which took into account the total size of the nucleus.

They confirmed that there is a statistically significant
relationship between the nuclear grade and patient survival. Furthermore, Sommers (1969) showed that intraductal
carcinomas have more small nuclei neoplastic cells than
invasive carcinomas, and Eichner et al. (1970) believed
that nuclear size is an important factor in the survival
of breast cancer patients.

Atkin (1972) studied the DNA content of breast cancers
in 67 patients and, comparing their survival, observed
that the group of patients with near normal DNA content
(near-diploid) had a significantly better prognosis than
patients with a higher DNA content (triploid-tetraploid).
He thought that the cancers with subnormal DNA (near-
diploid) could be "small nucleus carcinomas" and those
with high DNA "large nucleus carcinomas".

Estimating the sex chromatin content in tumor cells
can also have a prognostic value. Thus, Savino and Koss
(1971) showed a correlation between the number of nuclei
with sex chromatin and the prognosis of breast cancer.

Other authors, such as Castelain (1958) and more
recently Mouriquand et al. (1979) have drawn attention to
the importance of the size and the color of the nucleoli
in the neoplastic nucleus in the survival of breast cancer patients. They show that malignancy increases with
the size of the nucleolus or nucleoli and with their
difference in staining properties. Wallegren et al.
(1976) measured the nuclei of neoplastic cells from cytological aspirates of breast cancers and studied patient
survival ; their results are very similar to ours.

In a retrospective study, we measured the diameter
of the cell nuclei of neoplastic cells using an ocular
micrometer and an oil immersion lens (100 x), (Zajdela
et al., 1979).

The measurements were done on aspirate smears stained
with the May-Grunwald-Giemsa method. We measured at
least 100 round nuclei for each case (Carcinoma and benign tumors). Neither pycnotic nor unshapely nuclei have
been taken into consideration. The samples were taken
from 245 patients with histologically proved invasive
breast cancer. Some special type carcinomas were excluded
from the study : mucoid, medullary, apocrine, comedo,
adenocystic ca. and Paget's disease. The age limits of the
patients were 29-75 years, with a mean age of 52 years.
All the patients had a five year follow-up. We excluded
all those patients from the study who had been lost

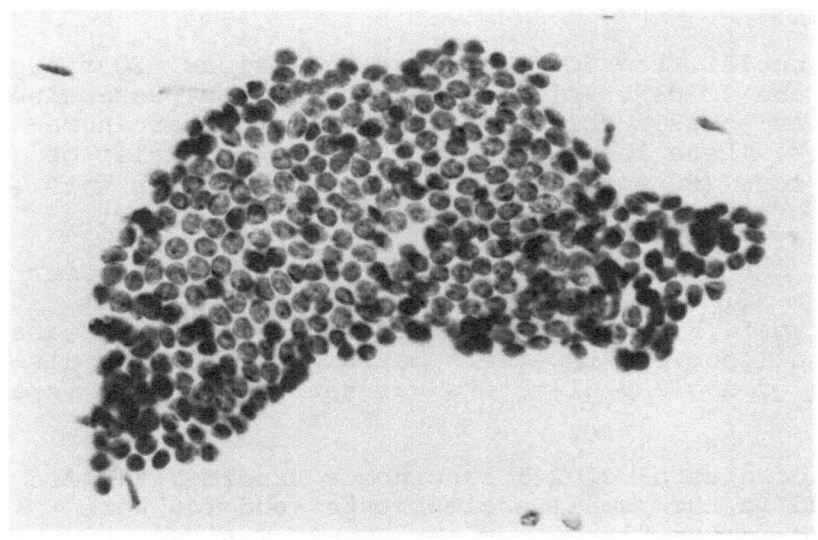

Fig. 1. <u>Aspiration smear</u>
        Group of cells from a breast adenoma. Most
        cells have nuclei 11 μ m or less.
        (Magnification x 400).

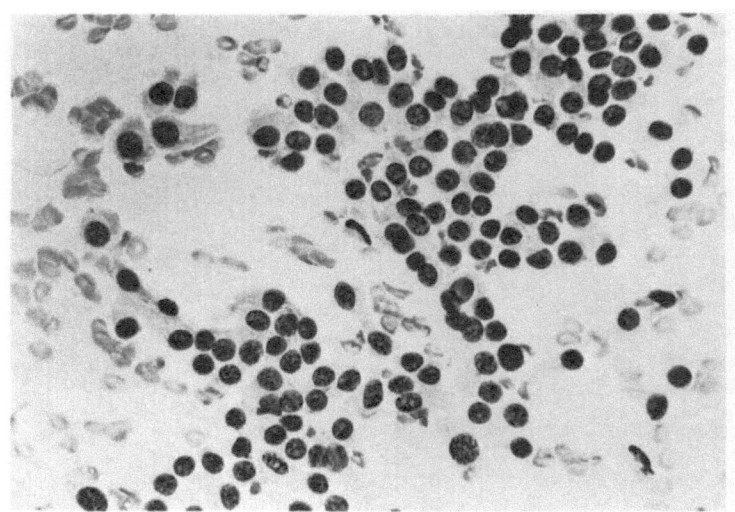

Fig. 2. <u>Aspiration smear</u>
        Small nuclear type carcinoma. Most cells
        have nuclei 12 μm or less.
        (Magnification x 400).

before the end of this interval. The patients were treated
by surgery alone, by radiotherapy alone, or by both
methods.

The nuclei from 50 benign breast lesions, 20 fibroadenomas and 30 cases of fibrocystic disease, were also
measured as a basis for comparison with the carcinomatous cells. These lesions had a majority of nuclei of
11 μm or less (80 % or more) (Fig.1). Carcinomas with a
majority of nuclei of less than 12 μm (80 % or more)
were classified in the category "small nuclear type"
(Fig. 2). Carcinomas with a majority of nuclei greater
than 12 μm (80 % or more) were classified as "large
nuclear type" (Fig. 3). The nuclei in 10 carcinoma cases
of the small nuclear type were measured twice. The distribution of nuclear diameters was nearly the same in all
10 cases.

Out of a total of 245 carcinomas studied, 96 were
classified in the "small nuclear type" and 149 were
classified in the "large nuclear type". The two groups
of carcinomas were divided according to the clinical
stage of the primary lesion, using the T.N.M. classification (1973). The mean survival at 5 years of 96 patients

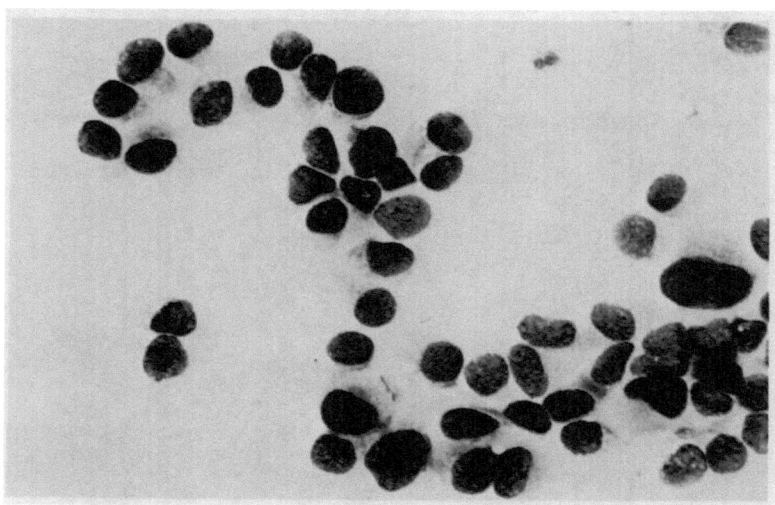

Fig. 3.   <u>Aspiration smear</u>
          Large nuclear type carcinoma.
          Presence of pleomorphic nuclei of diameters
          varying from 13 to 25 μm.
          (Magnification x 400).

TABLE V

SMALL NUCLEAR TYPE CARCINOMA - 96 CASES

DIAM. 9 μm - 12 μm

TUMOR	TOTAL	Alive 5 years with no signs of cancer	%
T_1	37	33	89
T_2	40	35	88
$T_3 + T_4$	19	18	94

TABLE VI

LARGE NUCLEAR TYPE CARCINOMA - 149 CASES

DIAM. 12 μm - 25 μm

TUMOR	TOTAL	Alive 5 years with no signs of cancer	%
T_1	30	22	73
T_2	85	52	61
$T_3 + T_4$	34	12	35

with small nuclear type carcinomas (diameters 9 µm to
12 µm) for all the 4 clinical stages was 90 % (86/96).
The mean 5 year survival of 149 patients with large
nuclear type carcinomas (diameters 12 µm to 25 µm) for
all the 4 clinical stages was 58 % (89/149).

The patients survival within each T.N.M. clinical
stage was as follows for the small nuclear type carcinomas (diameters 9 µm to 12 µm) : 89 % for T_1, 88 % for
T_2 and 94 % for T_3 and T_4 (Table V). This study shows
that, based on the diameter of the nuclei of the neoplastic cells, one can isolate the category of patients with
small nuclear type carcinomas, whose survival proves to
be better than that predicted by the T.N.M. classification. Indeed, their prognosis seems to be independent of
their T category and is not made worse, even if the
lesions are classified T_2 and T_3- T_4. Thus, the 5 year
survival predicted by the T.N.M. classification of 45 %
for T_3 and T_4 is, in reality, 94 % at 5 years for small
nuclear type carcinomas. In contrast, large nuclear type
carcinomas have a much poorer prognosis, in that it
remains related to their T category (Table VI).

Application of the Scarff, Bloom and Richardson histo-prognosis method to aspiration breast cytology

The histological prognosis of breast cancers, as
established by Scarff, Bloom and Richardson (Patey and
Scarff, 1928 ; Bloom and Richardson, 1957), was recognized
and introduced by the World Health Organization in 1968
(Scarff and Torloni, 1968) as an important index in the
prediction of malignancy.

The histological criteria of the Scarff, Bloom and
Richardson (S.B.R.) method are based on the following
parameters :
    I - Differentiation of the tumor,
   II - Volume, shape and staining affinities of the nuclei,
  III - Nuclear hyperchromatism and mitoses.

Points from 1 to 3 are given for a worse prognosis
within each of the three parameters. Then all the points
are added : a total of 3 to 5 points is considered an
index of low malignancy (grade I) ; a total of 6 to 7
points is considered an index of moderate malignancy
(grade II) ; a total of 8 to 9 points is considered an
index of high malignancy (grade III).

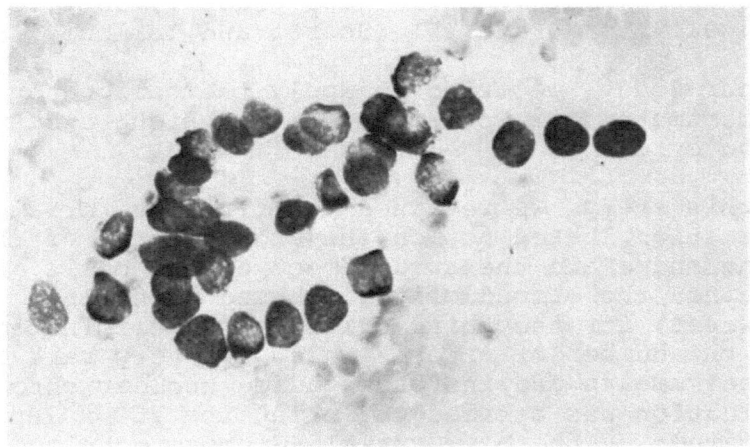

Fig. 4. Cytologic pattern of grade I carcinoma.
(Magnification x 400).

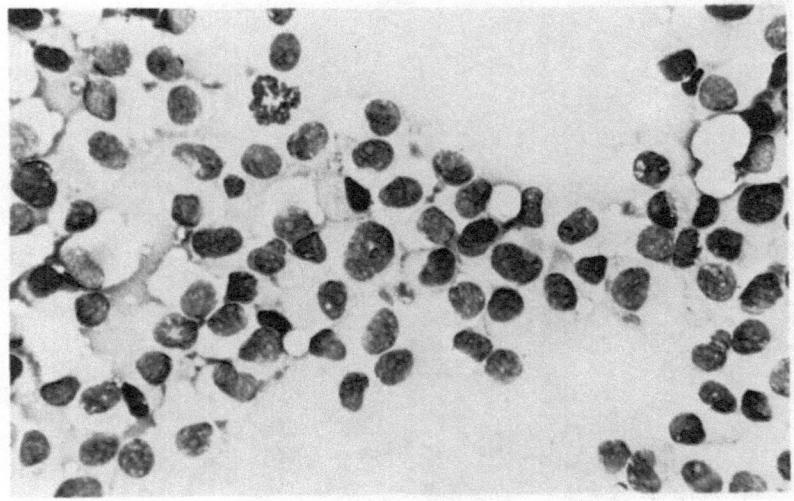

Fig. 5. Cytologic pattern of grade II carcinoma.
(Magnification x 400).

The 5 year survival rate of patients with breast
cancer is approximately : 75 % for grade I, 53 % for
grade II, 31 % for grade III (Scarff and Torloni, 1968).

In our study, we tried to apply the malignancy pre-
dicting parameters of Scarff, Bloom and Richardson to
aspiration cytology.

In this study, we retained the first criteria of
differentiation, based not on the architecture of the cell
but on the shape and the arrangement of the cells. We
also retained the second criteria based on nuclear volume. However, for the third criteria, we eliminated the
value of the number of mitoses which are very rare in
cytological smears and instead studied nuclear chromatin.
This evaluation was carried out using the 250 x lens on
smears stained by the May-Grunwald-Giemsa technique
containing a minimum of 3,000 neoplastic cells per
patient.

122 breast tumors were graded cytologically. The
cytological grade was compared with the histological
grade attributed by the histopathology department.

The cyto-histological concordance was as follows :
96 % for grade I (52 cases) (Fig. 4) ; 85 % for grade II
(46 cases) (Fig. 5) ; 92 % for grade III (24 cases)
(Fig. 6).

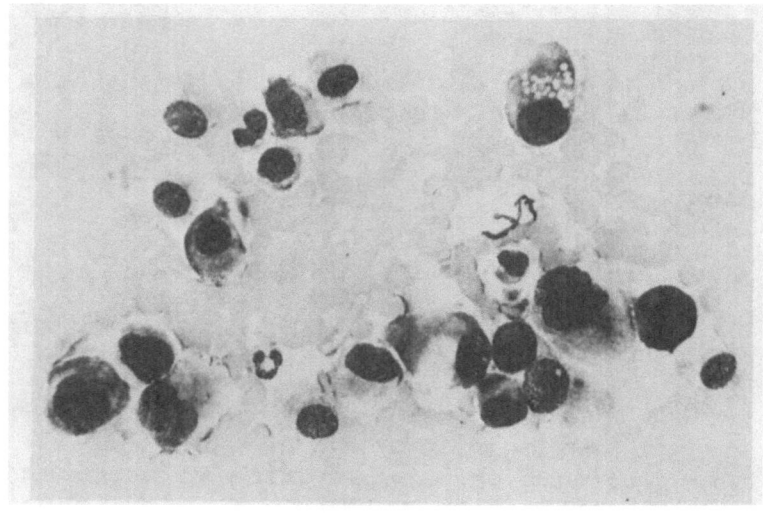

Fig. 6.   Cytologic pattern of grade III carcinoma.
          (Magnification x 400).

This study shows that the appreciation of the degree of malignancy from a prognostic point of view, according to Scarff, Bloom and Richardson, can also be applied to cytology.

These studies prove that there are several cytological criteria for evaluating the malignancy of a breast cancer. The cytological data, which have not all been completely studied, could be useful complements to the histological results already obtained.

REFERENCES

Atkin, N.B., 1972, Modal deoxyribonucleic acid value and survival in carcinoma of the breast. Brit. Med. J., 1, 271-272.

Black, M.M., and Speer, F.D., 1957, Nuclear Structure in cancer tissues. Surg. Gynec. et Obst., 105, 97-105.

Bloom, H.J.G., and Richardson, W.W., 1957, Histological grading and prognosis in breast cancer. Brit. J. Cancer, 11, 359-377.

Burn, J.I., and Malakar, K., 1968, Drill biopsy and the dissemination of cancer, Brit. J. Surg., 55, 628-634.

Castelain, G., 1958, Cytodiagnostic extemporané et cyto-pronostic des tumeurs du sein. Path. Biol., 34, 235-239.

Cornillot, M., and Verhaeghe, M., 1955, Confrontation clinique et cytologique dans les tumeurs du sein, Cancérologie, 2, 204-214.

Cornillot, M., Verhaeghe, M., Cappelaere, P., and Clay, A., 1971, Place de la cytologie par ponction dans le diagnostic des tumeurs du sein (2267 examens cytologiques). Lille Med., 16, 1027-1031.

Eichner, W.J., Lemon, H.M., and Friedell, G., 1970, Tumor grade in the prognosis of breast cancer. Nebr. Med. J., 55, 405-409.

Franzen, S., and Zajicek, J., 1968, Aspiration biopsy in diagnosis of palpable lesions of the breast. Acta Radiol., 7, 241-262.

Godwin, J.T., 1956, Aspiration biopsy : technique and application. Ann. N.Y. Acad. Sci., 63, 1348-1373.

Hajdu, S.I., and Melamed, M.R., 1973, The diagnostic value of aspiration smears, Am. J. Clin. Path., 59, 350-356.

Kister, S.J., Sommers, S.C., Haagensen, C.D., Friedell, G.H., Cooley, E., and Varma, A., 1969, Nuclear grade and sinus histiocytosis in cancer of the breast. Cancer, 23, 570-575.

Kreuzer, G., and Zajicek, J., 1972, Cytologic diagnosis
    of mammary tumors from aspiration biopsy smear,
    Acta Cytol., 16, 249-252.
Lopes Cardozo, P., 1976, Atlas of clinical cytology.
    Targa Hertogenbosch, The Netherlands, 477-508.
Martin, H.E., and Ellis, E.B., 1930, Biopsy by needle
    puncture and aspiration. Ann. Surg., 92, 169-181.
Martin, H.E., and Ellis, E.B., 1934, Aspiration biopsy.
    Surg. Gynecol. Obstet., 52, 578-589.
Mouriquand, J., Bodin, J.P., Sage, J.C., Egal-Boulard, V.,
    Peralta, J.L., Bouchet, Y., 1979, Cyto-pronostic
    préthérapeutique du cancer du sein. Nouv. Pr. Med.,
    36, 2877-2880.
Patey, D.H., and Scarff, R.W., 1928, Position of histolo-
    gy in the prognosis of cancer of the breast. Lancet,
    1, 801-804.
Robbins, G.F., Brothers, J.H., III, Eberhart, W.F., and
    Quan, S., 1954, Is aspiration biopsy of breast
    cancer dangerous to the patient ?. Cancer, 7,
    774-778.
Savino, A., and Koss, L.G., 1971, The evaluation of
    sex chromatin as a prognostic factor in carcinoma
    of the breast. Acta Cytol., 15, 372-375.
Scarff, R.W., and Torloni, H., 1968, International
    Histological Classification of tumours. Histolo-
    gical typing of breast tumours. World Health
    Organization, Fascicule 2, Geneva, 19-20.
Sommers, S.C., 1969, Histologic changes in incipient
    carcinoma of the breast. Cancer, 23, 822-825.
T.N.M., Classification of malignant tumors, 1973,
    U.I.C.C., A.J.C., (Suppl.), Geneva.
Wallegren, A., Silfversward, C., and Zajicek, J., 1976,
    Evaluation of Needle aspirates and tissue sections
    as prognostic factors in mammary carcinoma. Acta
    Cytol., 20, 313-327.
Zajdela, A., 1963, Valeur et intérêt du diagnostic cyto-
    logique dans les tumeurs du sein par ponction.
    Etude de 600 cas confrontés cytologiquement et
    histologiquement. Arch. Ana. Path., 11, 85-87.
Zajdela, A., Ghossein, N.A., Pilleron, J.P., Ennuyer, A.,
    1975, The value of aspiration cytology in the diag-
    nosis of breast cancer : experience at the Fondation
    Curie. Cancer, 35, 499-506.
Zajdela, A., et de Maublanc, M.A., 1979, Valeur et intérêt
    de la ponction cytologique dans la surveillance des
    cancers mammaires irradiés. Bull. Cancer (Paris),
    66, n° 2, 107-112.
Zajdela, A., Saravia de la Riva, L., Ghossein, N.A.,
    1979, The relation of prognosis to the nuclear
    diameter of breast cancer cells obtained by

cytologic aspiration. Acta Cytol., 23, 75-80.
Zajicek, J., 1974, "Aspiration biopsy cytology" Part I
        in : Monographs in clinical cytology. Karger, Basel,
        Munchen, Paris, London, New York, Sydney, 136-194.

HETEROTRANSPLANTATION OF HUMAN MAMMARY CARCINOMA CELLS

Luciano Ozzello[*] and Martine Sordat

Department of Pathology, University of Lausanne
School of Medicine, Lausanne, Switzerland
[*] New address : Div. of Surgical Pathology,
Columbia-Presbyterian Medical Center,
630 West 168th Street, New York, N.Y. 10032

The experimental study of factors regulating the
behavior and the evolution of human mammary carcinomas
has long been hindered by the lack of appropriate models
Indeed, multiple differences in the physiopathology of
mammary neoplasms of various species limit the utilization of spontaneous tumors of experimental animals. Tissue
culture techniques, although very useful in investigations of mammary cell biology, are not applicable to the
study of such processes as recurrences and metastases.
Therefore, transplantation of human neoplasms into
appropriate hosts appears to offer a more suitable
approach as an in vivo system to verify and elucidate
clinical and pathological observations on humans.

In recent years the nude thymus-deficient mouse has
proved to be a better model for heterotransplantation
than others used previously. Nevertheless, contrary to
expectation, it was soon found that the rate of successful takes differed greatly from one tissue to another,
and that some human tumors were particularly difficult
to transplant.

Primary transplantation of human breast carcinomas
into nude mice so far has given inconstant results.
Giovanella et al.(1978) reported 53 % of successful takes,
but only a few tumors could be serially passaged. In our

experience, intraductal carcinomas have survived transplantation better than invasive carcinomas, but tumor
growth has been minimal (Ozzello, 1980). On the contrary,
human mammary carcinoma cells previously cultured in
vitro often produce tumors when injected into nude mice,
and most of these tumors can be serially passaged. In a
recent review Engel and Young (1978) have pointed out
that 14 of 17 human mammary carcinoma cell lines have
been successfully transplanted into nude mice. Such tumors, composed of human mammary carcinoma cells supported
by murine vessels and stroma, are a useful tool for the
experimental study of human breast cancer cells in vivo.
Their utilization in experimental oncology, however,
requires full knowledge of their behavior as the latter
varies according to the cell line and the experimental
conditions used (Ozzello, 1980 ; Ozzello and Sordat,
1980).

The purpose of this paper is to point out the potentials of this experimental model by illustrating the
behavior of tumors produced in nude mice by the subcutaneous (sc) transplantation of 3 mammary carcinoma cell
lines, which have been studied over numerous serial
passages. Part of this work has been reported elsewhere
(Ozzello, 1980 ; Ozzello and Sordat, 1980).

MATERIAL AND METHODS

Nude mice.

The animals used in these studies were adult inbred
BALB/c nu/nu mice raised in our laboratory from an original set of breeders kindly given to us by Dr. G.S.
Kistler (Department of Anatomy, University of Zurich,
Switzerland). Both breeders and experimental animals were
uninterruptedly kept under pathogen-limited conditions
(Gullino et al., 1976) without antibiotic coverage in
a room equipped with laminar flow and maintained at a
constant temperature of 26°C and 50 % relative humidity.
The cages, covered.by a lid, and the bedding material
were sterilized. The appropriate pelleted mouse diet was
sterilized by irradiation (4 MR, U.A.R., Villemoisson-
sur-Orge, France) and the drinking water autoclaved. The
animals were handled exclusively by personnel in sterile
attire. These precautions have proved to be of paramount
importance to insure a long survival and good health of
these mice as compared to those maintained under conventional conditions.

Cell lines.

The BT-20 cell line was originally started from a primary infiltrating ductal carcinoma in a 74-year-old woman (Lasfargues and Ozzello, 1958). Its karyotype and a growth pattern, including dome formation and ultrastructure (Buehring and Hackett, 1974 ; Ozzello, 1972) are typically epithelial and are in keeping with a human mammary epithelial origin. They are grown as monolayers in plastic flasks and fed with medium RPMI 1640 supplemented with 2 % fetal calf serum. The BT 20 cells do not synthetize milk proteins (Hurlimann and Dayal, 1978) and do not have estrogen or prolactin receptors (unpublished data).

The MCF-7 line was originated from a pleural effusion of a 69-year-old woman with metastatic mammary carcinoma (Soule et al., 1973). These cells have a typical epithelial morphology. They have been extensively characterized as being of human mammary origin, they have estrogen, progesterone, androgen and glucocorticoid receptors, and synthetize α-lactalbumin (Engel and Young, 1978). They were kindly sent to us by Dr. E.M. Jensen of the Mason Research Institute through the courtesy of the Breast Cancer Task Force (NCI). At the time of transplantation they were grown in this laboratory as monolayers in plastic flasks using Eagle's Minimal Essential Medium supplemented with 10 % fetal calf serum and insulin (10 µg/ml).

Cell line CaMa 15 was started by Dr. G. Fossati (Istituto Nazionale Tumori, Milan, Italy) from a primary infiltrating ductal carcinoma in a 45-year-old woman. Originally, these cells had typical epithelial features as judged by light and electron microscopic observations, but subsequently they became elongated and no longer displayed a mosaic-like pattern of growth (G. Fossati, personnal communication). Their precise nature requires further elucidation as some of the immunological, enzymatic, and Giemsa banding findings do not fit standard patterns and are difficult to interprete. Nevertheless, the material of origin, the history, the karyotypes prior to transplantation, the presence of α-lactalbumin in some of their tumors (see below) are in support of their human mammary epithelial nature.

HeLa cell contamination of these 3 lines was excluded by glucose-6-phosphate dehydrogenase mobility.

Transplantation

The cultured cells were trypsinized, washed, and then suspended in serum-free medium. The inocula, ranging from 5 to 7 x 10^6 cells in a few drops of medium, were injected s.c. in the dorso-lateral region of the mice next to the thoracic mammary glands. Such location was preferred to the mammary fat pad to avoid ventral tumors which may be cumbersome and are more easily traumatized. This is particularly important for sizable tumors and for long follow-up studies. For subsequent passages, 2-3 mm^3 of freshly excised tumor tissue were finely minced in culture medium and transplanted s.c. in the dorso-lateral region of 1 or more mice by means of a trocar.

Tumors

The tumors were allowed to grow for variable periods of time during which they were periodically measured. Some tumors were surgically excised and the mice allowed to survive. The operated tumors were used for serial passages and for various investigations. The other tumors, including those deemed inoperable, were allowed to grow until the death of the animals. A complete autopsy was then performed. Recurrences were excised when operable, otherwise they were left undisturbed.

Histological verification of all tumors and autopsy specimens was carried out using conventional techniques. In addition, selected tumors were studied by indirect immunofluorescence by Dr. J. Hurlimann (Dept of Pathology, University of Lausanne) to determine the presence of α -lactalbumin using antigens and antisera prepared as previously described (Hurlimann and Dayal, 1978).

The volume of the tumors was determined according to the formula :

$$V = \frac{\pi}{6} \times (d_1 \cdot d_2 \cdot d_3)$$

where $d_{1,2,3}$ represent the 3 largest diameters. For an approximate estimation of the daily increase in size of the tumors a growth index (GI) was calculated using the formula :

$$GI = \frac{Tumor\ volume}{Age\ of\ tumor\ in\ days} \times 100$$

Table 1

Tumors produced in nude mice by BT 20, MCF-7 and CaMa 15 cell lines

Cell line	Transplants/ takes	Passages in nude mice	Tumors			
			Histology	Volume (cm^3)[a]	Age of tumors (days)	Growth index[a]
BT 20	46/46	21	mod. diff. carcinoma	5.2+0.7	18-91	12.9+1.5
MCF-7	114/114	39	mod. diff. carcinoma	0.6+0.06	14-151	1.1+0.06
CaMa 15	123/123	59	undiffer. carcinoma	3.4+0.3	10-35	20.0+1.2

[a]Mean + S.E.

Table 2

Follow-up of tumors produced in nude mice by BT 20, MCF-7 and CaMa 15 cell lines

Cell line	Mice with metastases[a]	Metastatic sites				Recurrences/ excisions	Tumor-free survivals[b]
		Lymph nodes	Lungs	Mediastinum	Others		
BT 20	5/37	4	3	0	0	7/24	14/24
MCF-7	12/59	11	1	2	0	1/10	
CaMa 15	64/113	31	44	29	29[c]	58/92	14/92

[a] Expressed as number of mice with metastases/number of mice with adequate follow-up

[b] Expressed as number of mice free of recurrences and metastases/number of operated mice

[c] Pleura, pericardium, heart, peritoneum, retroperitoneum, mesentery, pancreas, liver, spine, soft tissues

RESULTS

Tables 1 and 2 summarize the salient features of the 3 groups of tumors.

BT 20

Fourty-six transplantations (original injections and 21 serial passages) induced the development of 1 or more tumors in 46 mice yielding a total of 50 neoplasms. The small lump of transplanted material faded away during the first 24 to 48 hours following transplantation to reappear in form of a growing tumor nodule after latent periods extending from 7 to 36 days.

The tumors grew to a size of 0.1 to 25.6 cm^3 (mean 5.2 $\pm$ 0.7) over periods of time of 18 to 91 days (Fig. 1). their mean GI was 12.9 $\pm$ 1.5 (0.5-61.0). It must be noted, however, that many tumors, particularly the large ones, presented extensive areas of necrosis leading to the formation of pseudocysts. They were composed of carcinoma cells arranged in cords and ill-defined masses separated by scanty stroma (Fig. 2). Although most of them were seemingly well delimited on macroscopic examination, they

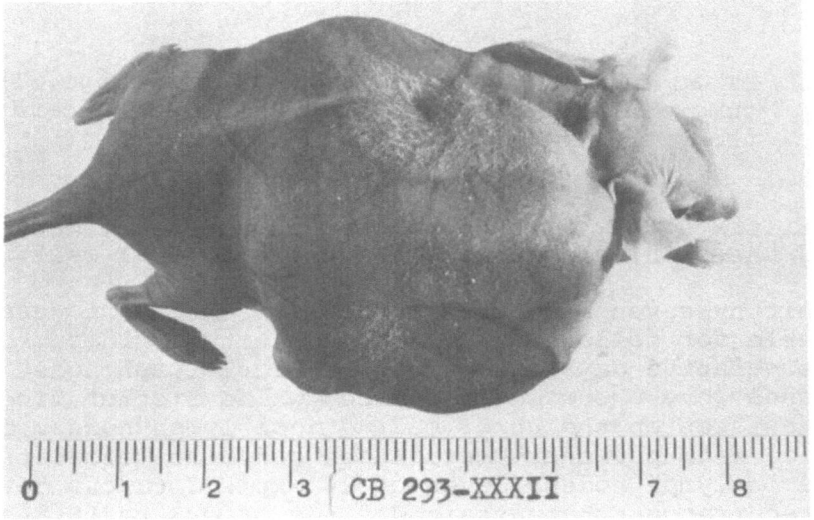

Fig. 1.   BT 20 tumor 42 days after the 7th passage in nudes. This tumor grew rapidly to a large size (GI : 61.0), but it contained large areas of necrosis.

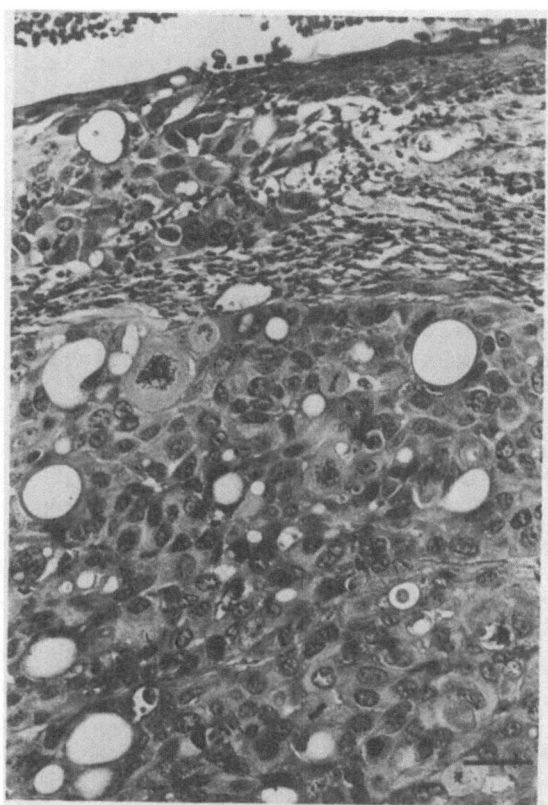

Fig. 2.   BT 20 tumor 35 days after the 1st passage. The
tumor infiltrates the s.c. tissue and ulcerates
the overlying skin. H et E.(Bar = 50 µm).

did infiltrate the surrounding tissues and sometimes
invaded the skin, the muscles and the abdominal wall.

Thirthy-seven mice with a total of 47 tumors were
acceptable for follow-up (28-304 days with a minimum of
14 postoperative days). Regional axillary lymph node
metastases were observed in 2 mice, while 2 other mice
had metastases in the upper mediastinal lymph nodes. Two
of 3 mice with pulmonary metastases had also metastatic
disease in lymph nodes. Seven of 24 excised tumors developed recurrences that attained sizes of 0.3 to 16.8 cm^3
with GIs from 0.6 to 22.1. No recurrences or metastases
were found in 14 mice followed to death, 14 to 280 days
after excision of the tumor. Most of these tumors did not
cause any serious impairment except for hemorrhages

secondary to skin ulcerations and disturbances of loco-
motion in the case of sizable masses.

MCF-7

     All of the 114 transplants performed unilaterally
or bilaterally in 64 virgin female mice produced tumors
after latency periods of 7 to 14 days. At the time of
transplantation these mice received the s.c. implant of a
pellet containing 1.25 mg 17- β-estradiol in cholesterol
since we had previously observed that original inoculations of MCF-7 cells in our mice without estrogen
treatment were unsuccessful (Ozello and Sordat, 1980).

     The tumors attained volumes of 0.01 to 4.5 cm^3
(mean 0.6 $\pm$ 0.06) in 14 to 151 days. The GI varied from
0.05 to 3.6 (mean 1.1 $\pm$ 0.06). The histological appearance
was that of an infiltrating carcinoma (Fig. 3) and was
comparable to that described by Russo et al. (1977).
Many neoplastic cells contained α-lactalbumin. Grossly,
most of these tumors appeared to be circumscribed. Such
circumscription, however, was deceptive in that the tumors
invaded the surrounding tissues and sometimes became
fixed to the skin and to the deep muscles. Furthermore,
MCF-7 tumors often showed perineural invasion.

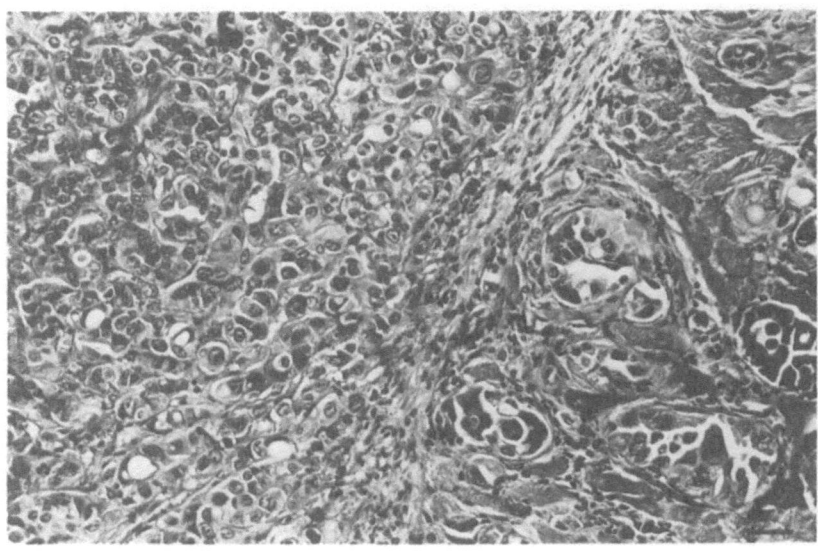

Fig. 3.   MCF-7 tumor, 81 days after the 10th passage,
          invading the adjacent soft tissues. H & E.
          Bar = 50 μm.

Adequate follow-up (27-184 days) was available for 59 mice with a total of 112 tumors. Twelve mice developed metastases : 7 in axillary lymph nodes only (Fig. 4), 3 in upper mediastinal nodes, 1 in the mediastinum, and 1 in the lungs, mediastinum and axillary lymph nodes. Ten tumors were excised, but only 1 recurred producing a nodule of 0.1 cm³ in 67 days (GI 0.15). No statement can be made as to tumor-free survivals since most of the mice had been transplanted bilaterally and only 1 of the 2 tumors was removed.

No complications attributable to the presence of the tumors were noted. On the other hand, the estrogen stimulation frequently led to severe secondary effects including thinness, early wasting, and extensive squamous metaplasia of the endometrium with plugging of the cervical canal and secondary marked dilatation of both cornua. As a result, the life span of the estradiol-treated animals was shorter than that of the other groups.

<u>CaMa 15</u>

All transplants, including the original inoculations and 59 serial passages, carried out on a total of 123 mice, induced tumors after no appreciable latency periods. Most tumors, perhaps all, began to grow within the first

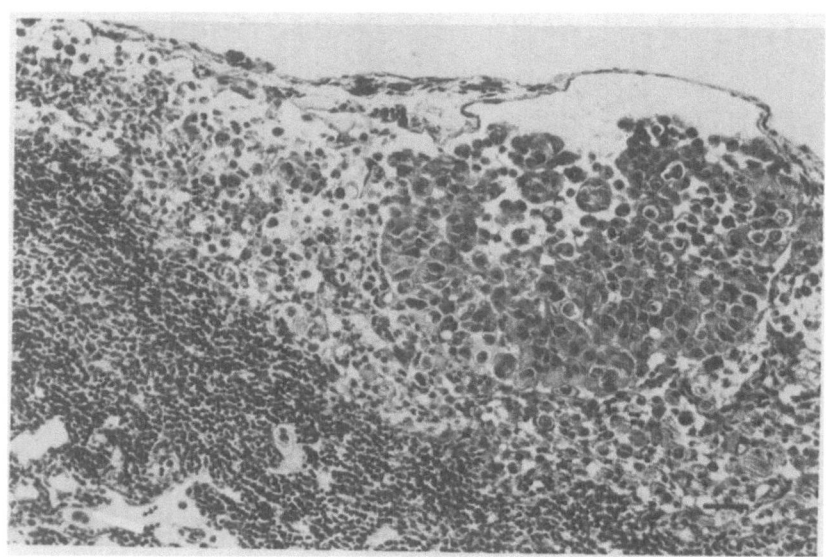

Fig. 4. Axillary lymph node metastasis of an MCF-7 tumor, 88 days after the 5th passage. H & E. Bar = 50 µm.

24 hours. In fact, the small s.c. lump of transplanted
material did not fade away and it showed mitotic activity
and invasion of fat and muscle as early as 10 hours
after grafting (Tobon and Ozzello : in preparation). The
tumors attained volumes ranging from 0.1 to 21.0 cm^3
(mean 3.4 ± 0.3) over periods of time that varied from
10 to 35 days. Their GI ranged from 0.5 to 75.0 (mean
20.0 ± 1.2).

The tumors rapidly infiltrated the surrounding
tissues frequently ulcerating the skin or invading
through the abdominal wall. Invasion through the thoracic wall occurred less frequently. They were composed of
undifferentiated round or spindle cells arranged in ill-
defined bundles or in no particular pattern (Fig. 5 and
6). Their nuclei showed marked atypia, prominent nucleoli and numerous mitoses. α-lactalbumin was demonstrable
in the cytoplasm of occasional neoplastic cells by
immunofluorescence. At the periphery of the tumors the
cells were mostly round and penetrated into the tissues
singly rather than forming compact cords or masses with
pushing margins. Round separate cells were especially
noticeable where the tumor invaded loose connective
tissues (Fig. 7).

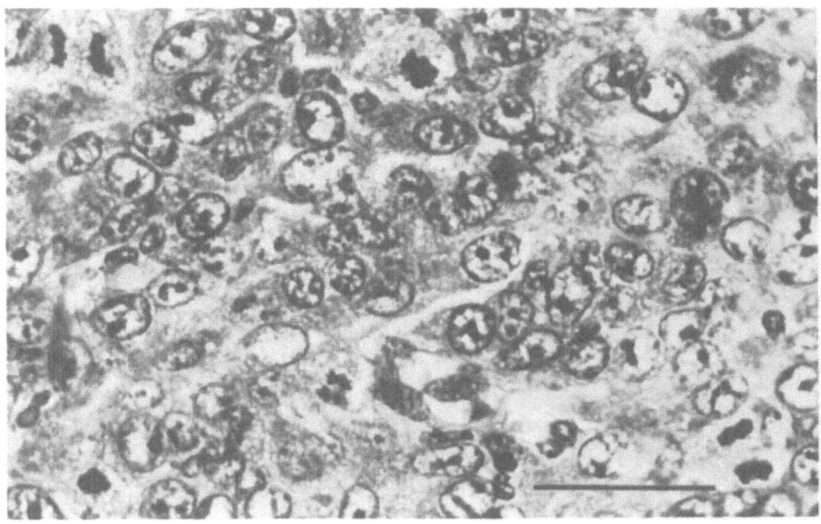

Fig. 5.   CaMa 15 tumor 11 days after 43rd passage
          featuring undifferentiated cells arranged in
          no particular pattern. H & E. Bar = 50 μm.

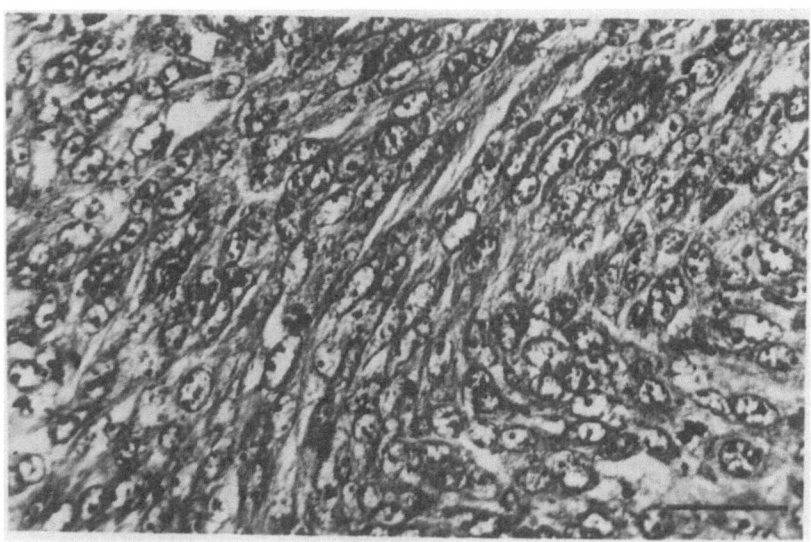

Fig. 6.   Another area of the same fumor of Fig. 5 in
           which the cells become elongated. H & E.
           Bar = 50 μm.

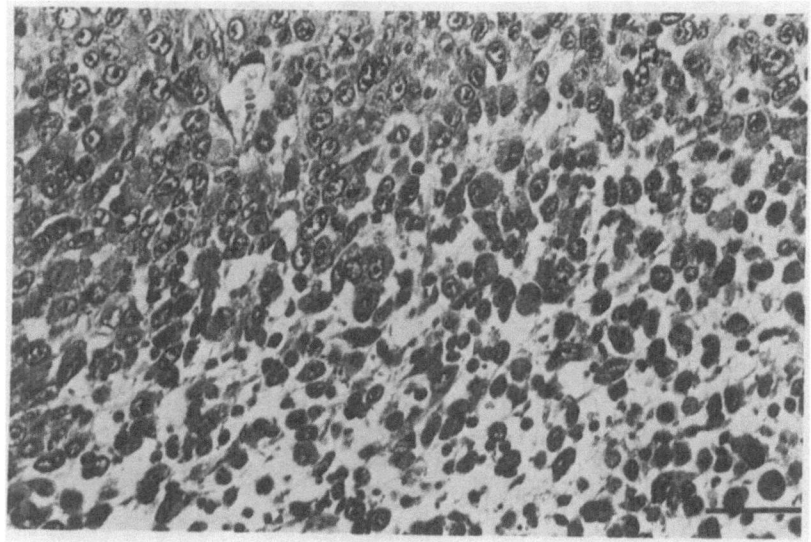

Fig. 7.   Same tumor as Figs. 5 and 6. Invasion of loose
           connective tissue at the edge of the tumor by
           round single cells. Bar = 50 μm.

One hundred and thirteen mice were followed to death, 14 to 364 days with a minimum of 10 postoperative days. Ten were excluded from follow-up because they died unexpectedly and no autopsy was performed. Of 92 mice whose tumor was surgically removed, 58 developed recurrences which were multiple (2 to 7) in 26 mice. Recurrent tumors varied in volume from 0.002 to 14.0 cm^3 (mean 3.4 $\pm$ 0.4) after periods of growth extending from 7 to 54 days. Their GI ranged from 0.01 to 93.6 (mean 15.3 $\pm$ 1.7).

Metastases occured in 64 mice. Their location is given in table 2. It should be noted that in 37 animals metastases were found in several locations, and that in the lungs and in the mediastinum they were frequently multiple. Pulmonary metastases were frequently peribronchial and invaded the wall of blood vessels (Fig. 8) occasionally producing a complete occlusion of the vascular lumen and consequent pulmonary infarction. Lymphatic metastases were found in the axillary (15), mediastinal (15), and retroperitoneal (1) nodes. It is also possible that some of the metastases involving the soft tissues of the mediastinum started in lymph nodes. Of the 58 mice whose tumor recurred, 42 had metastases, but only 8 of the 22 mice without recurrences developed metastases 10 to 59 days after excision. Among the 31 mice that were not operated, 17 were free of metastases, but their

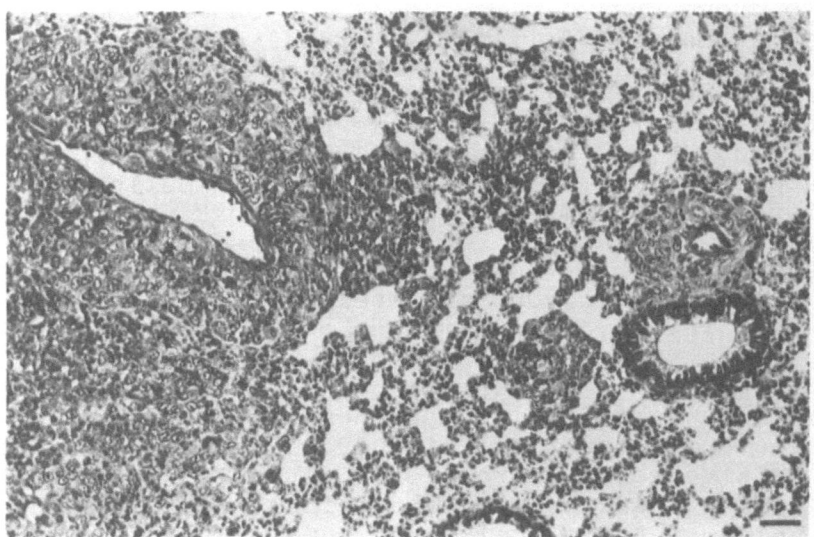

Fig. 8.   Perivascular pulmonary metastases from a
           CaMa 15 tumor 42 days after the 48th passage.
           Bar = 50 μm.

follow-up was short as they died or were sacrificed 14
to 35 days after grafting. Fourteen mice had tumor-free
survivals of 53 to 364 postoperative days.

With the exception of early wasting and anemia,
secondary effects caused by the main tumors were unim-
portant. Metastases on the other hand were responsible
for respiratory distress and, occasionally, of neuro-
logical complications such as paralysis and disturbances
of equilibrium.

DISCUSSION

The cell lines used in this study and the tumors
that they produce are a useful tool for the experimental
study of human mammary neoplastic cells in vivo. When
tumors of this kind are to be used for experimental
studies it is important that the malignancy and the
putative human mammary nature of the cultured cells be
ascertained.

The malignancy of the cell lines used here is attes-
ted to by their tumorigenicity which at the present time
is considered to be the most meaningful criterion to test
the malignant transformation of cultured cells (Fogh
et al., 1977 ; Stiles et al., 1976).

To prove that a given cell line is of human mammary
nature may be more difficult. Several criteria have been
outlined by Engel and Young (1978) and the reader is
referred to their excellent publication for the details.
In our opinion the most reliable criterion to determine
the mammary nature of tumor cells in vitro or in vivo
is the presence of milk fractions in the cells in
questions. Immunohistochemical demonstration of α-lac-
talbumin is very useful for this purpose particularly
if the antisera have been shown to be specific for
human α-lactalbumin. Unfortunately, milk proteins may
be present in very small amounts and only in some cells
of any given tumor. Furthermore, carcinoma cells of
unquestionable mammary origin, as for instance BT 20
cells, under certain circumstances may not synthetize
any detectable amounts of milk proteins. Consequently
only positive results are useful for this purpose. Morphological criteria are more difficult to evaluate. Histological features of cells and tumors are useful only
when typical of carcinoma cells by standard diagnostic
criteria as is the case with BT 20 and MCF-7 tumors.

On the other hand, the morphology of undifferentiated
carcinomas may be misleading and suggest the erroneous
conclusion that an induced neoplasm made up "fibroblast-
like" cells is a sarcoma. Indeed, a variety of undifferentiated carcinomas may present a pseudosarcomatous
appearance as, for instance, the rare human mammary carcinomas with spindle cell metaplasia, and as shown by
the CaMa 15 tumors which are composed of spindle cells
some of which contain α -lactalbumin. Furthermore, the
spindle cell appearance of cultured tumor cells does not
exclude their epithelial nature. Some BT 20 cultures
showed a change from an epithelial to a fibroblast-like
pattern when folic acid was withdrawn from the medium
and spontaneously reverted to the original epithelial
morphology a few months later (Lasfargues and Ozzello,
1958). Transformation from an epithelial to a spindle
cell morphology could also be induced in cultures of
another human mammary carcinoma (SK-BR-3) and in the
tumors that they produced in nude mice by prolonged
exposure to a medium rich in L-cysteine (Ozzello and
Leuchtenberger : in preparation). Ultrastructural parameters, such as intracellular lumens, secretory granules,
variable distribution of organelles, microfilaments and
desmosomes are supportive evidence of the mammary nature
of tumor cells in vivo (Ozzello, 1980) and in vitro
(Buehring and Hackett, 1974 ; Ozzello, 1972). Nevertheless they are not entirely specific as they may be
present in other cell types and be missing in some
mammary carcinomas.

We have previously pointed out that differences in
the behavior of tumors produced in nude mice by human
cell lines cannot be considered as fixed characteristics
of any given cell population as these tumors may be influenced by host factors beyond our control (Ozzello,
1980 ; Ozzello and Sordat, 1980). This is documented by
the wide variations in the growth rate of tumors in
each group. Nevertheless, comparisons between series of
tumors produced by different cell lines are justified
when the transplantations are carried out under the
same experimental conditions. From our results we can
therefore say that the behavior of these tumors is at
least in part dependent on the cell line of origin. Of
the 3 reported here only the MCF-7 tumors proved to be
estrogen dependent. We can also say that, when compared
to the BT 20 and MCF-7 tumors, those produced by CaMa 15
cells are undifferentiated and far more aggressive.
Likewise, their metastases are more numerous and are
more frequently blood born. As to the metastatic spread,

we were surprised by the rarity of hepatic metastases
(only 1 case in the present series) even when the tumors
invaded the abdominal viscera and had access to the
portal circulation.

Surgical excision of the tumors offers a good model
to investigate the formation and the evolution of recurrences, a subject which deserves to be studied on a
larger scale. As to the effectiveness of tumor excision
in preventing metastases the figures are too small and
allow only a tentative interpretation at this time. In
the CaMa 15 tumors studied thus far more metastases
occurred in mice whose neoplasms recurred than in mice
free of recurrences. It would then appear that in these
animals surgery could be effective in preventing metastases when recurrences are controlled. Furthermore, since
recurrences were more frequent after excision of tumors
allowed to attain a large size, early excision of small
tumors might reduce the incidence of recurrences and
consequently of metastases. However, 16 of 58 mice with
recurrent CaMa 15 tumors did not develop metastases
suggesting that in these animals surgery was presumably
of no particular benefit. In addition, 8 of 22 mice with
nonrecurring CaMa 15 tumors were found to have metastases
indicating that the metastatic spread occurred before
the tumor was removed and that surgery was therefore
ineffective in preventing the development of metastases
in these animals.

In conclusion :

1. Tumors produced by transplantation of human
mammary carcinoma cell lines in nude mice are a suitable
model for the experimental study of human breast cancers
in vivo.

2. The behavior of these tumors varies to some extent according to the cell line of origin and to the
experimental conditions used.

3. These tumors are malignant as they invade and
give rise to lymphatic and hematogenous metastases.

4. As in the human, the metastatic spread occurs
early and is probably greater in undifferentiated neoplasms.

5. Functional characteristics of the cells (synthesis of milk proteins, such as α-lactalbumin ; hormone
dependency) are retained by the transplanted tumors.

ACKNOWLEDGEMENTS

Supported by Grant FOR.136.AK.79(2) from the Swiss League against Cancer.

REFERENCES

Buehring, G.C., and Hackett, A.J., 1974, Human breast tumor cell lines : identity evaluation by ultra-structure. J. Natl. Cancer Inst., 53, 621-629.

Engel, L.W., and Young, N.A., 1978, Human breast carcinoma cells in continuous culture. Cancer Res., 38, 4327-4339.

Fogh, J., Fogh, J.M., and Orfeo, T., 1977, One hundred and twenty-seven cultured human tumor cell lines producing tumors in nude mice. J. Natl. Cancer Inst., 59, 221-225.

Giovanella, B.C., Stehlin, J.S. Jr.,Williams, L.J. Jr., Lee, S.S., and Shepard,R.C., 1978, Heterotrans-plantation of human cancers into nude mice. A model system for human chemotherapy. Cancer, 42, 2269-2281.

Gullino, P.M., Ediger, R.D., Giovanella, B., Merchant,B., Outzen, H.C. Jr., Reed, N.D., and Wortis, H.H., 1976, Guide for the care and use of the nude (thymus-deficient) mouse in biomedical research, LAR News, 19, M1-M20.

Hurlimann, J., and Dayal, R., 1978, Antigens of a human breast carcinoma cell line (BT 20). I. Synthesis of serum proteins, membrane-associated antigens, and onco-fetal-associated antigens. J. Natl. Cancer Inst., 61, 677-686.

Lasfargues, E.Y., and Ozzello, L., 1958, Cultivation of human breast carcinomas. J. Natl. Cancer Inst., 21, 1131-1147.

Ozzello, L., 1972, Ultrastructure of human mammary car-cinoma cells in vivo and in vitro. J. Natl. Cancer Inst., 48, 1043-1050.

Ozzello, L., 1980, The breast, in "Electron Microscopy in Human Medicine", J.W. Johannessen ed., McGraw Hill International, Düsseldorf, vol. 9, in press.

Ozzello, L., 1980, Tissue culture and transplantation applied to breast diseases, in "Advances in Surgical Pathology", C.M. Fenoglio and M. Wolff eds., Masson Publishing U.S.A., New York, in press.

Ozzello, L., and Sordat, M., 1980, Behavior of tumors produced by transplantation of human mammary cell lines in athymic nude mice. Eur. J. Cancer, in press.

Russo, J., McGrath, C., Russo, I.H., and Rich, M.A.,
        1977, Tumoral growth of human breast cancer cell
        line (MCF-7) in athymic mice, in "International
        Symposium on Detection and Prevention of Cancer",
        H.E. Nieburgs ed., M. Dekker, Inc., New York,
        Vol. 1, pp. 617-626.
Soule, H.D., Vazquez, J., Long, A., Albert, S.,and
        Brennan, M., 1973, A human cell line from a
        pleural effusion derived from a breast carcino-
        ma. J. Natl. Cancer Inst., 51, 1409-1416.
Stiles, C.D., Desmond, W., Chuman, L.M., Sato, G., and
        Saier, M.H. Jr., 1976, Relationship of cell
        growth behavior in vitro to tumorigenicity in
        athymic nude mice. Cancer Res., 36, 3300-3305.

HUMAN BREAST TUMOR CELLS IN CULTURE ; NEW CONCEPTS IN

MAMMARY CARCINOGENESIS

E.Y. Lasfargues and W.G. Coutinho

Tumor Cell Biology Laboratory, Institute for
Medical Research, Camden, N.J. 08103

INTRODUCTION

The cultivation of human breast tumor cells has
been, over the years, a subject of intensive efforts.
It still is, but the aims and objectives which originally motivated the isolation of tumor cells have
changed.

Until the mid 70's the major drive underlaying all
efforts, was the belief that a virus was the major cause
of human breast cancers. This belief became more and
more strongly entranched following the overwhelming
experimental evidence which accumulated from studies on
the mouse mammary tumors. It is while cross-breeding
various strains of mice in search for the possible
genetic roots of mammary tumors that Bittner (1936) came
across an infectious agent, transmitted through milk and
which appeared to be the inducer of this disease. Indeed,
cultivation of mouse mammary tumors and their observation
by electron microscopy revealed the unquestionable presence of a virus produced at the cell membrane
(Lasfargues et al., 1959). This virus was also generated
by tissue culture cell lines established from mouse
mammary tumors and whose cell-free supernatant induced
tumors in receptive mouse strains (Sykes et al., 1968).
It is only after the extensive analysis of infective
milks by ultracentrifugation, electron microscopy and
elaborate biochemical assays that the mouse mammary
tumor virus (MuMTV) was finally characterized. It is
an RNA particle with a very distinct physical appearance

(Dalton et al., 1975) and very specific chemical properties (Dion and Moore, 1977). An exhaustive review of
the experimental evidence leading to MuMTV identification
was recently published by Moore et al. (1979a). This
massive accumulation of data spanning several decades,
expresses more than anything else the strong needs for
a fundamental model that could help to understand the
human disease. Even today, however the complete etiology of breast cancer is far from being understood.

In the mouse, and despite the relative importance of
the hormonal, genetic and environmental factors, a specific virus is certainly involved. In the same way as
it is possible to immunize against many virus diseases,
C57BL mice which do not secrete virus in their milk, have
been successfully vaccinated with a killed MuMTV and
been fully protected against tumor development when
challenged with a live virus (Charney and Moore, 1972).

Such results strongly stimulated the cultivation of
human breast tumor cells and the desire to establish
permanent cell lines that would reproduce under strictly
controlled conditions. One of the great advantages of
established cell lines is their potentially inexhaustible
capability to replicate. If a virus was involved they
would provide the virus necessary for the preparation of
vaccines as well as specific tumor antigens to be used
in a variety of diagnostic tests. The tremendous practical value of such concepts received support from the
finding, in some human milks, of virus particles resembling MuMTV (Seman et al., 1969 ; Moore et al., 1971)
and from the presence, in human sera, of antibodies
capable of binding to the surface of virus-producing
mouse tumor cells (Miller et al., 1977 ; Mesa-Tejeda
et al., 1978). If indeed a virus comparable to that of
the mouse really existed in human breast carcinomas, its
demonstration and characterization appeared as a relatively simple matter if the tissue culture methods that
proved so successful in the mouse were to be utilized.

MuMTV IN MOUSE MAMMARY CULTURES

Mouse mammary tumors grow well in tissue culture.
Following their explantation in vitro sheets of epithelium migrate on the glass or plastic surface of the
culture vessel, then can be maintained indefinitely
through successive passages. Cell replication requires
a relatively simple commercial medium such as Eagle's

MEM (1963) or RPMI-1640 (Moore et al., 1966) complemented
with 10 % fetal bovine serum (FBS) and 0.25 i.u. insulin
per ml. No other hormonal additive seems to be necessary.
In this manner cell lines were easily established
(Lasfargues et al., 1972 ; Lasfargues and Lasfargues,
1975) in which MuMTV was abundantly produced.

The detection and identification of virus particles
presented no difficulties. Electron microscopy of thin
sections, either through cell cultures or tumors, showed
the presence of small vesicles about 100 nanometers in
diameter with an internal, excentric nucleoid (Bernhard,
1960). The vesicles were limited by one or several membranes, the most external one presenting characteristic
spikes as described by Sarkar and Moore, (1974). The
nucleoid contained a specific RNA and an enzyme, the
RNA-directed DNA polymerase (RDDP), with which the viral
RNA transcribes a complementary DNA (Schlom and Spiegelman, 1971). The complementary viral DNA is known to migrate to the cell nucleus and to integrate into the
chromosomal material ; surprisingly Varmus et al.
(1973) demonstrated that all mouse cells (not specifically
the mammary cells) do contain DNA sequences related to
MuMTV-RNA. Furthermore, tissues from high as well as from
low tumor-incidence mouse strains equally contain complementary viral DNA. The virus particles are mainly produced by the alveolar epithelium even in the absence of
well defined mammary tumor (Pitelka et al., 1958). In
culture, the isolated cells are generally of alveolar
origin. They release the virus in the culture supernatant
where RDDP can be detected and from which intact virions
can be retrieved. In turn these virions induce mammary
tumors when inoculated into low-cancer strains of mice.
Thus, the mechanisms of viral carcinogenesis in the mouse
follow a specific pattern which should be easy to recognize in a duplicate human model.

CULTURES OF HUMAN BREAST TUMORS

From the very first attempts, however, the cultivation of human breast tissues was impaired by serious
technical problems. For instance, unlike the mouse
tumors, the human neoplasms are not dissociated by
trypsin. In the rare cases of a comedo or medullary carcinoma, slicing the specimen in culture medium caused
viable tumor cells to spill out of the tumor stroma.
These, eventually initiated small epithelial colonies
exhibiting an extremely slow growth rate. The "spilling"
method with which the first continous line of human

breast carcinoma was established (Lasfargues and Ozzello,
1958) prevailed for several years but was totally ineffi-
cient to isolate tumor cells from scirrhous carcinomas,
by far the most frequent.

Collagenase dissociation

In scirrhous carcinomas the tumor cells are assembled
in relatively small nests surrounded by fibroblasts,
large amounts of collagen, elastic fibers and adipose
tissue ; they also might appear as single rows of cells
lined up within lymph spaces. When scirrhous specimens
come to the tissue culture laboratory they often contain
such a small number of tumor cells that explantation
of fragments or of spilled material are completely
unsuccessful.

The use of collagenases to isolate the epithelial
cells from their surrounding stroma was first introduced
by our laboratory in attempts to separate normal mammary
cells from the rest of the glandular tissues (Lasfargues,
1957). The collagenases are non-toxic proteolytic enzymes
derived from Clostridium Histolyticum. Unlike trypsin and
versene routinely used for tissue dissociation, their
maximum efficiency is obtained in presence of calcium
and magnesium ions ; moreover, they are not inactivated
by small concentrations of serum. Because of these
properties there is no critical restrictions concerning
the length of enzymatic dissociation or enzyme concentration. Fragments of tumors with heavy collagen matrices have therefore been incubated at 37°C for
several hours, often overnight, in complete culture
media containing up to 1 mg collagenase per ml without
noticeable damage to the cell viability (Fig. 1). The
cells released during the stromal breakdown can, in
fact, begin to replicate in a medium that is already
compatible with their growth. After 24 hours or longer
in a collagenase medium the tumor fragments are entirely
dissociated. The viable cells, heavier, can be separated
from the debris by sedimentation, washed and be explanted in culture vessels with the appropriate medium. The
collagenase procedure now permits to extract viable
tumor cells from all breast specimens that contain them.

Isolation of the epithelium

Following explantation, a very heterogeneous cell
population that includes lymphoid cells, fibroblasts
and epithelial cells is obtained. Lymphoid cells and

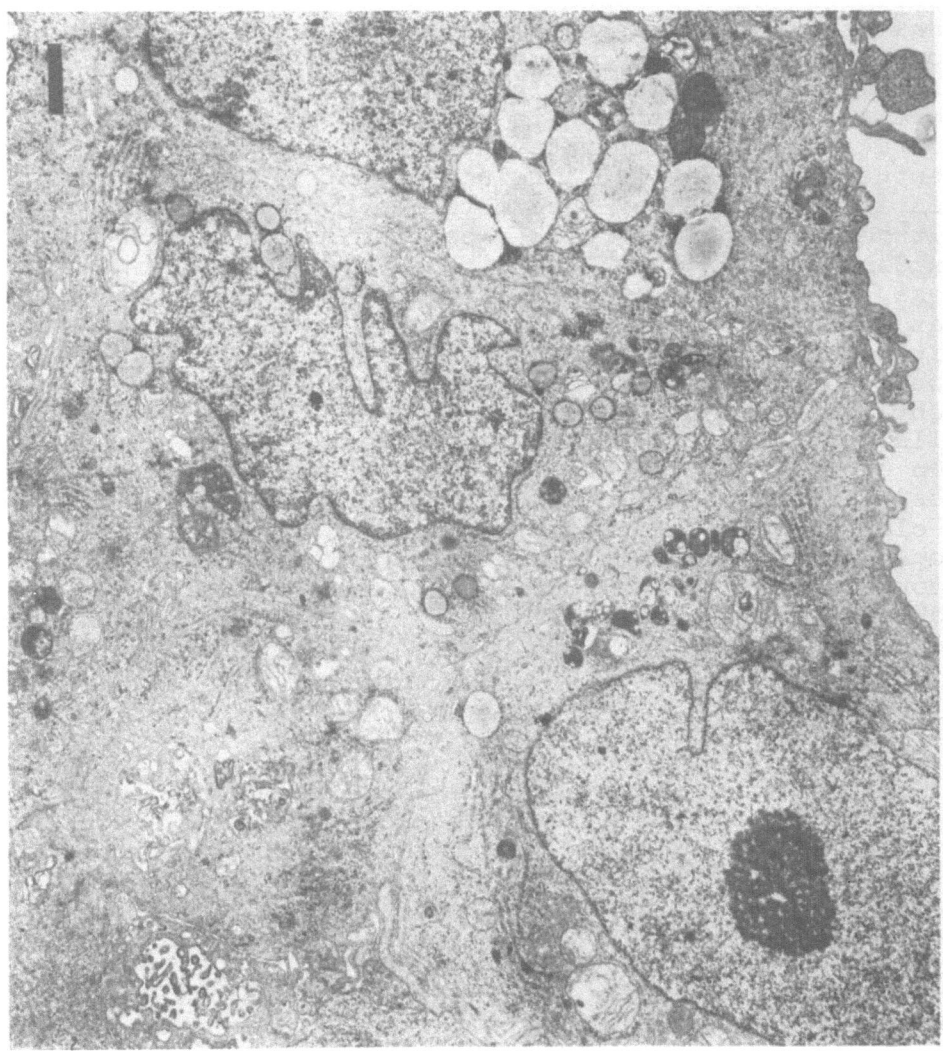

Fig. 1. Electron micrograph of primary breast tumor cells immediately following their isolation by collagenase dissociation. It can be seen that the cells were not damaged by this procedure. The indented nuclei, the reduced endoplasmic reticulum, atypical mitochondria and intracytoplasmic lumina are all characteristics of tumor cells. Bar = 1 micron.

fibroblasts attach rapidly to the glass or plastic
whereas the epithelial cells remain as floating grape-
like aggregates of very refractile cells. It is therefore
easy to effect a primary selection of the epithelium by
transferring the suspended aggregates into a new culture
flask after 48 hours. Attachment of the epithelium is
slow. When it finally occurs one can ofter observe some
fibroblasts which had not been noticed in the free-
floating aggregates. Once in culture, the fibroblasts
grow at a much faster rate than the epithelium and
eventually smother it. A relative control of this fibroblastic outgrowth has been obtained by washing the
cultures periodically with a calcium-magnesium-free saline
containing 0.02 % EDTA and 0.04 % trypsin (Lasfargues
et al., 1979). Following a 1 to 2 minute exposure to
that mixture at 37°C the fibroblasts detach but the
epithelium does not. Fibroblasts also die out spontaneously after a time in culture. This phenomenon which
might result from the limited life span of human diploid
cells (Hayflick, 1975) helps to obtain a total elimina-
tion of that cell type. With some care, it is therefore
possible to isolate mammary epithelial cells which, short
of cloning, are relatively pure. When, therefore, the
biopsy specimens contain a significant proportion of
tumor tissues the above techniques eliminate all major
problems in the isolation of healthy, viable, epithelial
cells.

Maintenance and replication

Once isolated however, the human epithelial cells
do not grow. The media used for the cultivation of
mouse mammary tumors do not maintain the viability of
human tumor cells longer than 6 to 8 weeks. Increasing
the proportion of serum from 10 to 25 % resulted in
even shorter life spans (3-4 w). Mitoses are rare and
observed only in the few hours following explantation.

Nutritional studies have shown that one of the
reasons for this, is that commercial sera contained
hormonal combinations which might strongly inhibit
growth. In effect, the use of a serum substitute increased the life span of the isolated epithelial cells up
to 6 months and longer (Lasfargues et al., 1973) but
cell replication was not stimulated. Recently, a culture
medium was designed that permits a slow but nevertheless
positive growth of the isolated cells (Lasfargues et
al., 1979). The main features of that medium when
compared to media currently used for the cultivation of

mouse mammary tissues are a) a 2 to 3-fold higher concentration in some amino acids and vitamins ; b) a 4
times increase in glucose ; c) insulin (10 micrograms/
ml) ; d) 10 % of a commercial fetal bovine serum (FBS)
heat-inactivated and charcoal-absorbed for the removal
of steroid hormones (Armelin et al., 1974). With this
medium, primary cultures initiated from solid carcinomas have been maintained up to a year and have shown
a positive mitotic activity. Continuous cell lines now
fully established are already used as a source of human
material for experimental purposes.

Other sources of tumor cells

Human breast tumor cells appear to have been isolated with much greater ease from pleural effusions. In
this case there is no tumor stroma. The tumor cells
sedimented by centrifugation of the fluids collected by
thoracocentesis, are usually recognizible in culture at
their large nucleus and high refractibility. They grow
more rapidly than other cells derived from primary
solid carcinomas and only require standard culture media supplemented with untreated commercial FBS. To date,
there exist about 4 times as many cell lines from metastasis and pleural effusions than from solid tumors.
Tables 1 and 2 show a list of the best characterized
cell lines actually available from cell banks or from
the original investigators. A surprising observation
is that no common characteristic could be found between
these cell lines (Engel and Young, 1978) : each one is
morphologically different from the next. Some are fast
growing (MCF-7, BOT-2), some others are very slow
(BT-483 ; MDA-MB-157), some have a very large array of
hormone receptors (MCF-7), some others one or two
(BT-474 ; BT-483) or none at all. In the same manner
functional activity as expressed by the production of
casein and alphalactalbumin is found only in a few cell
lines. There is evidence therefore, that if differences
exist in the adaptative ability of primary and metastatic mammary tumor cells to tissue culture, there are
also qualitative differences that distinguish tumor
cells within each category even from tumor to tumor.

The reason why primary tumor cells are more fas-
tidious to grow than metastatic cells is not known but
it is possible that a suitable medium has not yet been
found. New techniques using collagen matrices as a
culture substrate appear to give encouraging results
with neoplastic as well as with normal mammary cells

Table 1

Cell lines derived from :

A - Solid Primary Tumors of the Breast

Cell line	Pathology	Reference	
BT-20	IDC[*]	Lasfargues & Ozzello	1958
BOT-2	IDC	Nordquist et al.	1975
HS578T	IDC	Hackett et al.	1977
BT-474	IDC	Lasfargues et al.	1979
BT-483	IDC	" " "	1978a
BT-549	AC	Lasfargues	1978b

B - Solid Metastasis of the Breast

Cell line	Pathology	Reference	
ALAB(Lung)	AC	Reed & Gey	1963
MDA-MB-361(Brain)	AC	Cailleau et al.	1978
DU475(Skin)	IDC	Langlois et al.	1979

---

[*]IDC : intraductal carcinoma ; AC : adenocarcinoma

(Emerman and Pitelka, 1977 ; Emerman et al., 1979 ; Yang et al., 1979). A major advantage of the collagen matrices is that they are conducive to a 3-dimensional organization. Unlike the observations made in non-organized monolayer cultures, collagen permits to follow the effects of specific growth factors and of selected hormones on the differentiation and functional activity of mammary cells assembled in a reconstructed organ. Another advantage of this technique is that one can recognize the various cell types participating to specific structures. Even though electron microscopy is of considerable help to recognize the fine structure of mammary cells, there still exist problems to distinguish, in a dispersed cell population, a mammary epithelial cell from a myoepithelial or an endothelial cell. An organized growth in a collagen gel helps to make that distinction and lends itself to the isolation of one particular cell type.

SEARCH FOR VIRUSES IN HUMAN MAMMARY CULTURES

Despite the difficulties in obtaining rapidly replicating cultures of breast epithelium, the major

Table II
Cell lines derived from
A - Breast metastasis in Ascitic Fluids

Cell line	Pathology	Reference	
ZR-75-1	IDC[*]	Engel et al	1978
ZR-75-30	IDC	" " "	

B - Breast Metastasis in Pleural Effusions

Cell line	Pathology	Reference	
MCF-7	IDC	Soule et al	1973
MDA-MB-134	IDC	Cailleau et al	1974a
" " 175	IDC	" " "	"
" " 231	AC	" " "	"
" " 253	IDC	Cailleau et al	1974b
" " 309	IDC	" " "	"
MDA-MB-331	AC	" " "	"
" " 390	AC	" " "	"
MDA-MB-157	MC	Young et al	1974
MDA-MB-330	ILC	Cailleau	1978
" " 415	AC	"	1978
SK-Br-3	AC	Fogh and Trempe	1975
MDA-MB-415	AC	Cailleau et al	1978
" " 416	AC	" " "	"
MDA-MB-431	AC	" " "	"
MDA-MB-436	AC	" " "	"
T-47D	IDC	Keydar et al	1978
ZR-75-27	IDC	Engel et al	1978
AR-75-31	IDC	" " "	"

[*]IDC : intraductal carcinoma
  AC : adenocarcinoma
  MC : medulary carcinoma
 ILC : intralobular carcinoma

objective that was to develop a culture system dupli-
cating that of the mouse has been achieved. The most
serious problem in dealing with human material was the
rarity of viable tumor cells. The isolation of epithelial
cells from human specimen either by the spilling or the
collagenase methods, efficiently resolved that problem.
The epithelial structures collected from sedimentation
pellets contained a high proportion of viable cells
through which thin sections could reveal, like in the
mouse, the existence of a budding virus if there was
one. On the other hand, the laboriously established
human cell lines are a good duplication of the mouse
model. Like the mouse lines, the human cells are a
highly selected population of epithelium in which necrosis is reduced at a minimum. Their identification and
characterization exhaustively challenged by the continuous testing of their ultrastructure, cytogenetics,
biochemical enzymology, clonal growth and transplantation abilities in nude mice is the strongest assurance
that these lines are not contaminated by other cell types.

Despite these prime conditions, however, the search
for a virus particle in more than 600 specimen pellets
has been unsuccessful. In the same manner, a search
through all human breast tumor cell lines established
to date has failed to demonstrate the presence of a
budding virus. The absence of virus particles in cell
lines could be explained by an inhibition of virus expression resulting from long-term cultivation. This
has been a common observation in mouse cultures (Sanford
et al., 1961 ; Tsubura et al., 1968) where the initialy
abundant virus production can dwindle to very low or
nonexistent rates after 1 to 6 months of continuous
cultivation. But this argument is not valid for the
primary cells. In this case the lack of budding virions
could no longer be attributed to the gross interference
of atypical cells from the glandular stroma or to physical cell damage : all primary cultures initiated from
sediment pellets showed a healthy population of predominantly epithelial cells that metabolized correctly.
The repeated absence of budding viruses in these specimen as opposed to their high frequency in mouse
material strongly suggested that a human breast tumor
virus did not exist.

Similar observations reported over the years by
several other laboratories have reached a concensus
with only one exception : MCF-7, a cell line derived from
a pleural effusion has provided indirect evidence for
the existence of a virus comparable to MuMTV (McGrath

et al., 1974 ; Yang et al., 1978). This conclusion, based mainly on the biochemical analysis of cell extracts rather than on electron microscope visualization, is supported by the finding of an RNA-containing particulate that sediments at the same density level as MuMTV particles in sucrose-density gradients. This particulate band also contains RDDP, the specific enzyme found in oncogenic viruses. The RNA itself is related to MuMTV-RNA as demonstrated by nucleic acid hybridization techniques. The crux of the matter is, however, that no typical virus has been identified in the sucrose band and no actual budding was seen at the cell membrane.

Possibilities for a "silent" MuMTV genome

Even though a virion cannot be found in MCF-7 the biochemical results are tantalizing enough to suggest a possible inapparent infection of the cells by MuMTV. Such infection could involve the integration of only a small part of the viral genome into the cell, which though defective to code for a complete virion, would be able to generate viral constituants responsible for the observed cross-reactions. This hypothesis appears to be supported by the finding in the serum of breast cancer patients, of an antigen precipitable with anti-MuMTV sera (Müller et al., 1972) and of antibodies capable of binding murine cells that produce MuMTV (Hoshino and Dmochowski, 1973). Furthermore, migration of leukocytes from about one-third of breast cancer patients is inhibited by MuMTV and this was found to correlate with inhibition by a component present in some breast tumors (Zachrau et al., 1978). Some human tumors have also been shown to contain RNA sequences that were homologous to the MuMTV genome (Vaidya et al., 1974). It is interesting to note, however, that these RNA sequences could not be equated with an integrated viral DNA and did not correlate with the cellular immune response of patients to MuMTV antigens (Vaidya, unpublished).

Taking advantage of a technique developed in our laboratory which permits to introduce MuMTV into xenogenic cells (Lasfargues et al., 1976a et b), attempts were made to infect several human breast tumor cell lines with a MuMTV extracted and purified from RIII mouse milk. Two lines derived from solid invasive ductal carcinomas (BT-474 and BT-483) and MCF-7, originally derived from a metastatic pleural effusion, were successfully infected. Infection was monitored

by membrane immunofluorescence using a rabbit antiserum
prepared against purified RIII-MuMTV. A month after their
experimental infection, 60 % of the BT-474 cells and
15 % of BT-483 cells had virus antigen at their surface
but 90 % of the MCF-7 cells reacted positively. Even
though 5 to 10 % of the MCF-7 cells already posessed a
surface glycoprotein which naturally cross-reacted with
MuMTV antiserum prior to infection (Yang et al., 1977)
the response was obviously greatly amplified following
cell inoculation with RIII-MuMTV. BT-474 and BT-483 cells
did not react with the MuMTV antiserum prior to inoculation. After infection, the BT-474 cells did not only
show the viral antigen demonstratable by immunofluorescence but virions budding from the plasma membrane
and clusters of intracytoplasmic A particles in several
cells. Moreover, the culture supernatant that contained
a RDDP specific for MuMTV was able to induce mammary
tumors in test mice thus demonstrating the release of
an infectious virus (Lasfargues et al., 1979). It was
clear, then, that human cells were susceptible to
infection by the mouse virus. In this particular case,
however, since the host cells were neoplastic before
their experimental infection, it is unlikely that a
mouse virus could have initiated this neoplasia. Furthermore none of the available techniques had been able to
detect a virus presence before the experiment. After
infection, no doubts could be left about the competence
of the cells to support the mouse virus replication.
Obviously, if a virus had been the etiologic agent it
would have been seen, at least in the early stages of
cultivation. However, since human cells are sensitive to
MuMTV and have the ability to support its replication,
the integration of partial sequences of viral DNA into
the cell genome becomes a real possibility.

VIRUS - CELL RELATIONSHIPS

        Following the experimental infection of BT-474 cells
with RIII-MuMTV there was no immediate difference, either
morphologically or in growth rate between the inoculated
and control cultures. After 4 to 6 weeks, the growth rate
of the inoculated cells dropped below that of the controls
as expressed by a lag of 48 hours or longer in reaching
confluency, and furthermore the BT-474 cells lost their
ability to grow in soft agar.

        A widely accepted property of tumor cells is their
characteristic growth in clonal colonies when suspended

in a soft-agar medium (McPherson, 1973). BT-474 cells
did develop large colonies when explanted in soft agar
(Fig. 2) ; moreover, their inoculation into BALB/c Nu/Nu
athymic mice produced tumor nodules whose size increased
in time. The combination of these two parameters is generally considered as a reliable proof of the tumorigenic
properties of a cell (Shin et al., 1975). After inoculation with RIII-MuMTV, however, BT-474 cells ceased to
form colonies in soft agar (Fig. 3) and did not produce
tumor nodules in nude mice. These observations confirmed
through four independent attempts to infect BT-474 cells
with MuMTV suggest a loss of tumorigenic properties.
Nevertheless, the ability of the cells to produce a
virus antigen at their surface was not lost : a membrane
immunofluorescence test revealed that 40 to 60 % of the
cells were still capable to produce this antigen.

The loss of tumorigenic properties by the BT-474
cells might after all, be circumstantial. If a correlation of clonal growth in agar and tumor induction in
nude mice is, in effect, solid evidence for the neoplasia of cells, a lack of growth in agar and a transplantation rejection is not an equally strong evidence
for the loss of their tumorigenic properties. Indeed,
some "normal" lines have shown an ability to grow in
soft-agar ; vice-versa some "tumor lines" did not grow
(Marshall et al., 1977). Furthermore it is difficult
to rely entirely on the "take" of an heterotransplant
when it is already known that only 30 % of breast tumors
can give rise to a tumor nodule when transplanted into
nude mice (Giovanella et al., 1976 ; Sebesteny et al.,
1979). Confirmation for a loss of tumorigenic activity
must therefore be obtained from a syngeneic system in
which, either take or rejection would be equally
significant. The BALB/c mouse offered such an ideal
system.

BALB/c spontaneous mammary tumors

BALB/c mice have been classified as a low incidence
strain because they rarely develop mammary tumors. When
these occur, generally around 19 months of age or later,
there is no detectable sign of virus expression either
in the animal or in its tumor (Moore et al., 1979b). A
cell line, BALB/c ST, derived from one of these tumors
was established. The isolated epithelial cells did not
shed virions, had no surface viral antigen, no RDDP in
the culture supernatant, but produced clonal growth in
soft agar. The cultures were, therefore, comparable in
all respects to the human breast tumor lines.

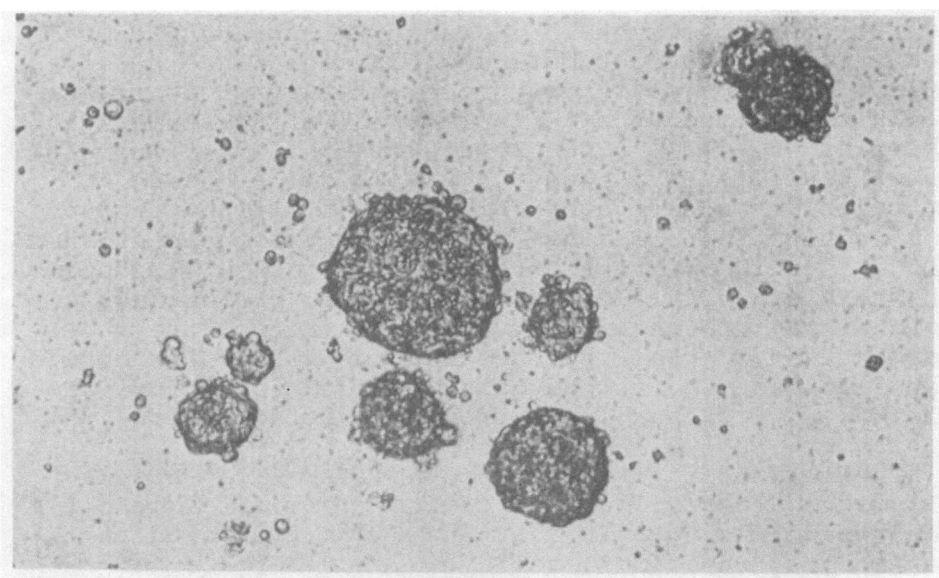

Fig. 2.   Human breast tumor cells BT-474 produce clonal
colonies when suspended in a soft-agar medium.
Bar = 50 microns.

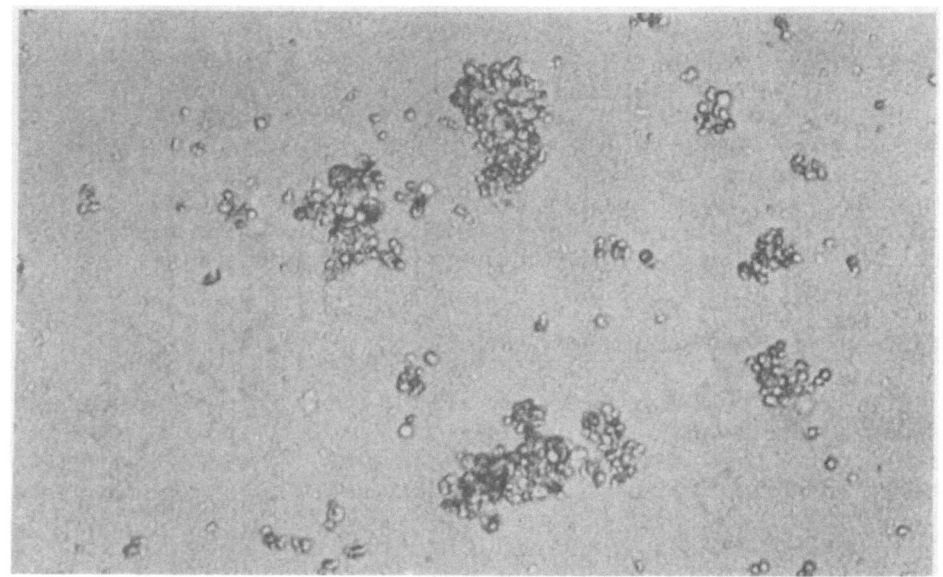

Fig. 3.   Some human breast tumor cells (BT-474) after
inoculation with RIII-MuMTV. Colonies of viable
cells do not form in soft agar. Bar = 50 microns.

When BALB/c ST cells were experimentally exposed
to RIII-MuMTV their sensitivity to the virus was signaled
by the appearance of a surface viral antigen in 80 % of
the cell population. Following infection, the ability of
the cells to form colonies in soft agar became considerably reduced. In contrast with human cells, however,
the BALB/c ST cells could be tested for tumorigenicity
by direct transplantation into syngeneic recipients.
When this was done, it was observed that inoculation of
4×10^6 BALB/c ST cells into all BALB/c test animals
resulted in infinite growth while the same number of
cells implanted after infection with MuMTV did not
induce a single tumor nodule.

It would therefore appear that MuMTV had brought
about a "reversion" of the tumorigenic process perhaps
by interfering with a regulatory mechanisms which controls cell growth. Whether or not this resulted from
the integration of the viral DNA at specific sites in
the cell genome, or more simply from the production
of a "repressor" by the virus itself remains to be determined.

DISCUSSION AND CONCLUSIONS

These observations are somehow startling considering
that MuMTV can induce mammary tumors in 40 to 60 % of
C57BL mice inoculated with purified preparations. Nevertheless, several attempts to bring about the transformation of normal mouse mammary cells infected with
MuMTV in tissue culture have consistently failed. Furthermore normal mouse mammary cell lines maintained in a
state of continuous cultivation have spontaneously
transformed without help of an oncogenic virus (Lasfargues
and Lasfargues, 1980). Cells of rodent origin (mouse,
rat, hamster) are noted to be particularly "unstable"
and to acquire, spontaneously, a potential for endless
multiplication (Ponten, 1974). A variable proportion of
genetically defective cells might therefore be the
reason for high and low incidence strains of mice. In
humans where some families have been observed to be
more prone to develop breast cancer than others, a genetic predisposition rather than a virus etiology should
be considered.

Several arguments can support this statement : one
is that a virus comparable to that of the mouse has not
been found in human breast tumors. Evidence obtained
from hundreds of specimens is overwhelming. Furthermore

the competence shown by human cells to support MuMTV
replication is no less convincing of the initial absence
of such a virus. Because human cells are susceptible to
MuMTV, however, the eventuality of an accidental infection by the mouse virus cannot be completely dismissed
but it is difficult to prove that the neoplastic transformation resulted from such an event. The leukocyte
migration inhibition (LMI) assay provided an early and
most serious clue that some breast carcinomas possessed
a MuMTV-related antigen (Black et al., 1974). A major
viral envelope antigen from RIII-MuMTV, glycoprotein
gp55, appeared to be involved in that response, but a
similar glycoprotein from A-MuMTV (gp50) did not elicit
comparable results even though gp55 and gp50 are immunologically cross-reactive (Dion et al., 1980). This
suggests that the reacting protein found at the surface
of some human tumor cells might not be, after all, of
MuMTV origin. It is of interest to note, however, that
finding this specific protein in a patient is a good
prognostic for an eventual control of the disease (Black
et al., 1978).

Another argument is that all mammary tumors, even
in mice, are not necessarily of viral origin. Evidence
is mounting that specific genetic defects affecting the
regulatory mechanisms of the cell genome are prerequisite
for the emergence of a fully developed cancer cell. We
can reasonably assume on the basis of studies by
Knudson (1977) that an initial genetic damage in some
cells of the mammary gland might result into a mutation
when primed by a secondary event such as an hormonal
inbalance, an environmental carcinogen, a diet deficiency
or even a virus. It should be kept in mind that the
mammary cell is a very complex unit submitted to frequent
physiological changes. Several times in the life of the
host, the mammary cell is stimulated by specific hormones,
from a state of rest to one of replication, then to
secretion and again to rest. If in the chain of events
which characterize the mammary cycle, some of the genes
that regulate the delicate switching mechanisms are
defective, the cell either die or give rise to a new
population in which these changes, reflected by chromosomal variations, can be analyzed by banding methods.
It has already been shown that loss of specific chromosomes in initially non-malignant hybrids initiate the
appearance of tumorigenic properties (Wiener et al.,
1974). In the same vein, the appearance of neoplasia in
cells treated with carcinogens has been linked to the
loss of growth-controlling genes (Yamamoto et al., 1973 ;
Benedict et al., 1975). Other reports concerning the

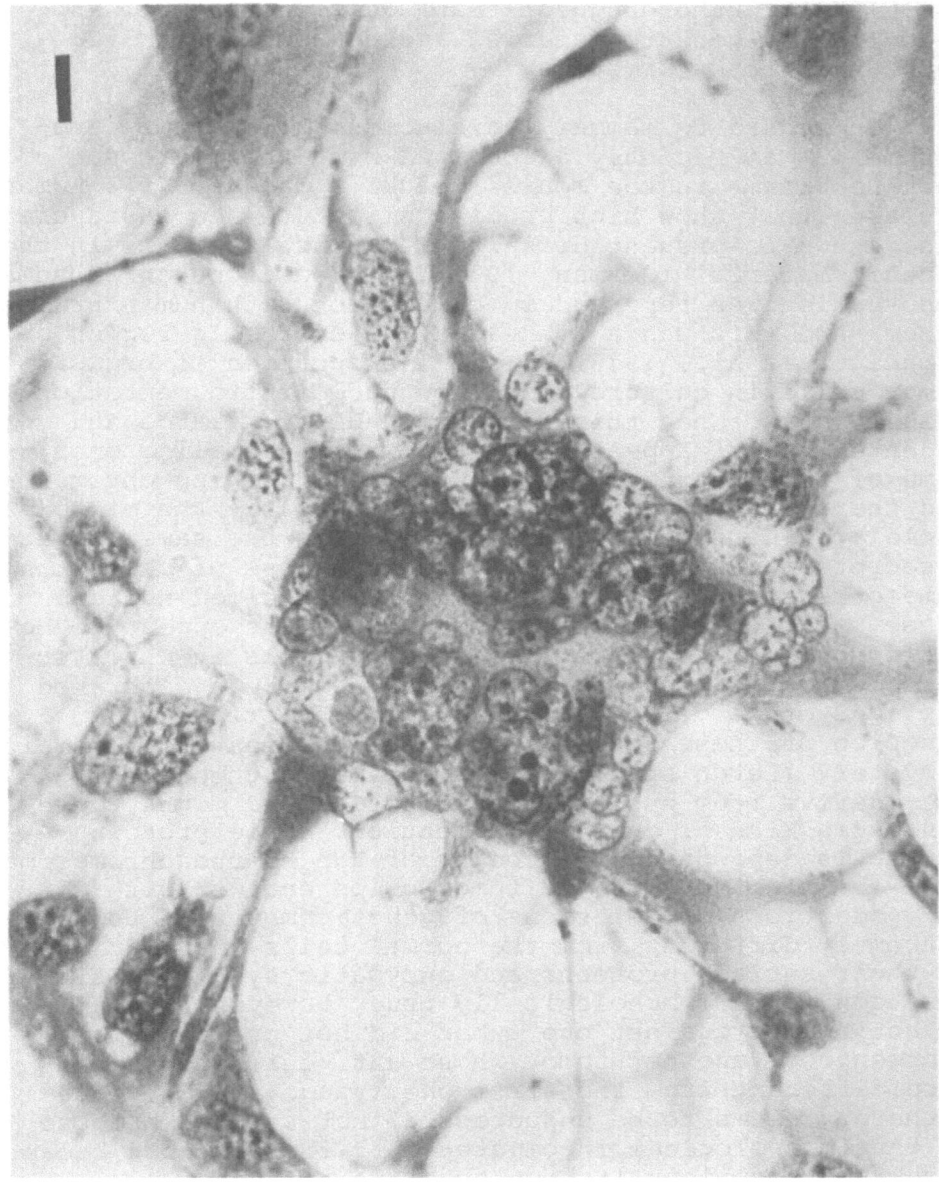

Fig. 4. A multinucleated cells from BT-474 isolated from
an intraductal breast carcinoma. The variety in
size of the nuclei does not result from mitotic
divisions but from nucleus fragmentation.
Bar = 5 microns.

frequency with which specific trisomies occur in mice
developing leukemias (Dofuku et al., 1975 ; Wiener et
al., 1978) further suggest that additions as well as
deletions of genetic material ,are connected with the
neoplastic transformation.

In regard to mammary carcinomas, trisomy of chromosome 13 was recently associated with the emergence of
such neoplasms in the mouse (Dofuku et al., 1979). Human
diseases that show high predisposition to neoplasia are
also known to present definite structural changes in their
genetic material (German, 1972). At least one chromosomal
observation was reported in connection with human breast
cancer and this was a translocation of the 1q region
(Cruciger et al., 1976). A small proportion of breast
tumor cells in culture also show nuclear fragmentation
(Figs. 4, 5). When this happens, unusually large and
indented nuclei appear to breakdown into smaller ones,
some of them extremely tiny but all containing chromatin
and therefore, genetic material. Eventually the micro-
nuclei can be expelled from the cell in the same way as
a secretory vesicle thus resulting in loss of chromatin.
Some others fuse together forming re-arranged nuclei.
These spectacular morphological variations appear to be
reflected in the karyotypes of tumor cells in which so-
called "double minute" chromosomes have been described
(Spriggs et al., 1962). Even though the origin and
function of these double minute chromosomes still remain
a mystery (Levan et al., 1976) one might theorize that
they derive from nuclear fragmentation and might represent some kind of gene amplification. Since protein
synthesis depends on the coding of RNA by the chromosomal
DNA, one might expect the tumor cells endowed with so
many additions or deletions of genetic material to be
extremely different from the normal cells in relation
to their surface proteins and enzymatic systems. This
has been found immunologically true, however, building
up antibodies against one tumor did not prevent the
emergence of another tumor whose antigenic properties
were different from the first one (Vaage, 1978). Immunotherapy seems to be unsuccessful not so much because
of the immunological incompetence of the host but because
each tumor develops its own specific antigens.

Since it is difficult to detect a common unifying
factor between breast tumors the most promising approach
appears to be a genetic analysis. There exist techniques
of gene transfer from one cell to another consisting in
fusing cells containing complete or partial genomes to

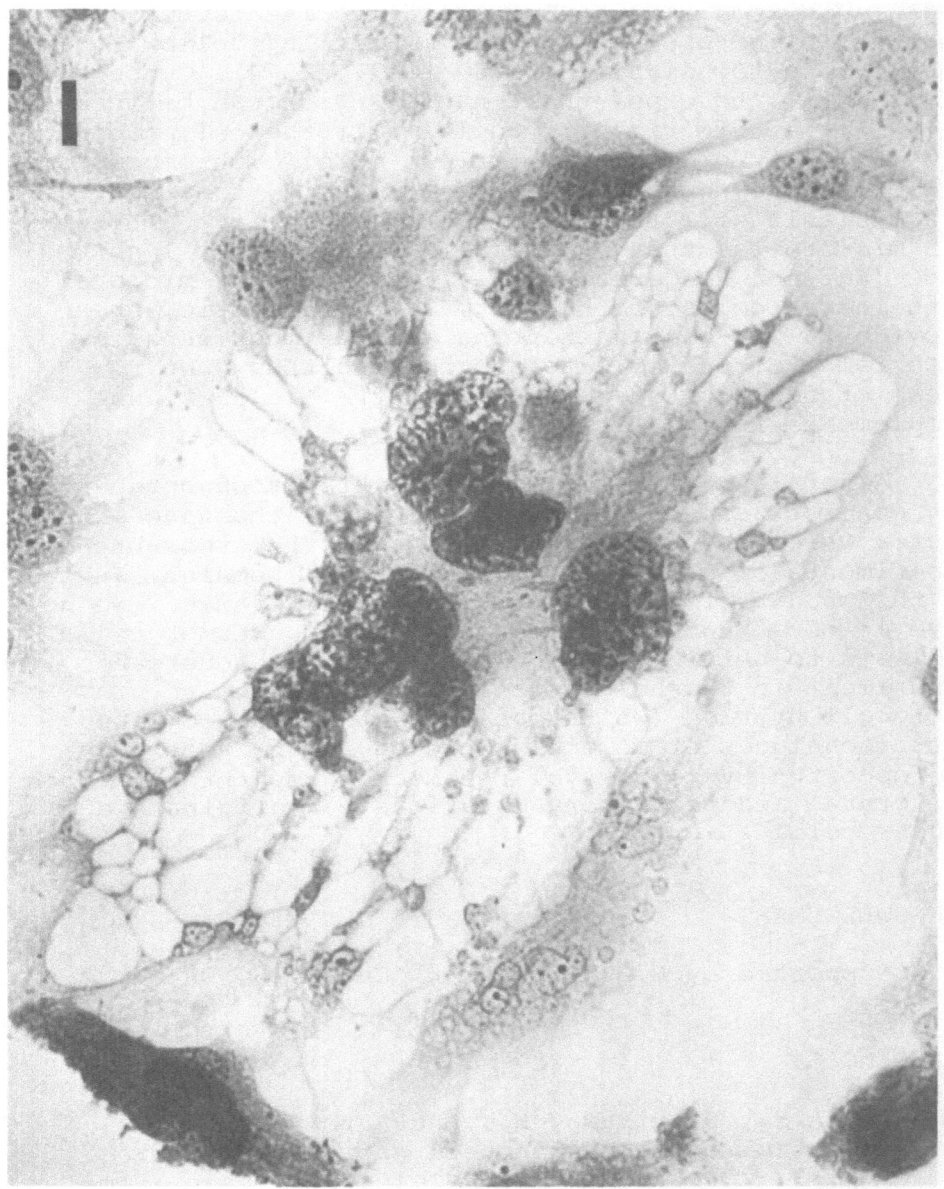

Fig. 5.   Another multinucleated cell from BT-549 breast
          carcinoma illustrating how the loss of genetic
          material might occur. Bar = 5 microns.

form cell hybrids. Interspecific cell hybrids have made it possible to map genes to specific chromosomes of several mammalian species including man (Weiss and Green, 1967 ; Davidson, 1978). Even more precise techniques now consist in the preparation of "minicells" following exposure to cytochalasin B (Ege et al., 1974). Cytochalasin causes cells to expel their nuclei which can be isolated with only a thin rim of cytoplasm. If the cell nucleus is already fragmented in multiple mitotic chromosomes following prolonged exposure to colcemid, treatment with cytochalasin will result in the formation of a multitude of "microcells" that may contain as little as 1 chromosome (Ege and Ringertz, 1974). Fusion of the microcells with intact cells, either normal or neoplastic, then provides a way of transferring well defined genetic material from one cell to another and thus open new areas of research particularly in the field of gene complementation analysis.

After long years of research, breast cancer has not concretized as a viral disease, but the genetic factor which originally had motivated the cross-breeding experiments of J. Bittner (1936), still remains. Instead of the crude animal models which then prevailed, we now have at our disposal collections of human tumor cells and ways to obtain normal cells with which one can experiment in tissue culture. The extensive use of microcell hybrids (which has not yet begun) combined with techniques of molecular biology might soon give the opportunity to unravel the mechanisms through which structural and regulatory mutations can originate a cancer cell.

ACKNOWLEDGMENTS

Supported by N.C.I. Grant n° CA-08515, DHEW.

REFERENCES

Armelin, A.H., Nishikawa, K., and Sato, G.H., 1974, Control of mammalian cell growth in culture p. 97-104. "Control of proliferation in animal cells (Clarkson and Baserga eds.), Cold Spring Harbor Laboratories, Cold Spring Harbor.

Benedict, W.F., Rucker, N., and Mark, C., 1975, Correlation between balance of specific chromosomes and expression of malignancy in hamster cells. J. Natl. Cancer Inst., 54, 157-162.

Bernhard, W., 1960, The detection and study of tumor

viruses with the electron microscope. Cancer
Research, 20, 712-727.

Bittner, J.J., 1936, Some possible effects of nursing
on the mammary gland tumor incidence in mice
(preliminary report). Science, 84, 162-163.

Black, M.M., Moore, D.H., Shore, B., Zachrau, R.E., and
Leis, H.P., 1974, Effect of murine milk samples
and human breast tissues on human leukocyte migration indices. Cancer Research, 34, 1054-1060.

Black, M.M., Zachrau, R.E., Shore, B., Dion, A.S., and
Leis, H.P., 1978, Cellular immunity to autologous
breast cancer and RIII-murine mammary tumor virus
preparations. Cancer Research, 38, 2068-2076.

Cailleau, R., Mackay, B., Young, R.K., and Reeves, W.J.,
1974a, Tissue culture studies on pleural effusions
from breast carcinoma patients. Cancer Res., 34,
801-809.

Cailleau, R., Olive, M., and Cruciger, Q.V., 1978, Long
term human breast carcinoma cell lines of metastatic origin : preliminary characterization.
In Vitro, 14, 911-915.

Cailleau, R., Young, R., Olive, M., and Reeves, W.J.,
1974b, Breast tumor cell lines from pleural
effusions. J. Natl. Cancer Inst., 53, 661-674.

Charney, J., and Moore, D.H., 1972, Immunization studies
with mammary tumor virus. J. Natl. Cancer Inst.,
48, 1125-1129.

Cruciger, Q.V., Pathak, S., and Cailleau, R., 1976, Human
breast carcinomas : marker chromosomes involving
19 in seven cases. Cytogenet. Cell Genet., 17,
231-235.

Dalton, A.J., Heine, U.I., and Melnick, J.L., 1975,
Symposium : Characterization of oncornaviruses
and related viruses : a report. J. Natl. Cancer
Inst., 55, 941-942.

Davidson, R.L., 1978. Genetics of cultured mammalian cells
as studied by somatic cell hybrydization. Natl.
cancer Inst. Monogr., 48, 21-30.

Dion, A.S., and Moore, D.H., 1977, Some biochemical
aspects of murine mammary tumor virus and the
putative human mammary tumor virus. In : Recent
Advances in Cancer Research : Cell Biology, Molecular Biology and Tumor Virology (Gallo R.C. ed.)
CRC Press, Cleveland,69-87.

Dion, A.S., Farwell, D.C., Pomenti, A.A., and Girardi,
A.J., 1980, A human protein related to the major
envelope protein of murine mammary tumor virus :
identification and characterization. Proc. Natl.
Acad. Sci. U.S.A. in press.

Dofuku, R., Biedler, J.R., and Splengler, B.A., 1975, Trisomy of chromosome 15 in spontaneous leukemia of AKR mice. Proc. Natl. Acad. Sci. U.S.A., 72, 1515-1517.

Dofuku, R., Utakoji, T., and Matsuzawa, A., 1979, Trisomy of chromosome ≠ 13 in spontaneous mammary tumors of GR, C3H and noninbred Swiss mice. J. Natl. Cancer Inst., 63, 651-656.

Eagle, H., 1963, Amino acid metabolism in mammalian cell cultures. Science, 130, 432-437.

Ege, T., Hamberg, H., and Krondahl, U., 1974, Characterization of minicells (nuclei) obtained by cytochalasis enucleation. Exp. Cell Res., 87, 365-377.

Ege, T., and Ringertz, N.R., 1974, Preparation of microcells by enucleation of micronucleate cells. Exp. Cell Res., 87, 378-382.

Emerman, J.T., and Pitelka, D.R., 1977, Maintenance and induction of morphological differentiation in disassociated mammary epithelium cells on floating collagen membranes. In Vitro, 13, 316-328.

Emerman, J.T., Burwen, S.J., and Pitelka, D.R., 1979, Substrate properties influencing ultra-structural differentiation of mammary epithelial cell cultures. Tissue and Cell, 11, 109-119.

Engel, L.W., and Young, N.A., 1978, Human breast carcinoma cells in continuous culture : a review. Cancer Res., 38, 4327-4339.

Engel, L.W., Young, N.A., Tralka, T.S., Lippman, M.E., O'Brien, S.J., and Joyce, M.J., 1978, Establishment and characterization of three new continuous cell lines derived from human breast carcinomas. Cancer Res., 38, 3352-3364.

Fogh, J., and Trempe, G., 1975, New human tumor cell lines. Human tumor cells in vitro (Fogh ed.) Plenum Press, New York.

German, J., 1972, Genes which increase chromosomal instability in somatic cells and predispose to cancer. Prog. Med. Genet., 8, 61-102.

Giovanella, B.C., Stehlin, J.S., Lee, S.S., Shepart, R., and Williams, L.J., 1976, Heterotransplantation of human breast carcinomas in "nude" thymus defficient mice. Proc. Am. Assoc. Cancer Res., 17, 124 (494).

Hackett, A.J., Smith, H.S., Springer, E.L., Owens, R.B., Nelson-Rees, W.A., Riggs, J.L., and Gardner, M.B., 1977, Two syngeneic cell lines from human breast tissue : the aneuploid mammary epithelial (HS578T) and the diploid myoepithelial (Hs 578 Bst) cell lines. J. Natl. Cancer Inst., 58, 1795-1806.

Hayflick, L., 1975, Cell biology of aging. Bio. Science,

25, 624-637.

Hoshino, M., and Dmochowski, L., 1973, Electron microscopy study of antigens in cells of mouse mammary
tumor cell lines by peroxydase-labeled antibodies
in sera of mammary tumor-bearing mice and of
patients with breast cancer. Cancer Res., 33,
2551-2561.

Keydar, I., Chen, L., Karby, S., Delarea, Y., Ramanara-
mayan, M., Mesa-Tejada, R., Spiegelman, S.,
Hager, J.C., and Calabresi, P., 1978, Detection of
an antigen in a human breast cancer cell line
(T-47D) immunologically related to the mouse
mammary tumor virus. Proc. 11th Meeting on
Mammary Cancer in Exp. Animals and Man. p. 66.

Knudson, A.G., 1977, Genetic predisposition to cancer.
Cold Spring Harbor Symposia. Cold Spring Harbor.
pp. 45-52.

Langlois, A.J., Holder, W.D., Iglehart, J.D., Nelson-
Rees, W.A., Wells, S.A., and Bolognesi, D.T.
1979, Morphological biochemical properties of a
new human breast cancer cell line. Cancer Res.,
39, 2604-2613.

Lasfargues, E.Y., 1957, Cultivation and behavior in
vitro of the normal mammary epithelium of the
adult mouse. Anat. Rec., 127, 117-129.

Lasfargues, E.Y., and Ozzello, L., 1958, Cultivation of
human breast carcinomas. J. Natl. Cancer Inst.,
21, 1131-1147.

Lasfargues, E.Y., Moore, D.H., Murray, M.R., Haagensen,
C.D., and Pollard, E.C., 1959, Production of the
milk agent in cultures of mouse mammary carcinoma. J. Biophys. Biochem. Cytol., 5, 93-96.

Lasfargues, E.Y., Kramarsky, B., Sarkar, N.H., Lasfargues,
J.C., and Moore, D.H., 1972, An established RIII
mouse mammary tumor cell line ; kinetics of
mammary tumor virus (MTV) production. Proc. Soc.
Exp. Biol. Med., 139, 242-247.

Lasfargues, E.Y., Coutinho, W.G., Lasfargues, J.C., and
Moore, D.H., 1973, A serum substitute that can
support the continuous growth of mammary tumor
cells. In Vitro, 8, 494-500.

Lasfargues, E.Y., and Lasfargues, J.C., 1975, Production
of the mouse mammary tumor virus in cultures of
BALB/cfC3H strain. Biotech. and Bioeng., 17,
733-743.

Lasfargues, E.Y., Lasfargues, J.C., Dion, A.S., Greene,
A.E., and Moore, D.H., 1976a, Experimental infection of a cat kidney cell line with the mouse
mammary tumor virus. Cancer Res., 36, 67-72.

Lasfargues, E.Y., Vaidya, A.B., Lasfargues, J.C., and Moore, D.H., 1976b, In vitro susceptibility of mink lung cells to the mouse mammary tumor virus. J. Natl. Cancer Inst., 57, 447-449.

Lasfargues, E.Y., Coutinho, W.G., and Redfield, E.S., 1978a, Isolation of two human tumor epithelial cell lines from solid breast carcinomas. J. Natl. Cancer Inst., 61, 967-978.

Lasfargues, E.Y., 1978b, BT-549 ; Breast Cancer Task Force Cell Culture Bank, Rockville, MD : EGLG Mason Research Institute.

Lasfargues, E.Y., Coutinho, W.G., and Dion, A.S., 1979, A human breast tumor cell line (BT-474) that supports mouse mammary tumor virus replication. In Vitro, 15, 723-729.

Lasfargues, E.Y., and Lasfargues, J.C., 1980, Mouse mammary carcinogenesis ; genetic basis of cell transformation. Proc. Am. Assoc. Cancer Res., 21, in press.

Levan, G., Mandahl, N., Bregula, U., Klein, G., and Levan, A., 1976, Double minute chromosomes are not centromeric regions of the host chromosome. Hereditas, 83, 83-90.

McGrath, C.M., Grant, P.M., Soule, H.D., Clancy, T., and Rich, M.A., 1974, Replication of oncorna virus-like particles in human breast carcinoma cell line MCF-7. Nature, 252, 247-250.

McPherson, I., 1973, Soft agar techniques 276-280. In Tissue Culture Methods and Application (Kruse P.F. and Patterson, M.K. eds), Academic Press, New York.

Marshall, C.J., Franks, L.M., and Carbonell, A.W., 1977, Markers of neoplastic transformation in epithelial cell lines derived from human carcinomas. J. Natl. Cancer Inst., 58, 1743-1751.

Mesa-Tejada, R., Keydar, I., Ramarayanan, T., Ohno, T., Fenoglio, C., and Spiegelman, S., 1978, Detection in human breast carcinomas of an antigen immuno-logically related to a group specific antigen of mouse mammary tumor virus. Proc. Nat. Ac. Sci. USA, 75, 15-29, 1533.

Miller, M.F., Dmochowski, L., and Bowen, J.M., 1977, Immunoelectron microscope studies of antibodies in mouse sera directed against mouse mammary tumor virus. Cancer Res., 37, 2086-2091.

Moore, G.E., Sandberg, A.A., and Ulrich, K., 1966, Sus-pension cell culture and in vivo and in vitro chromosome constitution of mouse leukemia L1210. J. Natl. Cancer Inst., 36, 405-421.

Moore, D.H., Charney, J., Kramarsky, B., Lasfargues, E.Y.,

Sarkar, N.H., Brennan, M.J., Burrows, J.H., Sirsat, S.M., Paymaster, J.C., and Vaidya, A.B., 1971, Search for a human breast cancer virus. Nature (London), 229, 611-614.

Moore, D.H., Holben, J.A., and Charney, J., 1976, Biologic characteristics of some mouse mammary tumor viruses. J. Natl. Cancer Inst., 57, 889-896.

Moore, D.H., Long, C.A., Vaidya, A.B., Sheffield, J.B., Dion, A.S., and Lasfargues, E.Y., 1979a, Mammary tumor viruses. Advances in Cancer Research (G. Klein and S. Weinhouse eds.), Academic Press, 29, 347-418.

Moore, D.H., Sarkar, N.H., Holben, J.A., and Sheffield, J.B., 1979b, Idiopathic mammary tumors in BALB/c mice. Int. J. Cancer, 23, 713-717.

Müller, M., Hageman, P.C., and Daams, J.S., 1972, On antigens in human breast cancer sera related to the murine mammary tumor virus. Nature-New Biology, 237, 116-117.

Nordquist, R.E., Ishmael, D.R., Lovig, C.A., Hyder, D.M., and Hoge, A.F., 1975, The tissue culture and morphology of human breast tumor cell line BOT-2. Cancer Res., 35, 3100-3105.

Pitelka, D.R., Bern, H.A., DeOme, K.B., Schooley, C.M., and Wellings, S.R., 1958, Virus-like particles in hyperplastic alveolar nodules of the mammary gland of the C3H/He CRGL mouse. J. Natl. Cancer Inst., 20, 541-553.

Ponten, J., 1974, Carcinogenesis in vitro. Recent Results in Cancer Research (E. Grundmann ed.), V. 44, p. 98-102. Springer Verlag, Berlin, Heidelberg, New York.

Reed, M.V., and Gey, G.O., 1963, Cultivation of normal and malignant lung tissue . I. The establishment of three adenocarcinoma cell strains. Lab. Invest., 11, 638-653.

Sanford, K.K., Andervont, H.B., Hobbs, G.L., and Earle, W.R., 1961, Maintenance of the mammary tumor agent in long-term cultures of mouse mammary carcinoma. J. Natl. Cancer Inst., 26, 1275-1288.

Sarkar, N.H., and Moore, D.H., 1974, Surface structure of mouse mammary tumor virus. Virology, 61, 38-55.

Sarkar, N.H., Holben, J.A., and Sheffield, J.B., 1979b, Idiopathic mammary tumors in BALB/c mice. Int. J. of Cancer, 23, 713-717.

Schlom, J., and Spiegelman, S., 1971, Simultaneous detection of the reverse transcriptase and high molecular weight RNA unique to the oncogenic RNA viruses. Science, 174, 840-843.

Sebesteny, A., Taylor-Papadimitrion, J., Ceriani, R., Millis, R., Schmidt, C., and Trevan, D., 1979, Primary human carcinomas transplantable in nude mice. J. Natl. Cancer Inst., 63, 1331-1337.

Seman, G., Myers, B., Williams, W.C., Gallager, H.S., and Dmochowski, L., 1969, Studies on the relationship of viruses to the origin of human breast cancer. II. Virus-like particles in human breast tumors. Texas Rep. Biol. Med., 27, 839-866.

Shin, S., Friedman, V.H., and Risser, R., 1975, Tumorigenicity of virus-transformed cells in nude mice is correlated specifically with anchorage independent growth in vitro. Proc. Natl. Ac. Sci. USA, 72, 4435-4439.

Soule, H.D., Vazquez, A., Long, A., Albert, S., and Brennan, M.A., 1973, Human cell lines from a pleural effusion derived from a breast carcinoma. J. Natl. Cancer Inst., 51, 1409-1413.

Spriggs, A.L., Boddington, M.M., and Clarke, C.M., 1962, Chromosomes of human cancer cells. Brit. Med. J., 36, 1431-1435.

Sykes, J.A., Whitescarver, J., and Briggs, J., 1968, Observations on a cell line producing the mammary tumor virus. J. Natl. Cancer Inst., 41, 1315-1327.

Tsubura, Y., Toyoshima, K., Sano, S., and Watanabe, T., 1968, Fate of B particles of mouse mammary tumor in vivo and in vitro. In : "Cancer cells in culture" (H. Katsuta ed) pp. 216-230. University of Tokyo Press, Tokyo.

Vaage, J., 1978, A survey of the growth characteristics of and the host reactions to one hundred C3H/He mammary carcinomas. Cancer Res., 38, 331-338.

Vaidya, A.B., Black, M.M., Dion, A.S., and Moore, D.H., 1974, Homology between human breast tumor RNA and mouse mammary tumor virus genome. Nature (London), 249,565.

Varmus, H.E., Quintrell, N., Medeiros, E., Bishop, J.M., Nowinski, R.C., and Sarkar, N.H., 1973, Transcription of mouse mammary tumor virus genes in tissues from high and low tumor incidence mouse strains. J. Mol. Biol., 79, 663-679.

Weiss, M., and Green, H., 1967, Human-mouse hybrid cell lines containing partial complements of human chromosomes and functioning human genes. Proc. Nat. Ac. Sci., USA, 58, 1104-1111.

Wiener, F., Klein, G. and Harris, H., 1974, The analysis of malignancy by cell-fusion. V. Further evidence of the ability of normal diploid cells to suppress malignancy. J. Cell Sci., 15, 177-183.

Wiener, F., Ohno, S., Spira, J., Haran-Ghera, N., and
Klein, G., 1978, Chromosome changes (Trisomies
≠ 15 and 17) associated with tumor progression
in leukemias induced by leukemia radiation virus.
J. Natl. Cancer Inst., 60, 227-237.

Yamamoto, T., Rabinowitz, Z., and Sachs, L., 1973, Identification of chromosomes that control malignancy.
Nature, 243, 247-250.

Yang, N.S., Soule, H.D., and McGrath, C.M., 1977, Expression of murine mammary tumor virus-related
antigens in human breast carcinoma (MCF-7) cells.
J. Natl. Cancer Inst., 59, 1357-1367.

Yang, N.S., McGrath, C.M., and Furmanski, P., 1978, Presence of a mouse mammary tumor virus-related
antigen in human breast carcinoma cells and its
absence from normal mammary epithelial cells.
J. Natl. Cancer Inst., 61, 1205-1208.

Yang, J., Bowman, P., Richards, J., Guzman, R., Evans,
J., McCormick, K., Hamamoto, S., Pitelka, D.,
and Nandi, S., 1979, Sustained growth and 3-
dimensional organization of primary cultures of
normal and neoplastic mammary cells in embedded
collagen gels. In Vitro, 15, 226(276).

Young, R.K., Cailleau, R., Mackay, B., and Reeves, W.J.,
1974, Establishment of epithelial cell line
MDA-MB-157 from metastatic pleural effusions of
human breast carcinoma. In Vitro, 9, 239-245.

Zachrau, R.E., Black, M.M., Dion, A.S., Shore, B.,
Williams, C.J., and Leis, H.P., 1978, Specificity
of the simultaneous cell-mediated immune reacti-
vity to RIII murine mammary tumor virus glycoprotein 55 and human breast cancer tissues.
Cancer Res., 38, 3414-3420.

ELASTOSIS IN HUMAN BREAST CANCER. PART I. MORPHOLOGICAL

STUDIES

J.J. Adnet[1], P. Birembaut[1], R. Sadrin[1],
D. Gaillard[1], C. Pastisson[2], L. Robert[3],
H. Dousset[4], and W.V. Bogomoletz[5]

1. Laboratoire Pol Bouin, Centre Hospitalier
   Universitaire, 51100 Reims, France
2. Departement de Biologie Cellulaire, Faculté
   des Sciences, 51100 Reims, France
3. Laboratoire de Biochimie du Tissu Conjonctif,
   94010 Créteil, France
4. Service de Chirurgie, Clinique de Courlancy,
   51100 Reims, France
5. Laboratoire d'Anatomie Pathologique, Institut
   Jean Godinot, 51100 Reims, France

INTRODUCTION

The presence of abundant elastic fibres or elastosis in human breast cancer has long been known
(Letulle, 1931 ; Cheatle and Cutler, 1931). Its macroscopic appearances are well established : elastosis is
visible as yellow or whitish streaks and flecks in the
fibrous stroma of the tumour and best seen in its central portion. In the past, the streaks of elastosis
had been mistaken for areas of necrosis.

Elastosis has also been described in other breast
diseases, in the absence of malignancy (Davies, 1973 ;
Hamperl, 1975). It has often been confused with other
stromal changes such as amyloidosis (Bernath, 1952) or
hylinosis (Baptist and al., 1973).

The histology (Lundmark, 1972 ; Schiødt et al.,
1972 ; Azzopardi and Laurini, 1974), the ultrastructure
(Tremblay, 1974, 1976, 1979 ; Martinez-Hernandez et al.,
1977), the origin (Douglas and Shivas, 1974) and the

pronostic significance of elastosis in breast cancer
have been investigated more thoroughly since 1972. The
correlation between elastosis and oestrogen receptors in
breast cancer has also been discussed (Masters et al.,
1976). The chemical composition of elastosis and the
presence of an elastinolytic activity in breast cancer
have been demonstrated (Hornebeck et al., 1977, 1978).
Two recent monographs on breast pathology have devoted
an entire section to elastosis in breast cancer (Ahmed,
1978 ; Azzoparti, 1979).

We have been investigating elastosis for the past
5 years in 250 cases of human breast cancer, using a
multiparameter approach : light and electron microscopy, cytology, enzyme histochemistry, biochemical
assays and autoradiography. Some of our preliminary
results have previously been reported (Adnet et al.,
1976a). We present here a detailed and updated account
of our findings.

MATERIAL AND METHODS

Our series of 250 cases of invasive carcinoma of
the breast included 240 excisional biopsies, submitted
initially for frozen section diagnosis and their related 240 mastectomy specimens, as well as 10 specimens
from directly performed mastectomy. None of the 250
patients had been treated either by chemotherapy or
radiotherapy prior to surgery.

From the histological point of view, and using
the criteria of recent nomenclatures (Fisher et al.,
1975), the 250 invasive carcinomas were classified as
follows : 200 (80 %) infiltrating duct carcinomas not
otherwise specified (IDC NOS), 25 (10 %) infiltrating
duct carcinomas special types and 25 (10 %) infiltrating
lobular carcinomas.

Light microscopy

In all the 250 cases the material had been fixed
in either Bouin's fluid or formalin. Multiple paraffin-
embedded sections were stained by conventional haema-
toxyline-eosin and haematoxylin-phloxine-saffron. The
following special stains were also used on these sections : orcein, Weigert's resorcin fuchsin, Gomori's
aldehyde fuchsin and Van Gieson trichrome.

The 200 cases of IDC NOS were grouped according to Bloom and Richardson's histological grading (Bloom and Richardson, 1957). Bloom and Richardson's histological grading was compared with the degree of elastosis in 83 IDC NOS cases. The degree of elastosis was graded in 3 categories, according to a semi-quantitative method as previously described by us (Adnet et al., 1976b) : "+" = minimal elastosis, "++" = moderate elastosis and "+++" = marked elastosis.

Smears were also prepared in 50 IDC NOS cases from fine needle aspiration performed directly on the excisional biopsy specimen and imprints were made parallely from the cut surface of the block used for frozen section diagnosis. The smears and imprints thus obtained were stained with Papanicolaou and May-Grunwald-Giemsa. The grade of elastosis, after appropriate staining of a paraffin-embedded section was compared with the nuclear diameter of neoplastic cells from the corresponding imprint in all 50 cases. The nuclear diameter of at least 100 well-preserved neoplastic cells was measured and a mean nuclear diameter obtained for each imprint. In order to avoid artefacts due to poor fixation or poor staining, the nuclear diameter of the neoplastic cells was measured in relation to the diameter of the red blood corpuscles present in the imprint i.e. expressed arbitrarily in RBC-units.

Paraffin-embedded whole mounted sections from 25 mastectomy specimens, following excisional biopsy submitted for frozen section and reported as IDC NOS, were also studied histologically. Elastosis of the remaining glandular tissue was compared with elastosis of the corresponding invasive carcinoma.

Electron microscopy

Material from 25 IDC NOS cases was prepared for ultrastructural study. Small blocks of neoplastic tissue, taken at the time of frozen section diagnosis, were fixed in phosphate-buffered 2 % glutaraldehyde, postfixed in 2 % osmic acid and embedded in epoxy resin. Ultrathin sections were cut on a Reichert OMU2 microtome, stained with uranyl acetate and lead citrate as well as with orcein (Adnet et al., 1976b) and tannic acid (Cotta Pereira et al., 1977) for specific demonstration of elastosis and examined under a JEOL 100 S electron microscope.

In 5 cases, aspiration material obtained by fine needle technique as well as small blocks of neoplastic tissue were fixed in phosphate-buffered 2 % glutaraldehyde and examined under a JEOL JSM 25 scanning electron microscope.

Enzyme histochemistry

Frozen sections from 50 IDC NOS cases were submitted to enzyme histochemistry. The following enzymes were studied : acid and alkaline phosphatases, 5-nucleotidase, alpha-n-esterase, peroxydase, DPNH, glucose-6-phosphatase, leucine aminopeptidase, lactate, malate and succinate deshydrogenases.

Autoradiography

Sections from 6 IDN NOS cases were studied by contact autoradiography. Small blocks of tissue were incubated for 5 to 72 hours with $30 \mu Ci/ml$ of tritium labelled valine or proline in calf serum. Valine and proline were selected because these amino-acids entered the composition of elastin. Semithin sections were examined by light microscopy and ultrathin sections by electron microscopy.

Biochemical assays

In 35 IDC NOS cases the excisional biopsy specimen was cut in half. A block from the cut surface of one half was used for frozen section diagnosis as well as for the grading of elastosis after paraffin embedding. A block from the cut surface of the other half was submitted to biochemical assays (see L. Robert, part II of this chapter).

RESULTS

Light microscopy

Elastosis in routinely stained sections appeared as an eosinophilic material, either pulverulent (as in the focal form) or fibrillar (as in the diffuse form). Similar aspects were observed after staining with orcein, Weigert's resorcin fuchsin and Gomori's aldehyde fuchsin.

Three forms of distribution of elastosis in breast cancer were identified :

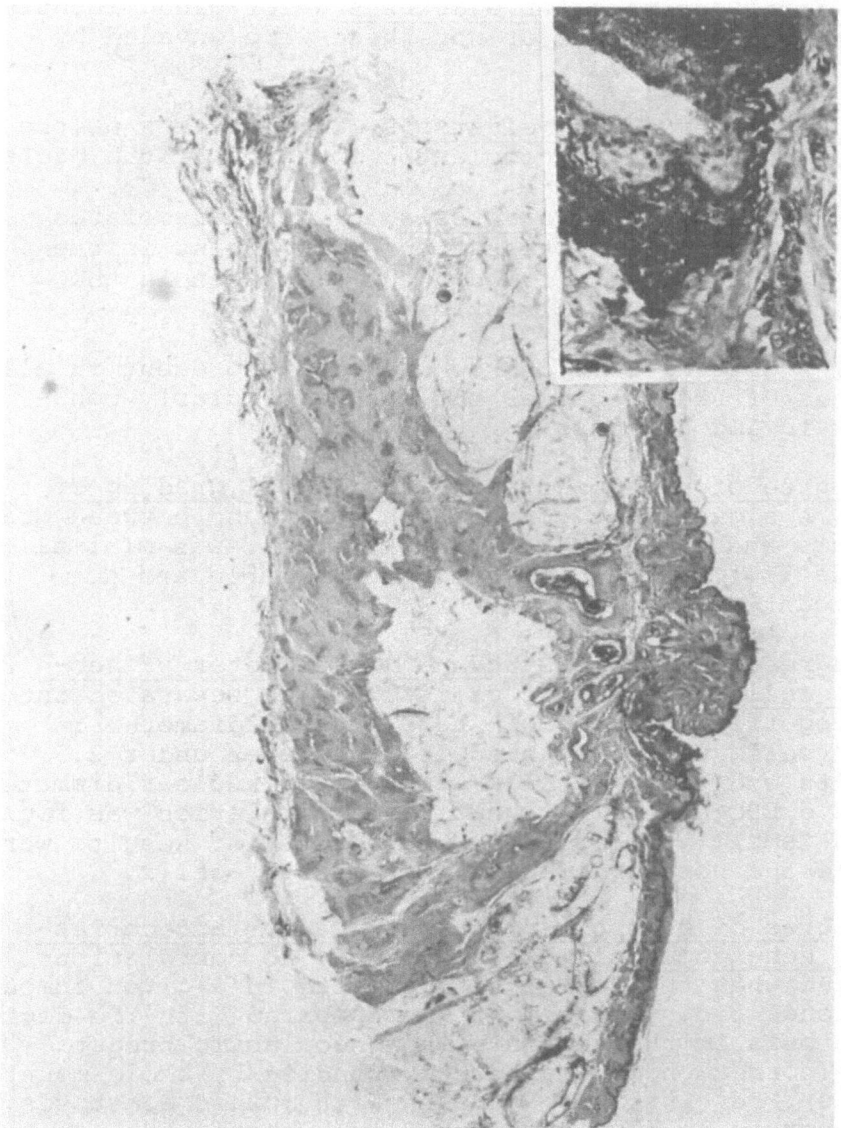

Fig. 1. Paraffin-embedded whole-mounted section of
        mastectomy specimen (following excisional
        biopsy) showing minimal elastosis in the non-
        neoplastic breast tissue. Orcein. Inset :
        marked periductal elastosis in an area of neo-
        plastic tissue of the corresponding excisional
        biopsy. Van Gieson.

A focal perivascular elastosis which predominantly
involved veins, whether or not these were invaded by
carcinoma ;

A focal periductal elastosis, irrespective of the
presence or absence of neoplastic invasion of the ducts ;

A diffuse stromal elastosis, closely associated
with the carcinomatous tissue and predominant in the
central portion of the tumour, but also seen in the
peripheral zone of infiltration.

Elastosis of some degree was always present in all
250 cases of breast cancer but was particularly cons-
picuous in IDC NOS cases.

Degree of elastosis and histological grading of
tumour. A significant correlation was found between Grade
I tumours and marked elastosis. Elastosis was minimal
in Grade III tumours. Results were variable and not
significant in Grade II tumours.

Degree of elastosis and nuclear diameter of neoplastic cells. Neoplastic cells could be separated into
two categories in terms of their nuclear diameter :
"small" cells with a mean nuclear diameter under 2.5
RBC-units and "large" cells with a mean nuclear diameter
above 2.5 RBC-units. A significant correlation was found
between "small" cells and marked elastosis. Results were
variable and not significant with "large" cells.

Degree of elastosis in breast cancer and corresponding non-neoplastic breast tissue. No correlation
was found when the degree of elastosis in a given tumour
(excisional biopsy specimen) was compared with the degree
of elastosis in the remaining non-neoplastic breast
tissue (corresponding mastectomy studied by whole mounted
sections). For instance, tumours with marked elastosis
were observed to have originated in breasts, the non-
neoplastic tissue of which showed minimal elastosis ;
the reverse situation was also seen. (Fig. 1).

Electron microscopy

Ultrastructural studies confirmed the 3 forms of
elastosis seen with conventional microscopy :

Periductal elastosis. (Fig. 2). Elastin was observed
to be in close contact with the basement membrane of the
ducts as well as with the tapering processes of the

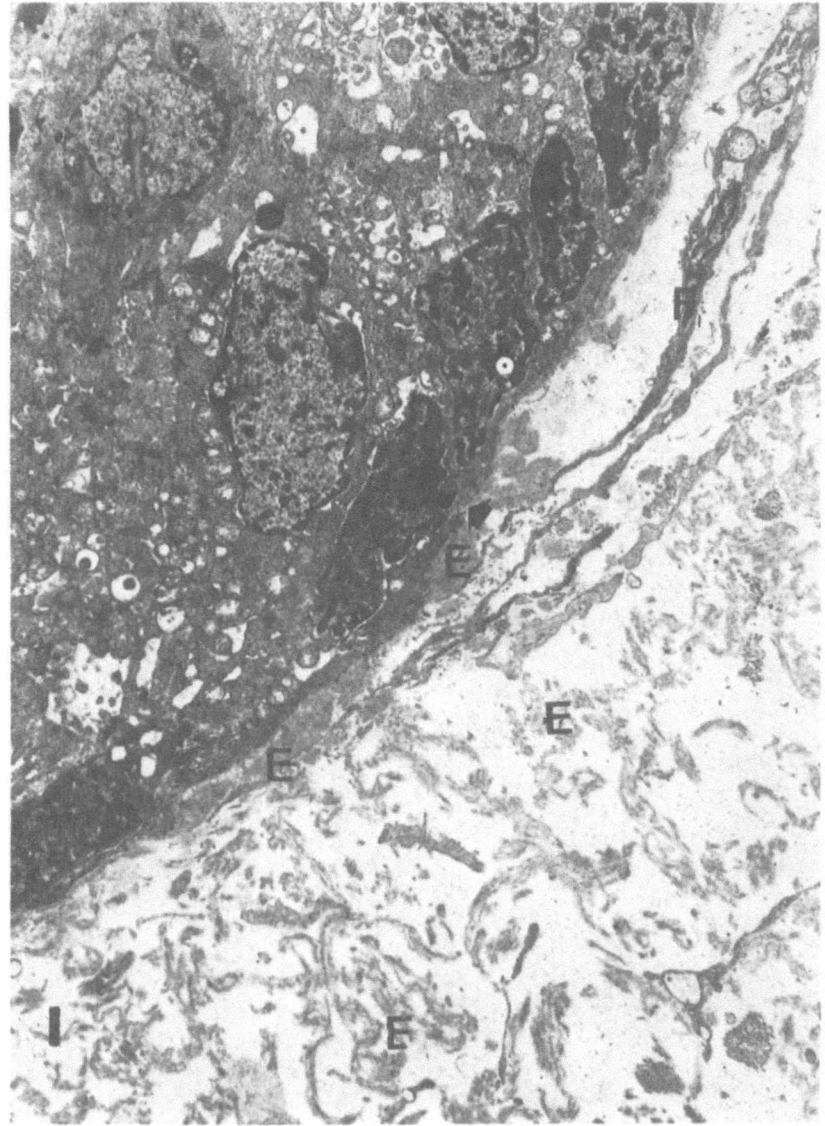

Fig. 2.   Electron micrograph of periductal elastosis.
Elastin (E) is present around the outer aspect
of the basement membrane of the duct (arrowed)
and is closely associated with the delimiting
fibroblasts (F). Uranyl acetate and lead
citrate.

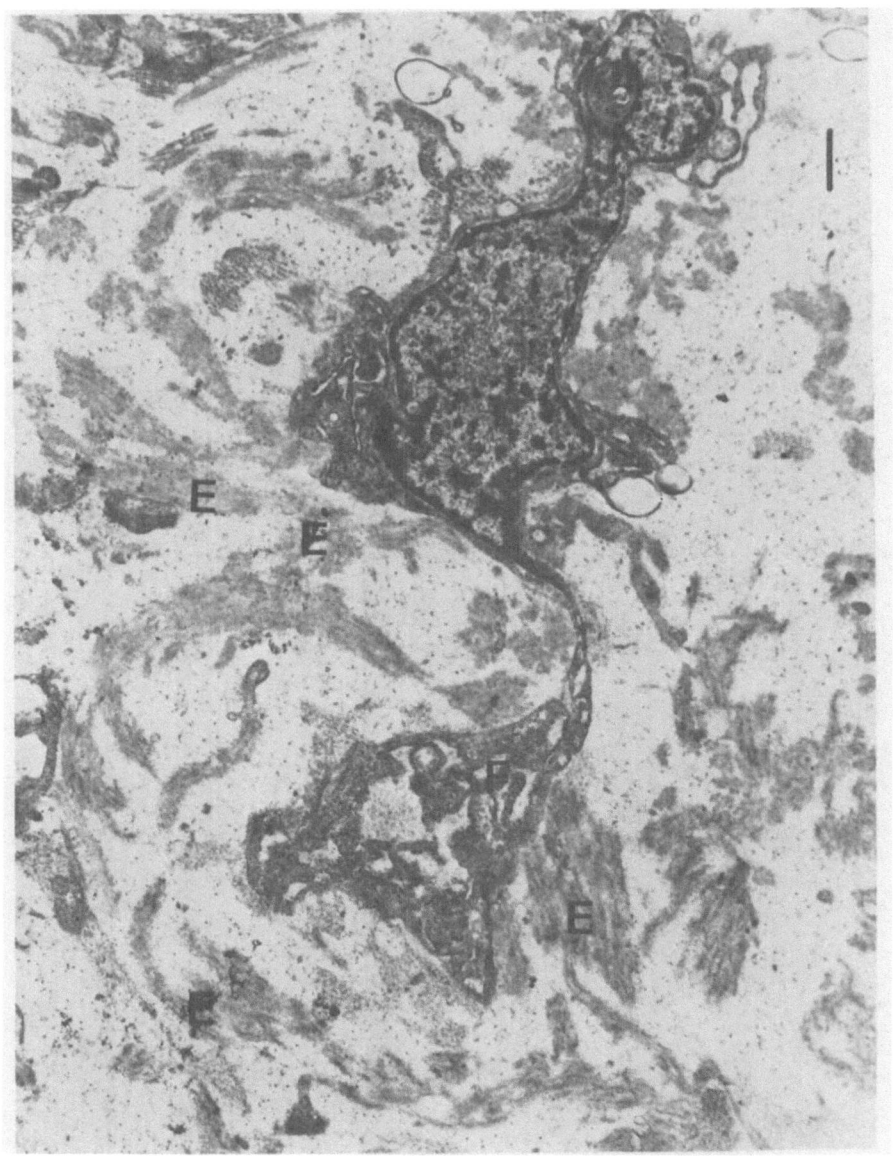

Fig. 3.   Electron micrograph of stromal elastosis.
          Abundant microfilamentous elastin (E) appears
          related to the stromal fibroblasts (F).
          Uranyl acetate and lead citrate.

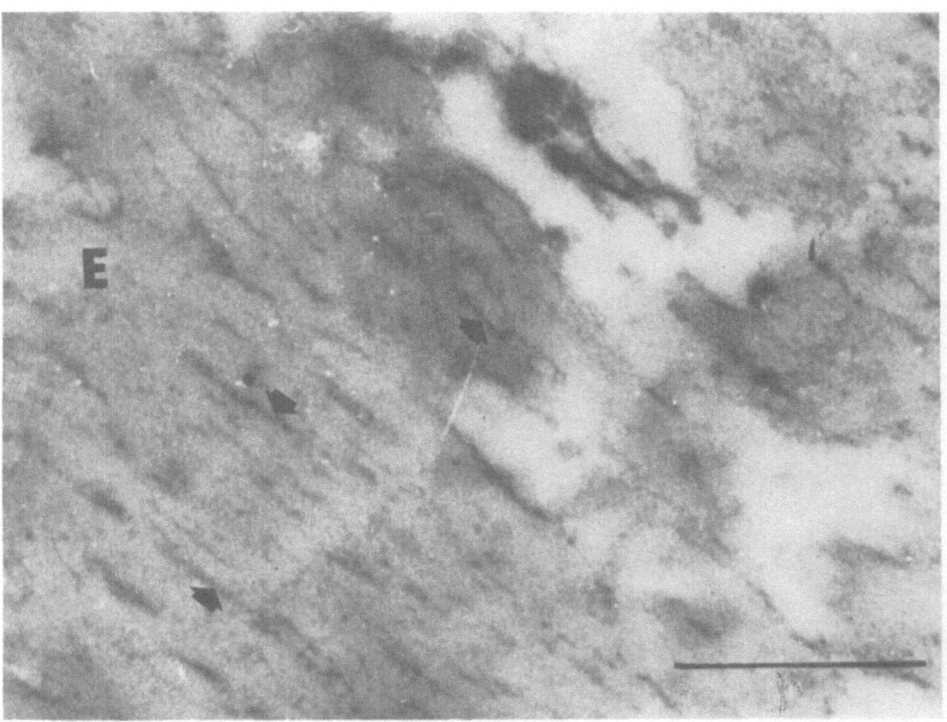

Fig. 4. Electron micrograph showing a typical pattern
         of normal elastin : glycoprotein microfibrils
         (arrowed) coated with elastin molecules (E).
         Uranyl acetate and lead citrate.

periductal fibroblasts, the latter corresponding to
the "delimiting fibroblasts" described in the breast
by Ozzello and Sanpitak (1970). In marked periductal
elastosis, these delimiting fibroblasts showed a well-
developed rough endoplasmic reticulum.

     Perivascular elastosis. The smooth muscle cells in
the tunica of the veins (Fig. 3.) underwent hypertrophy
and hyperplasia.

     Stromal elastosis. A prominent rough endoplasmic
reticulum was also observed in the cytoplasm of the
stromal fibroblasts.

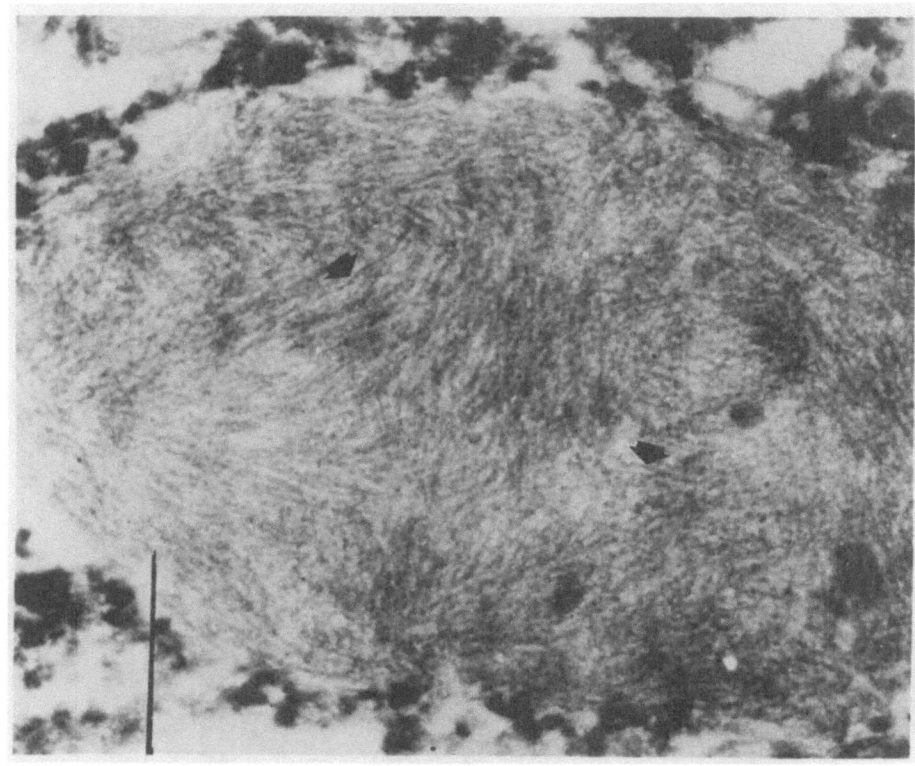

Fig. 5.   Electron micrograph of elastin which is
           entirely composed of microfibrils (arrowed).
           Uranyl acetate and lead citrate.

        No convincing image of elastin synthesis was seen
in neoplastic cells. The ultrastructure of the elastin
was variable. In some cases there was a typical pattern
of glycoprotein microfibrils coated with elastin molecules. (Fig. 4). More often the elastin appeared amorphous with fewer microfibrils and this pattern was
particularly observed in periductal elastosis. In rare
cases the elastin contained numerous microfibrils as
shown in Fig. 5. Staining with orcein and tannic acid
confirmed the histochemical nature of the elastin
material (Fig. 6). Microfibrils measuring 89 nm were
detected in some areas of periductal elastosis ; these
could represent oxytalan or elaunin fibres.

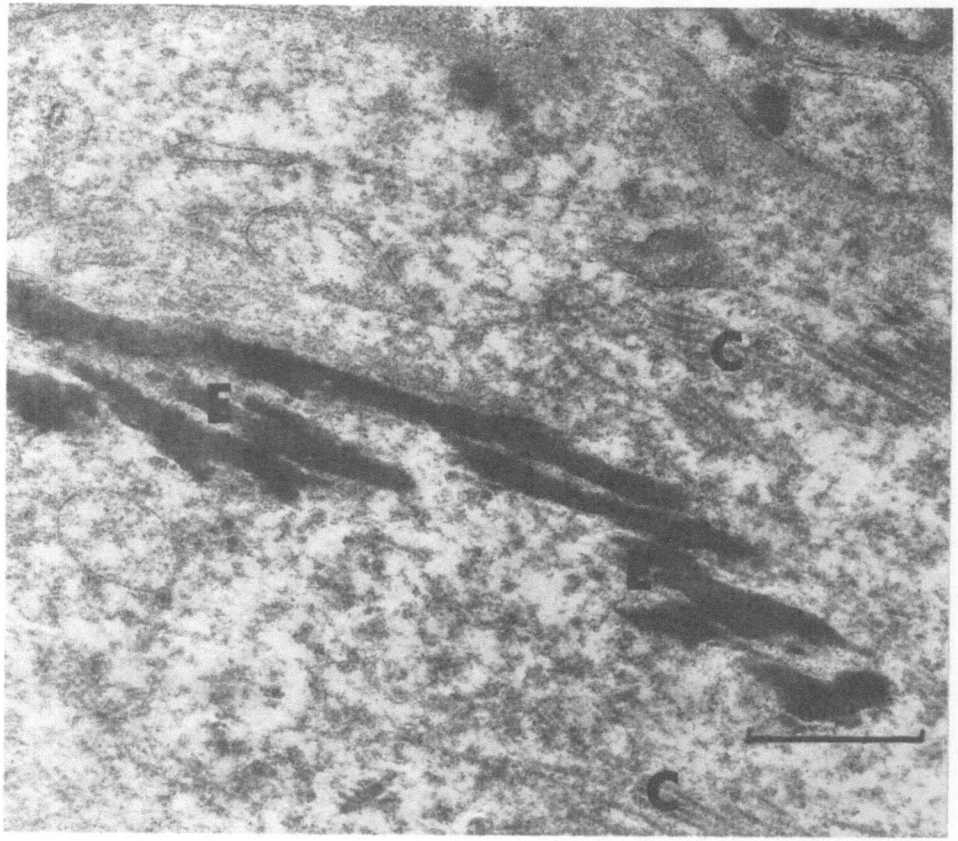

Fig. 6. High resolution electron micrograph showing
         the amorphous elastin (E) which is well
         contrasted amongst collagen fibres (C).
         Tannic acid.

Elastin was easily identified when present under
the scanning electron microscope (Fig. 7).

Neoplastic epithelial cells under the scanning
electron microscope showed prominent surface microvilli
and cytoplasmic pores suggestive of good cellular differentiation and secretion. No elastin synthesis was seen
in neoplastic cells (Fig. 8). However, synthesis of
elastin microfibrils was again observed to be associated
with fibroblasts in the fragments of neoplastic tissue,
thus confirming the preceding findings.

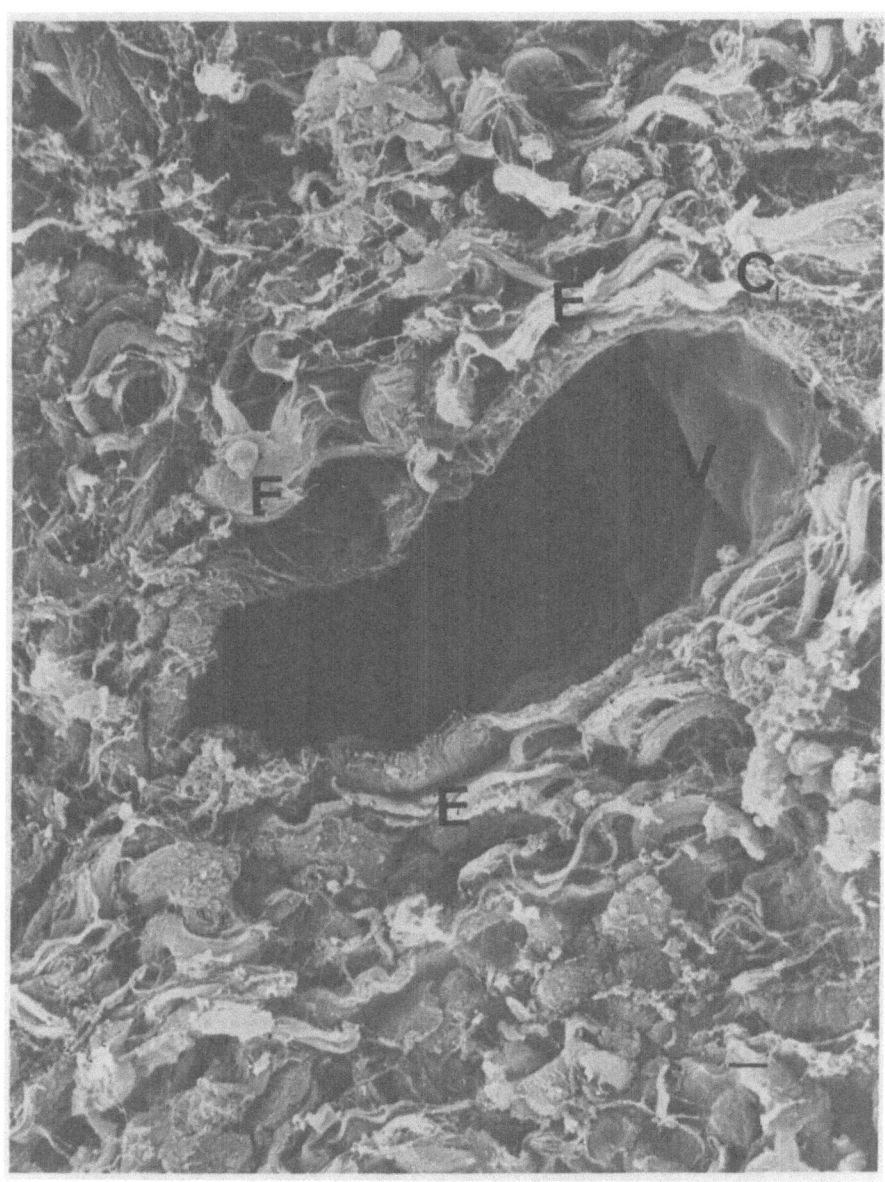

Fig. 7.   Scanning electron micrograph showing peri-
          vascular elastosis. Elastin (E), Fibroblast
          (F), Collagen fibres (C). Lumen of vein (V).

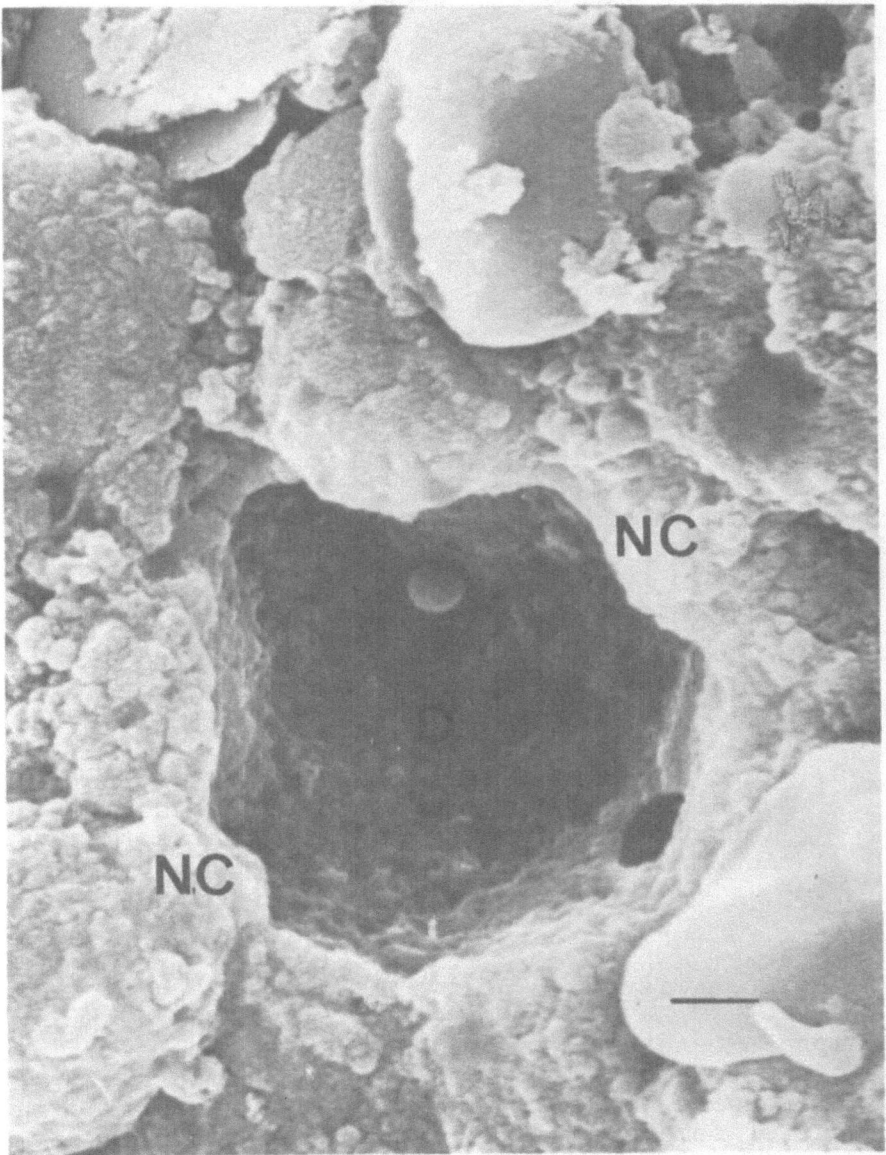

Fig. 8. Scanning electron micrograph of a fragment of neoplastic tissue from a grade I IDC NOS tumour with marked elastosis. No elastic fibres are identified around neoplastic cells. Duct (D), Neoplastic cells (NC).

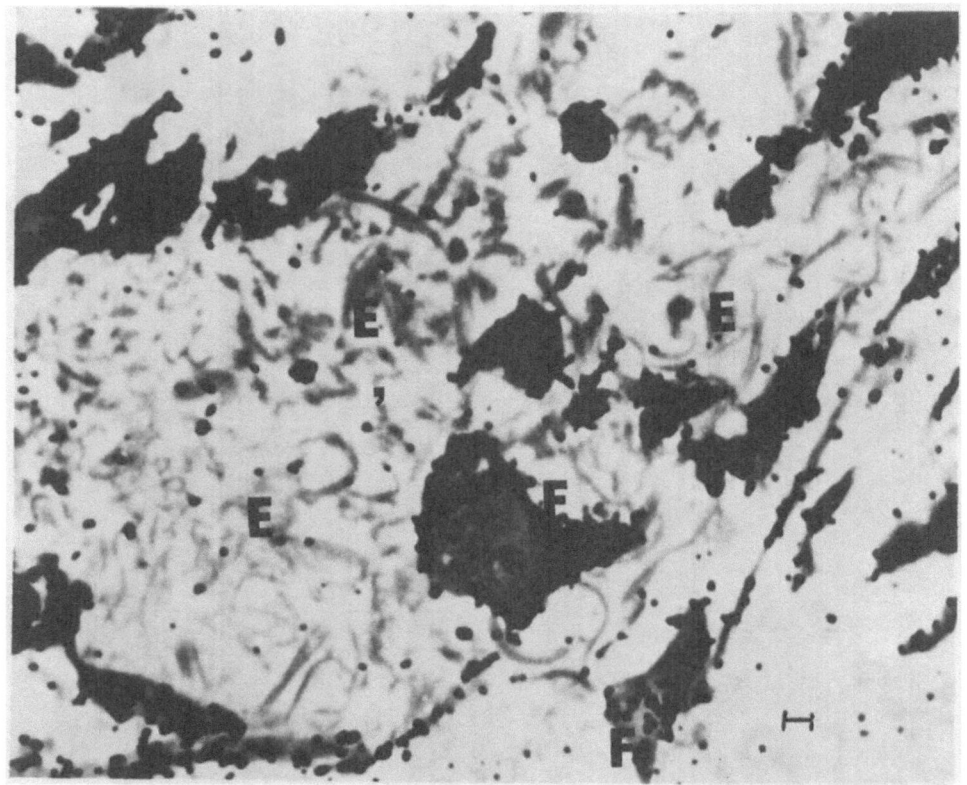

Fig. 9.   Autoradiograph of a semithin section from a
          grade II IDC NOS tumour. Fibroblasts have
          incorporated tritium-labelled Valine (72 hrs.
          incubation). Elastin (E), Fibroblast (F).

Enzyme histochemistry

     Alpha-n-esterase was present in the neoplastic
cells of most Grade I and some Grade II tumours of
IDC NOS. Leucine aminopeptidase was also identified in
the mucus of some special types of infiltrating duct
carcinoma (mucoid and apocrine carcinomas) as well as
in IDC NOS with "mucoid" areas.

Elastosis and autoradiography

     Stromal and delimiting fibroblasts as well as
vascular smooth muscle cells in the six IDC NOS cases

were seen to incorporate tritium-labelled valine and proline. These cases included two Grade I and two Grade II tumours, all four with marked elastosis, and two Grade III tumours with minimal elastosis. Neoplastic cells also incorporated the labelled amino-acids in the four Grade I + II tumours but not in the two Grade III tumours. (Fig. 9).

Degree of elastosis and biochemical assays

The results and corresponding discussion are presented in PART II of this chapter.

DISCUSSION

Our findings as regards the morphology of elastosis in breast cancer confirm those of Azzopardi and Laurini (1974), for light microscopy, and those of Tremblay (1974, 1976, 1979), for electron microscopy. In particular, we observe the three types of elastosis described by Azzopardi and Laurini (1974) and Azzopardi (1979), i.e. perivascular, periductal and stromal elastosis.

Our results throw further light on the concept of elastogenesis in IDC NOS, which constitute 80 % of our material ; the relationship between elastosis and neoplastic differentiation is noteworthy as regards prognosis. The abundant elastosis, which is significantly associated with IDC NOS grade I tumours (Bloom and Richardson's histological grading), may represent an additional and important histological parameter.

The cytological study, based on the nuclear diameter of neoplastic cells, corroborates our histological findings. It lends some support to the recent concept of Zajdela et al. (1975) who advocate a cytological classification based on "large nuclear type" and "small nuclear type".

There is also no apparent correlation between the degree of elastosis in IDC NOS and elastosis in the corresponding non-neoplastic breast tissue.

Enzyme-histochemistry of breast cancer does not appear to contribute any further significant information. Alpha-n-esterase and leucine aminopeptidase are present in neoplastic cells of well-differentiated and mucus-secreting infiltrating duct carcinomas. In addition to

our investigation of breast cancer cases, we have also
been able to demonstrate the presence of alkaline phos-
phatase and ATPases in myoepithelial cells, situated
close to the basement membrane of ducts, of normal breast
tissue. Benign breast tumours, such as fibroadenomas
and intraduct papillomas, show abundant alpha-n-esterase
and leucine aminopeptidase in their epithelial cells.

Our ultrastructural study highlights the variability in the pattern of elastin material, which is either
amorphous or contains abundant glycoprotein microfibrils.
This variability correlates well with the findings of
the biochemical assays, as demonstrated in the aminoacid composition of elastin (see Part II). It could
also be related to the metabolism of elastin and to the
presence of an elastinolytic activity.

With regard to the origin of elastosis, the cells
mainly responsible for the synthesis of the elastin
material appear to include (on morphological grounds
as well as based on autoradiographic findings) stromal
and delimiting periductal fibroblasts and smooth muscle
cells of vessels. We cannot entirely exclude any participation of neoplastic cells in elastin material synthesis because aminoacid precursors can also be demonstrated in these neoplastic cells by autoradiography.
However, synthesis, if present, of elastin material by
neoplastic cells must be comparatively low with that
by mesenchymal cells.

CONCLUDING REMARKS

Having been considered a morphological curiosity
for years, elastosis in breast cancer is assuming an
increasing importance.

The degree of elastosis is a significant parameter
which should be included, in our opinion, in any histological evaluation of breast cancer in terms of its
pathological grading. The study of larger series,
including survival rates, is mandatory in order to test
the prognostic significance of elastosis.

A more fundamental problem is that of the origin
of elastosis in breast cancer and the mechanism of
elastogenesis. The possibility of an "elastin-stimulating
factor", secreted by neoplastic cells and inducing
elastin synthesis by mesenchymal cells, needs further
investigation.

ACKNOWLEDGMENTS

   We wish to thank Mrs. H. Bobichon and Mrs. G. Evrard
for technical assistance, Mr. A. Guides for the photo-
graphy and Miss M-J. Bianchi for secretarial help.

REFERENCES

Adnet, J.J., Pinteaux, A., Caulet, T., Hibon, E., Petit,
     J., Pluot, M., and Roth, A., 1976a, L'élastose
     dans les cancers du sein. Etude anatomo-clinique,
     histochimique et ultra-structurale. Ann. Med.,
     Reims, 13, 147-153.
Adnet, J.J., Pinteaux, A., Pousse, G., and Caulet, T.,
     1976b, Caractérisation du tissu élastique normal
     et pathologique en microscopie électronique sur
     coupes semi-fines et coupes fines. Path. Biol.,
     24, 293-296.
Ahmed, A., 1978, Atlas of the ultrastructure of human
     breast diseases. Churchill-Livingstone, London,
     Vol. 1.
Azzopardi, J.G., and Laurini, R.N., 1974, Elastosis in
     breast cancer. Cancer, 33, 174-183.
Azzopardi, J.G., 1979, Problems in breast pathology, in :
     Major problems in pathology. W.B. Saunders Co.
     Ltd., London, Vol. II., 379-394.
Baptist, S.J., Thomas, J.A., and Kothare, S.N., 1973,
     Hyaline material in mammary cancer. Study of
     5 cases. Indian J. Cancer, 10, 317-321.
Bernath, G., 1952, Amyloidosis in malignant tumors. Acta
     Morphol. Acad. Scient. Hung., 2, 137-144.
Bloom, H.J.G., and Richardson, W.W., 1957, Histological
     grading and prognosis in breast cancer. Brit. J.
     of Cancer, 11, 359-377.
Cheatle, G.L., and Cutler, M.,1931, Tumours of the Breast.
     Their Pathology, Symptoms, Diagnosis and Treat-
     ment. Edward Arnold, London.
Cotta-Pereira, G., Guerra-Rodrigo, F., and David-Ferreira,
     J.F., 1977, Elastin and elastic tissue. Advances
     in experimental medicine and Biology. L.B. Sand-
     berg, W.R. Gray and C. Franzblau, eds., Plenum
     Press, New York, London, 79, 11-28.
Davies, J.D., 1973, Hyperelastosis, obliteration and
     fibrous plaques in major ducts of the human breast.
     J. Pathol., 110, 13-26.
Douglas, J.G., and Shivas, A.A., 1974, The origins of
     elastica in breast carcinoma. J. Royal Coll. Surg.
     Edinburgh, 19, 89-93.

Fisher, E.R., Gregoris, R.M., and Fisher, B., 1975, The pathology of invasive breast cancer. Cancer, 36, 1-85.

Hamperl, H., 1975, Strahlige Narben und obliterierende Mastopathie. Virchows Arch. A. Path. Anat. Histol., 369, 55-68.

Hornebeck, W., Derouette, J.C., Brechemier, D., Adnet, J.J., and Robert, L., 1977, Elastogenesis and elastinolytic activity in human breast cancer. Biomed., 26, 48-52.

Hornebeck, W., Adnet, J.J., and Robert, L., 1978, Age dependent variation of elastin and elastase in aorta and human breast cancer. Exp. Geront., 13, 293-298.

Letulle, M., 1931, Epitheliomas des glandes mammaires, in Anatomie Pathologique. T. III, Masson, Paris, pp. 21-29.

Lundmark, C., 1972, Breast cancer and elastosis. Cancer, 27, 1195-1201.

Martinez-Hernandez, A., Francis, D.J., and Silverberg, S.G., 1977, Elastosis and other stromal reactions in benign and malignant breast tissue. An ultrastructural study. Cancer, 40, 700-706.

Masters, J.R.W., Sangster, K., Hawkins, R.A., and Shivas, A.A., 1976, Elastosis and oestrogen receptors in human breast cancer. Brit. J. Cancer, 33, 342-343.

Ozzello, L., and Sanpitak, P., 1970, Epithelial stromal junction of intraductal carcinoma of the breast. Cancer, 26, 1186-1198.

Schiødt, T., Jensen, H., Nielsen, M., and Ranlov, P., 1972, On the nature of amyloid-like duct wall changes in carcinoma of the breast. Acta Pathol. Microbiol. Scand. Sect. A., 80, 151-157.

Tremblay, G., 1974, Elastosis in tubular carcinoma of the breast. Arch. Pathol., 98, 302-307.

Tremblay, G., 1976, Ultrastructure of elastosis in scirrhous carcinoma of the breast. Cancer, 37, 307-316.

Tremblay, G., 1979, Stromal aspects of breast carcinoma. Exp. Molecular. Pathol., 31, 248-260.

Zajdela, A., De Lariva, L.S., and Ghossein, N.A., 1975, The relation of prognosis to the nuclear diameter of breast cancer cells obtained by cytologic aspiration. Acta Cytol., 23, 75-81.

ELASTOSIS IN HUMAN BREAST CANCER. PART II. BIOCHEMICAL
STUDIES

L. Robert[1], W. Hornebeck[1], D. Brechemier[1],
and J.J. Adnet[2]

1. Laboratoire de Biochimie du Tissu Conjonctif,
   94010 Créteil, France
2. Laboratoire Pol Bouin, Centre Hospitalier
   Universitaire, 51100 Reims, France

INTRODUCTION

It is known since several decades that in many cases
of infiltrating epitheliomas of human breast variable
amounts of elastic fibers may appear. This finding was
reported and studied mainly by anatomo-pathologists
using morphological techniques (see Part I of this report
for the bibliography by Adnet et al., this volume). The
main problems which have been discussed concerned the
identity of these fibers with elastic fibers seen in
other parts of the organism and the possible diagnostic
or prognostic importance of this breast cancer elastosis.
In our knowledge however no detailed chemical investigation was undertaken on this interesting and important
subject. We started such an investigation a few years ago
and the purpose of this chapter is to summarize the
results we obtained and which were shortly reported
(Hornebeck and Robert, 1977 ; Hornebeck et al., 1977,
1978).

Our interest was drawn to this subject mainly because
of the fact that elastin is phylogenetically speaking
the "youngest" matrix protein which appears with certainty
only in vertebrates (Sage and Gray, 1977), in contradis-
tinction to collagens and structural glycoproteins, both
being present from the first metazoans, the Porifera or

sponges (Garrone, 1978) and the proteoglycans or glyco-
saminoglycans which were demonstrated to be present from
higher invertebrates. May be unrelated to this fact is
the observation that oriented structurally and functionally
valid elastic fibers are synthesised, led down, only
during the ontogenetic phase of human development (for a
review, see Robert, 1980). During maturation and aging
a progressive elastolytic process was observed in the
blood vessels as well as in the superficial layers of
the dermis (Bouissou et al., 1973, 1975 ; Hornebeck and
Robert, 1977 ; Hornebeck et al., 1978).

It was shown also, using rabbit aorta organ cultures
that the rate of synthesis of aorta matrix macromolecules
in general and of elastin in particular decrease nearly
exponentially with the age of the animal (Moczar et al.,
1976). Morphological studies showed however that elastogenesis remains possible to a detectable extent in the
arteriosclerotic process where the smooth muscle cells
migrate towards the intima and form the intimal cushion.
In this intimal proliferation smooth muscle cells were
observed to lay down fine randomly oriented elastic
fibrils. This observation as well as the morphological
studies carried out on aging rat aortas by Looker and
Berry (1972) showed that fine elastic fibrils can be
synthesised to a limited extent during the whole life
span.

The only example however of an important local elastogenesis, neosynthesis of elastic fibrils, is the observation of elastogenesis in human breast cancer. It was
therefore tempting to assume that as a result of the
malignant transformation of the epithelial cells some
factor(s) are liberated which somehow activate the silent
structural genes which code for both components of the
elastic fibers, namely the microfibrils which were shown
to be composed mainly of structural glycoproteins (Robert
et al., 1971) and polymeric elastin which is now considered
as being the cross-linked polymer of tropoelastin subunits
(for reviews see Sandberg et al., 1977 and Robert, 1980).
This "derepression" of silent genes can be considered as
a modification of the expression of the differentiated
state of some of the cells present in breast cancer and
can be taken therefore as a good model for the study of
the changes of differentiation resulting from the malignant
transformation.

On the other side, the detailed chemical study of
this phenomenon was thought to bring new facts to our
knowledge, which may be helpful for the interpretation

of the malignant process itself and throw new light on this debated problem of the prognostic and diagnostic value of breast cancer elastogenesis.

The morphological aspects of breast cancer elasto-genesis were discussed in the preceeding chapter (Adnet et al., 1980) and therefore we shall here concentrate only on the biochemical aspects of our investigations.

MATERIAL AND METHODS

Most of the methods used for the isolation of elastin and for the study of its aminoacid composition were described in previous papers (Robert and Hornebeck, 1976). Elastin was purified by the NaOH-extraction procedure (Hornebeck et al., 1977). Its aminoacid composition was determined after 48 h hydrolysis in 6N HCl on a 2-column aminoacid analyser. The extraction and quantitation of proteases capable to attack substrates considered as specific for elastases (elastolytic proteases) was carried out as described by Bieth (1979) and Bellon et al. (1978).

RESULTS

Using the simplest extraction procedure that is heating of defatted tissue in O.1N NaOH according to a modified Lansing procedure (Hornebeck et al., 1977) we could extract and purify polymeric elastin from about 50 different breast cancer samples. These purified elastin samples were washed in water and acetone and dried and weighed and an aliquote was solubilized with pancreatic elastase and its protein content determined. Using this quantification procedure, we could establish that the amount of elastin isolated from breast cancers and determined by this biochemical method correlated reasonably well with the amount of elastin determined by histochemical-morphometric procedures (Hornebeck et al., 1977). This is shown on Fig. 1.

This result lends further credit for the histochemi-cal-morphometric evaluation of elastogenesis in breast cancers.

Aminoacid composition of breast cancer elastin

The above mentioned procedure yielded elastin which was morphologically undistinguishable from elastin obtained

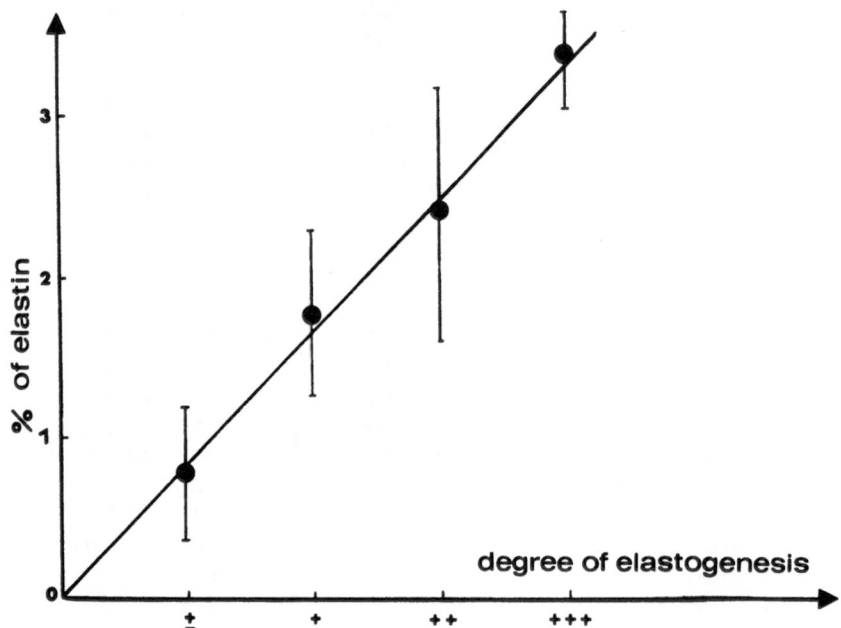

Fig. 1. Correlation between the elastin content deter-
        mined by microscopic evaluation and the chemical
        procedure.
        Abscissa : microscopic evaluation of the elastin
        content (for details see Hornebeck et al., 1977).
        Ordinates : % of elastin evaluated as mg of
        protein in the elastase extract per mg of dry
        tissue weight.
        The bars represent the standard error of the
        mean.

from human aorta samples. It was hydrolysed in 6N HCl for
48 h and submitted to aminoacid analysis and Table 1 shows
the results obtained as compared to the composition of
aorta elastin. It can be seen that the overall composition
of breast cancer elastin is similar to the one of aorta
elastin with however a few interesting differences. The
proline and hydroxyproline content, the glycine and
histidine content and also the desmosine content are
significantly lower than the one found in human aorta
elastin. The glutamic acid and histidine values are

TABLE 1

COMPARISON OF THE AMINO ACID COMPOSITION BETWEEN HUMAN
AORTA ELASTIN AND BREAST CANCER ELASTIN ISOLATED BY THE
HOT ALKALI PROCEDURE (from Hornebeck et al., 1977).

	Human breast cancer elastin (MUL +++)	Human aorta elastin
OH-PRO	5,0	13,9
ASP	4,0	3,3
THRE	10,0	7,4
SER	7,1	7,8
GLU	19,0	14,0
PRO	64,0	111,2
GLY	353,0	340,1
ALA	247,0	239,1
VAL	130,0	138,3
CYS	-	1,1
MET	-	0,5
ILE	21,0	24,2
LEU	58,0	55,5
TYR	4,0	6,6
PHE-ALA	17,0	26,4
LYS	4,1	3,8
HIS	1,0	0,4
ARG	5,1	5,5
(IDE-DES/4)	1,2	2,6

somewhat higher. These differences may be interpreted in
several ways. One of them is to assume the existence of
several types of genetically distinct elastins. It was
recently claimed that such different elastins exist, on
the basis of differences between the val-pro dipeptide
frequencies observed in elastin isolated from different
organs of the same species. Our results point also to the
possibility that genetically different elastins do exist.
It is therefore possible that the breast cancer elastin
represents a different genetic entity from aorta elastin.
This however needs further investigation.

The microfibrillar components

       As was shown in the preceeding chapter on the mor-
phology of breast cancer elastin, this elastin is relatively rich in microfibrillar components. The ultrastructural observations are in agreement with the chemical
findings, showing a high dicarboxylic acid content in
breast cancer elastin (Hornebeck et al., 1977). This is
in agreement with the finding supported by several teams
having investigated the ultrastructure of elastogenesis.
This starts with the deposition of a microfibrillar
scaffolding onto which tropoelastin is aggregated and
polymerized through the action of lysine-oxidase and
cross-link formation. The details of this process were
discussed in recent monographies and we shall not enter
these considerations in this chapter (see for references
Robert, 1980). We have only to underline the fact that
the dense microfibrillar structures detected in native
and purified mammary cancer elastin are in agreement with
the postulate that they represent freshly synthesized
young elastic fibers and that the maturation of elastic
fibers is accompanied by the increase of the elastin/
microfibril ratio.

Elastolytic protease in breast cancers

       Another interesting observation we made in respect
with elastogenesis in breast cancer is the presence in
saline extract of fresh biopsies or operation samples
of a protease having the characteristics of an elastase.
This protease could be quantified using the kappa-elastin
agarose gel procedure (Bellon et al., 1978). We could
detect this protease in every breast cancer sample we
studied (Hornebeck and Robert, 1977 ; Hornebeck et al.,
1978). It also could be shown that the activity of this
elastolytic protease is correlated with the elastin
content of a given breast sample. This correlation is

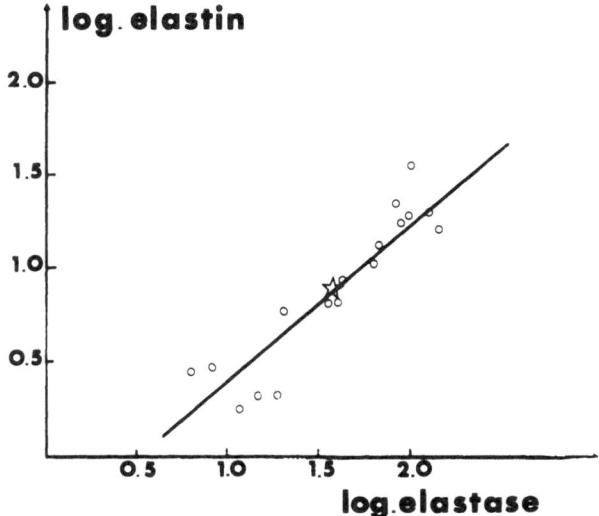

Fig. 2. Correlation between the elastin content of
human breast cancer samples and their elastolytic activity.
Abscissa : log of elastase activity determined
on K-elastin-agarose gels.
Ordinates : log of the elastin content of the
same tumors determined by the modified Lansing
procedure.
(Data from Hornebeck and Robert, 1977 and
Hornebeck et al., 1978).

shown on Fig. 2. The further purification and characterization of this elastolytic protease is now in progress.
Several cellular elements have to be considered as the
possible sources of this enzyme : endothelial cells,
myoepithelial cells, fibroblasts, smooth muscle cells
in vessel walls. All these cells were shown to be able to
elaborate elastolytic proteases (Bourdillon et al., 1980).
The contribution of infiltrating inflammatory elements
such as leukocytes or macrophages cannot be excluded but
they are not frequent and not regularly found in these
biopsy samples therefore their contribution to the elastase content of breast cancer extracts is improbable.

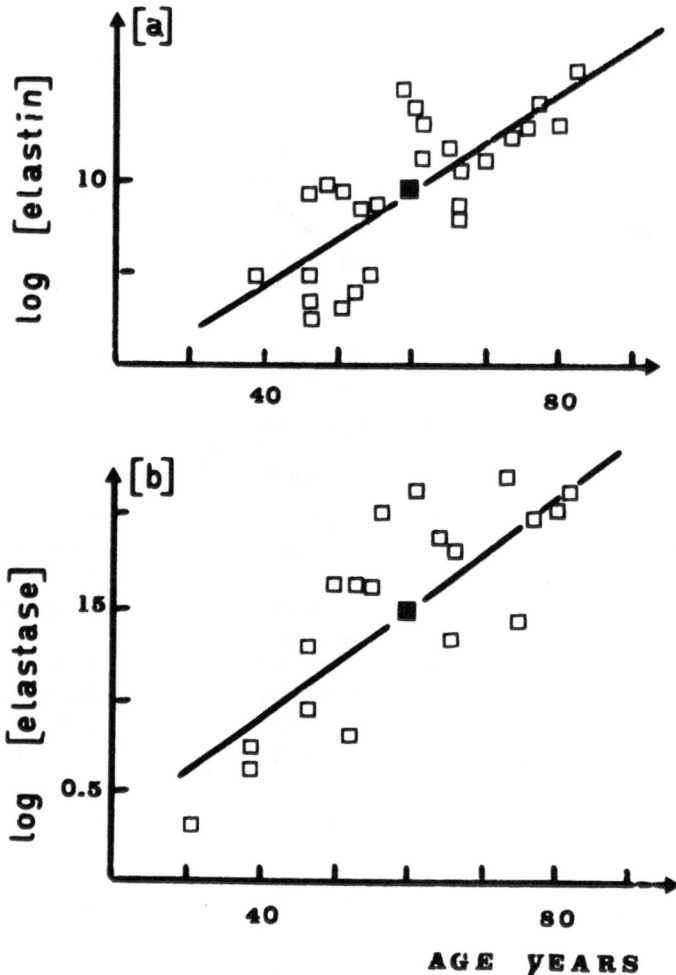

Fig. 3. (a) Variation of the elastin content of human
breast tumor samples with the age of the
patients. Abscissa : age in years. Ordinates : log of the elastin content expressed
as mg of protein in the elastase extract
per mg of dry tissue weight.

(b) Variation of the elastinolytic activity of
the breast tumor samples with age of the
patient. Abscissa : age in years. Ordinates : log of the elastinolytic activity
expressed as g equivalents of pancreatic
elastase per mg of dry tissue weight.

Effect of the age of patients on the elastin and elastase content of breast cancer

Figure 3 shows the age dependence of the elastin content and of the elastase content of about 50 different human breast cancer samples. It can be seen that there is a significant positive correlation between age and elastin content and age and elastase content. This means that the older a woman when she develops her breast cancer, the more elastin and the more elastase can be found in the cancer tissue. These results seem to be in agreement with the postulated correlation between the hormone-dependence of breast cancers and their elastogenic potential (Masters et al., 1976, 1979).

DISCUSSION

The above experiments confirm the presence of newly formed elastic tissue in human breast cancer and suggest several interpretations for this elastogenesis. The morphological observations showed already that the site of elastogenesis is variable. Newly formed and abundant elastic fibrils can be seen either in the stroma in the neighbourhood of fibroblast-like cells, around galacto-phores suggesting involvement of transformed epithelial cells as well as around blood vessels suggesting a possi-bility of a strong elasto-neogenesis by smooth muscle cells of vessel wall origin or by stromal fibroblasts.

These findings suggest that nearly any of the cellu-lar elements which were enumerated and are present in human breast cancers can be the source of the newly formed elastic fibrils. Immunochemical evidence was provided by McCullough and coworkers in favor of an elastogenesis by malignant epithelial cell clusters (personal communica-tion). The biochemical data suggest that the neoformed elastin is similar but not identical to the one found in human aorta. The reason of this difference needs further investigation. The possibility of the existence of several genetically distinct elastins is one of these explanations.

Another interesting finding is the presence of an elastolytic protease in these breast cancer extracts in quantities proportional to their elastin content. This suggests the possible correlation between the structural genes coding for elastin and for the elastolytic protease(s). Both genes may be "activated" through the same mechanism. This also suggests the hypothesis that this elastolytic protease may be involved in the "processing" of freshly synthesised elastin or in some other processes correlated to the biosynthesis of elastin and not only to its destruction or catabolism.

Finally the positive correlation between elastogenesi‍ and age strongly suggests a hormonal regulation of this "derepression" of the elastin and elastase genes in the malignant tissues.

All these facts are in agreement with the hypothesis we mentioned in the introduction and according to which the malignant cells may be at the origin of some factor(s) which we may call "differentiation factor(s)" and which would initiate the neosynthesis of elastic fibrils in a tissue which in its mature state has no or only very weak elastogenetic activity. Arguments in favor of this hypothesis were recently obtained in collaboration with Dr. Eugène Davidson (Hershley, USA) and will be published elsewhere.

REFERENCES

Adnet, J.J., Birembaut, P., Sadrin, R., Gaillard, D., Pastisson, C., Robert, L., Dousset, H., and Bogomoletz, W.V., 1980, Elastosis in breast cancer, Part I. Morphological study, in this volume.

Bieth, J., 1979, Elastases : structure, function and pathological role, in "Frontiers of Matrix Biology". Robert, L., ed., S. Karger, Basel, Vol. 6, pp 1-82.

Bellon, G., Hornebeck, W., and Robert, L., 1978, Méthodes simples pour quantifier l'élastase et ses inhibiteurs dans le sérum humain. Path. Biol., 26, 515-521.

Bouissou, H., Pieraggi, M.T., Julian, M., and Douste-Blasy, L., 1973, Cutaneous Aging. Its relation with arteriosclerosis and atheroma, in "Frontiers of Matrix Biology", Robert, L. and Robert, B., eds, S. Karger, Basel, Vol. 1, pp 190-211.

Bouissou, H., Pieraggi, M.T., Julian, M., and Douste-Blazy, L., 1976, Simultaneous degradation of elastin in dermis and in aorta, in "Frontiers of Matrix Biology", Robert, L. Ed., S. Karger, Basel, Vol. 3, pp 242-255.

Bourdillon, M.C., Brechemier, D., Blaes, N., Derouette, J.C., Hornebeck, W., and Robert, L., 1980,

Elastase-like enzymes in skin fibroblasts and rat
aorta smooth muscle cells. Cell. Biol. Intern.
Rep., 4, 313-320.

Garrone, R., 1978, Phylogenesis of connective tissue.
Morphological aspects and biosynthesis of sponge
intercellular matrix, in "Frontiers of Matrix
Biology", Robert, L. ed., S. Karger, Basel, Vol. 5.

Hornebeck, W., Derouette, J.C., Brechemier, D., Adnet,
J.J., and Robert, L., 1977, Elastogenesis and
elastinolytic activity in human breast cancer.
Biomédecine, 26, 48-52.

Hornebeck, W., and Robert, L., 1977, Elastase-like enzymes
in aortas and human breast carcinomas : quantita-
tive variations with age and pathology, in
"Elastin and Elastic Tissue". Sandberg, L.B.,
Gray, W.R. and Franzblau, C. eds., Plenum Press,
New York, pp 145-164.

Hornebeck, W., Adnet, J.J., and Robert, L., 1978, Age
dependant variation of elastin and elastase in
aorta and human breast cancers. Exp. Gerontol.,
13, 293-298.

Keith, D.A., Paz, M.A., and Gallop, P.M., 1979, Differences in valyl-proline sequence content in elastins from various bovine tissues. Biochem. Biophys.
Res. Comm., 87, 1214-1217.

Looker, T., and Berry, C.L., 1972, The growth and development of the rat aorta. II. Changes in nucleic
acid and scleroprotein content. J. Anat., Lond.
113, 17-34.

Masters, J.R.W., Sangster, K., Hawkins, R.A., and Shivas,
A.A., 1976, Elastosis and oestrogen receptors in
human breast cancer. Br. J. Cancer, 33, 342-343.

Masters, J.R.W., Millis, R.R., King, R.J.B., and Rubens,
R.D., 1979, Elastosis and response to endocrine
therapy in human breast cancer. Br. J. Cancer,
39, 536-539.

Moczar, M., Ouzilou, J., Courtois, Y., and Robert, L.,
1976, Age dependence of the biosynthesis of intercellular matrix macromolecules of rabbit aorta in
organ culture and cell culture. Gerontology, 22,
461-462.

Robert, B., Szigeti, M., Derouette, J.C., Robert, L.,
Bouissou, H., and Fabre, M.T., 1971, Studies on
the nature of the "microfibrillar" component of
elastic fibers. Eur. J. Biochem., 21, 507-516.

Robert, L., and Hornebeck, W., 1976, Preparation of
insoluble and soluble elastins, in "The Methodology
of Connective Tissue Research", Hall, D.A. ed.,
Joynson-Bruvvers Ltd, Oxford, pp 81-104.

Robert, L., 1980, Biology and pathology of elastic tissues,
       Vol. 8 of "Frontiers of Matrix Biology", S. Karger,
       Basel.
Sage, E.H., and Gray, W.R., 1977, Evolution of elastin
       structure, in "Elastin and Elastic Tissue".
       Sandberg, L.B., Gray, W.R. and Franzblau, C., eds.,
       Plenum Press, New York, 291-312.
Sandberg, L.B., Gray, W.R., and Franzblau, C., 1977,
       "Elastin and Elastic Tissue", Plenum Press,
       New York.

FIBRONECTIN IN BREAST CANCERS

P. Birembaut[1], J.J. Adnet[1], J. Labat-Robert[2],
F. Mercantini[2], and L. Robert[2]

1. Laboratoire Pol Bouin, Centre Hospitalier
   Universitaire, 51100 Reims, France
2. Laboratoire de Biochimie du Tissu Conjonctif,
   94010 Créteil, France

INTRODUCTION

Structural glycoproteins are among the phylogenetically oldest matrix components (for a review, see
Robert, 1980 ; Robert et al., 1976, 1980). They could
be detected together with collagen from the first metazoans, the Porifera (Labat-Robert et al., 1979 ; Junqua
et al., 1975 ; Junqua and Robert, 1979). Although these
matrix components were discovered and designated as
structural glycoproteins from the early 60's (Robert et
al., 1963, 1968), a great deal of interest was raised in
their investigation by the recent discoveries of fibronectin and laminin (for review, see Vaheri et al., 1980 ;
Timpl et al., 1980).

Fibronectin (or cold insoluble globulin, CIG, in
plasma) is one of the many different structural glycoproteins isolated and described in different animal
tissues (Vaheri and Mosher, 1978). Its aminoacid composition is similar to the one described for several other
structural glycoproteins (Robert et al., 1976 ; Yamada
et al., 1978). If this protein attracted so much interest
in the last years, this is because of the discovery of
its decrease or disappearance on the cell membrane of a
score of transformed malignant cells in culture (Hynes,
1973 ; Yamada and Olden, 1978 ; Vaheri and Mosher, 1978).
Although this observation concerns only the majority
but by no means all the transformed malignant cells,

it is still a pertinent observation which appears to be
related to the loss of histogenetic potential, anomalous
"social" behaviour, metastasis formation, etc, which are
considered as general characteristics of malignant cells.
This is partially due to the fact that cell membrane bound
fibronectin is considered as one of the (if not the most)
important factor(s) responsible for the anchoring of the
cells in a precise position in the intercellular matrix.
By this property, the membrane bound fibronectin may be
an important factor in the maintenance of the normal,
differentiated state, histogenetic potential and normal
"social" behaviour of differentiated cells (Yamada et al.,
1976 ; Ali et al., 1977 ; Hynes et al., 1979 ; Obrink
et al., 1980).

Although many observations were reported concerning
the loss of membrane bound fibronectin in transformed,
malignant cells, all of these observations were carried
out in tissue culture conditions. We therefore decided
to try to extend these observations to solid human tumors
in order to investigate the potential usefulness of the
qualitative and quantitative study of tissue and plasma
fibronectin in the detection and prognostic and diagnostic
evaluation of malignant tumors. We wish to report here
on our results obtained on human breast cancers (Labat-
Robert et al., 1980). Our studies on other solid human
tumors were also recently described (Birembaut et al.,
1980).

MATERIAL AND METHODS

Antibodies to human plasma cold insoluble globulin
were obtained as follows : CIG was isolated from human
plasma essentially as described by Vuento and Vaheri
(1979). The highly purified preparation gave only the
usual doublet on SDS-urea polyacrylamide gel electro-
phoresis, and gave one single line by immunodiffusion.

Antibodies to highly purified human plasma CIG were
raised in rabbits immunised by intradermal and subcutaneous injections of 1 mg of purified fibronectin in
complete Freund's adjuvant over one month, followed by
a booster injection and 5 days later exsanguination
through the carotide. We obtained immune sera giving
only one single line with a total human plasma and with
highly purified plasma fibronectin. The immune serum was
further purified, first on a gelatin-Sepharose column
in order to deplete it from the fibronectin present, then
on a fibronectin-deprived-plasma-protein ultragel column.

The purified antiserum was used in a dilution of 1:5 to
1:50 for immunofluorescence studies using the indirect
Coons technique. Fluorescein isothiocyanate labeled
antibodies to rabbit immunoglobulins, IgG, were obtained
from the Pasteur Institute, Paris.

Cryostat sections of the tumor tissue-samples were
prepared by the usual procedure and were incubated for
30 minutes with an appropriate dilution of the immune
serum, washed with sterile PBS and incubated with the
1:5 dilution of the fluorescent anti-rabbit IgG goat
serum. The sections were then examined in a fluorescent
microscope and photographs were taken on Ektachrome
films.

RESULTS

The normal breast tissue showed the presence of
fibronectin in three well defined locations : (a) around
the epithelial and myoepithelial cells in ductular
structures ; (b) in the basement membranes of the galactophores and blood vessels and (c) more weakly on the

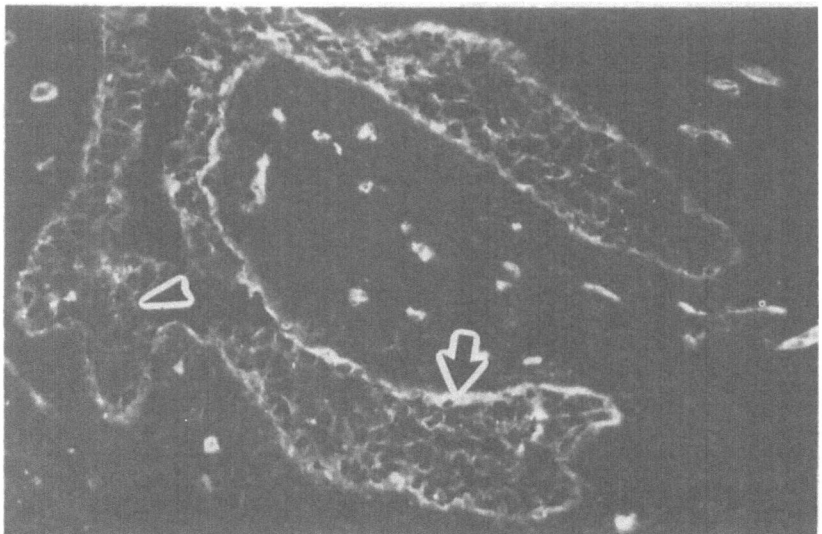

Fig. 1. Fibroadenoma of the mammary gland. Fibronectin
        is localized in the basement membranes (arrow)
        on the cellular surface of epithelial cells
        (head of arrow), of proliferative galactophoric
        ducts (x 200).

intercellular stroma. The fluorescent staining of the
first two sites, around the cell membranes and in basement
membranes, was continuous, clearly visible without any
patchy or discontinuous structures. The matrix localized
fibronectin was more irregular and followed usually the
outlines of the collagen bundles.

In benign breast tumors such as fibrocystic disease
and other benign breast conditions, this above mentioned
normal pattern was always present without any qualitative
modification (Fig. 1).

In malignant tumors such as infiltrating adenocarcinomas, the following modifications could be seen. First
the cell membrane localized staining disappeared ; this
was the earliest and constant finding. Then discontinuous
staining was observed in the periductal basement membranes. This could be seen in those parts of the mammary
gland which were not yed invaded by the tumor but were
in the proximity of malignant cell proliferation. When
this malignant proliferation became general and no distinct glandular structures could be seen, the specific
fibronectin staining disappeared around the tumoral cells.

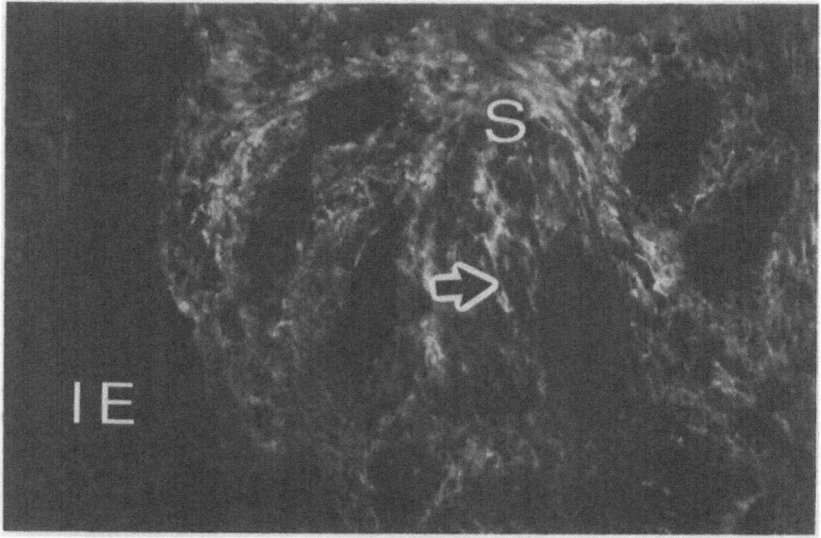

Fig. 2. Adenocarcinoma of the mammary gland. Fibronectin
        is seen as their strands (arrow) in the stroma
        (S). There is no definite border arround neo-
        plastic invasive epithelial clusters (IE)
        (x 200).

As a matter of fact, the basement membranes were no more present as could be shown using other specific staining techniques such as silver impregnation (Fig. 2).

The fibrous matrix bound staining was partially preserved at this stage, as well as the staining of vascular basement membranes.

The above mentioned modifications were progressive and could be followed from the earliest suspect dysplastic modifications (see Fig. 3) up to the completely invasive structureless tumors.

In one case of comedo-carcinoma and in one case of intraductal carcinoma, intermediary changes of the fibronectin distribution pattern could be seen : fibronectin staining disappears around the cell membranes but remains partially present in persisting glandular basement membranes and in the stroma (Fig. 4). In a case of medullary carcinoma, a slight pericellular staining was present but glandular basement membrane staining was lost. In a case of carcinoma with cartilagenous and bony metaplasia, both the pericellular and basement membrane stainings disappeared (see Table 1). Table 1 shows the

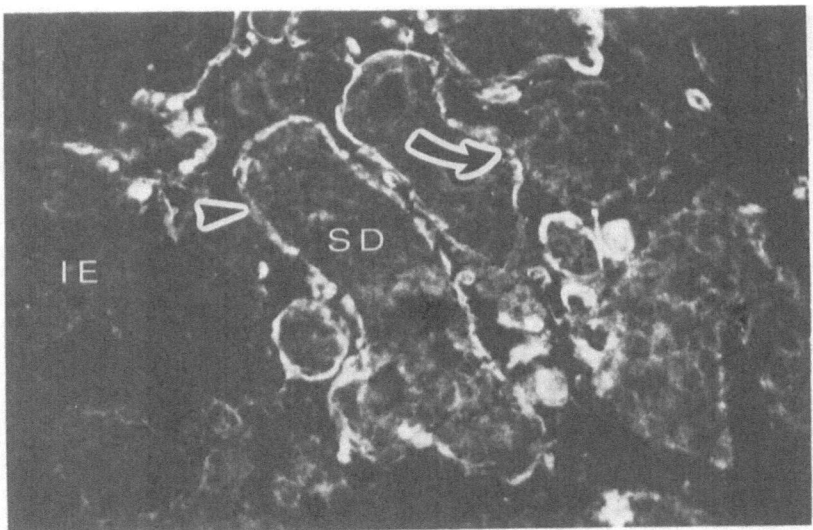

Fig. 3. Severe displastic modification (Fd) adjacent to
        infiltrating carcinoma (IC). Fibronectin is
        located in the basement membranes as irregular
        (head arrow). Loss of fibronectin (arrow) is
        related to infiltration (x 200).

TABLE 1

DISTRIBUTION OF FIBRONECTIN IN NORMAL HUMAN BREAST TISSUE, IN BENIGN AND MALIGNANT BREAST TUMORS.

Breast tissue taken from :	Intensity of immunofluorescence with antifibronectin antiserum		
	Glandular basement membranes	Pericellular (epithelial cells)	Fibrous stroma
Supernumerary gland	+++	++	++
Fibrocystic disease (5 cases)	+++	++	++
Fibroadenomas (5 cases)	+++	++	++
Invasive adenocarcinomas (16 cases)	-	-	+
Invasive lobular carcinoma	-	-	+
Comedo-carcinoma	++ (1)	-	++
Medullary carcinoma	-	+ (2)	++
Carcinoma with cartilagenous and bony metaplasia of the stroma	-	-	++
Non-invasive intraductal carcinoma	++ (3)	-	++

(1) Basement membrane staining is irregular and there is a loss of fibronectin in infiltrating areas in this case.

(2) Pericellular labeling is faintly positive and focal in this case.

(3) Basement membrane staining is also irregular.

breast tumors examined as well as the modifications of
the vibronectin staining observed.

DISCUSSION

    Because of the progressive nature of the above
mentioned modifications, the fibronectin staining of
breast tumors may be of diagnostic value. In severe dysplastic conditions and in non-infiltrating carcinomas,
the patchy staining of basement membranes and the partial
or total loss of fibronectin staining around the cell
membranes can be taken as a sign of the malignant nature
of the lesion. In all the benign tumors investigated
until now, no such changes could be found. Another interesting conclusion from the above observations is that
the behaviour of solid human tumors is similar to the
one which was found for a number of malignant cells in
tissue culture. This is shown by the progressive loss
of cell membrane bound and basement membrane bound fibronectin followed by its complete loss in typical infiltrating adenocarcinomas. Although the mechanism of this loss
is not yet known, it can be inferred from studies carried
out in tissue culture that fibronectin even if produced
by the malignant cells is faster degraded and/or cannot
be anchored and retained on the cell membrane and in

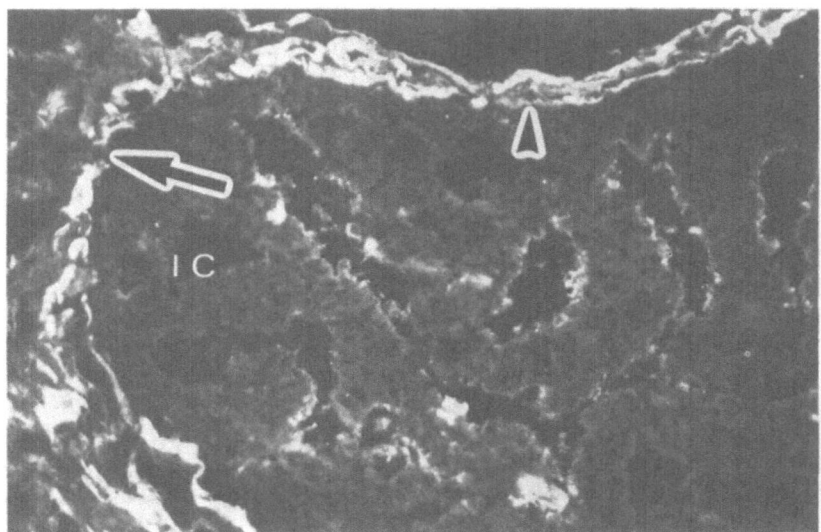

Fig. 4. Intraductal carcinoma (IC). Fibronectin is
        also localized within basal lamina (head of
        arrow) but staining is irregular and discon-
        tinuous (arrow) (x 200).

basement membrane (for a review, see Birembaut et al., 1980).

The presence of proteolytic enzymes as for instance the one which was described in the preceeding chapter (Robert et al., 1980) and which is capable to degrade elastin and other protein substrates may be one of those enzymes involved in the above mentioned accelerated catabolism and disappearance of fibronectin.

REFERENCES

Ali, I.U., Mautner, V., Lanza, R., and Hynes, R.D., 1977, Restoration of normal morphology, adhesion and cytoskeleton in transformed cells by addition of a transformation-sensitive surface protein. Cell, 11, 116-126.

Birembaut, P., Labat-Robert, J., Adnet, J.J., and Robert, L., 1980, Modification of the distribution pattern of fibronectin in solid human tumors. Invest. Cell Pathol., in print.

Hynes, R.O., 1973, Alteration of cell surface proteins by viral transformation and by proteolysis. Proc. Natl. Acad. Sci. USA, 70, 3170-3174.

Hynes, R.O., Destree, A.T., Perkins, M.E., and Wagner, D.D., 1979, Cell surface fibronectin and oncogenic transformation. J. Supramol. Struct., 11, 95-104.

Junqua, S., and Robert, L., 1979, Fractionation of sponge structural glycoproteins by affinity chromatography on lectins, in "Glycoconjugate Research". J. Gregory and R. Jeanloz eds., Acad. Press, New York, Vol. 1, pp. 177-197.

Junqua, S., Fayolle, J., and Robert, L., 1975, Isolation and characterization of structural glycoproteins from sponges, in "Protides of the Biological Fluids", Peeters, H. Eds., Pergamon Press, Oxford/N.Y., 22, 337-341.

Labat-Robert, J., Pavans de Ceccatty, M., Robert, L., Auger, C., Lethias, C., and Garrone, R., 1979, Surface glycoproteins of sponge cells : presence of a fibronectin-like protein on differentiated sponge cell membranes, its role in cell aggregation in "Glycoconjugates", Schauer, R., Boer, P., Buddecke, E., Kramer, M.F., Vliegenthart, J.F.G., Wiegandt, H. eds., Georg Thieme Pub., Stuttgart, pp 431-432.

Labat-Robert, J., Birembaut, P., Adnet, J.J., Mercantini, F., and Robert, L., 1980, Loss of fibronectin in human breast cancer. Cell Biol. Int. Rep., in print.

Obrink, B., Ocklind, K., Rubin, K., Hook, M., and Johansson, S., 1980, Cell-cell and cell-collagen adhesion, in "Biochemistry of Normal and Pathological Connective Tissue". Robert, A.M. and Robert, L., eds., CNRS, Paris, N° 287, Vol. II, pp 239-248.

Robert, L., Parlebas, J., Poullain, N., and Robert, B., 1963, Données nouvelles sur l'immunochimie des protéines fibreuses du tissu conjonctif, in "Protides of Biological Fluids", Elsevier, Amsterdam, 11, 109-113.

Robert, L., Robert, B., and Moczar, E., 1968, Structural glycoproteins of connective tissue : chemical and immunochemical properties, in "4th Int. Colloquium on Cystic Fibrosis of the Pancreas". Karger, Basel, part II, pp 309-317.

Robert, L., Junqua, S., and Moczar, M., 1976, Structural glycoproteins of the intercellular matrix, in "Frontiers of Matrix Biology", Robert, L. ed., S. Karger, Basel, Vol. 3, pp 113-142.

Robert, L., 1980, Structural glycoproteins : the fourth family of matrix macromolecules, in "Biochemistry of Normal and Pathological Connective Tissues". Robert, A.M. and Robert, L. eds., CNRS, Paris, N° 287, Vol. II, pp 189-194.

Robert, L., Hornebeck, W., Brechemier, D., and Adnet, J.J., 1980, Elastosis in breast cancer. II. Biochemical studies, in this volume.

Timpl, R., Rohde, H., Wick, G., Gehron-Robey, P., Rennard, S.I., Foidart, T.M., and Martin, G.R., 1980, Characterization of laminin, a major glycoprotein of basement membranes, in "Biochemistry of Normal and Pathological Connective Tissues". Robert, A.M. and Robert, L., eds., CNRS, Paris, N° 287, Vol. II, pp 225-228.

Vaheri, A., and Mosher, F., 1978, High molecular weight, cell surface associated glycoproteins (fibronectin) lost in malignant transformation. Biochim. Biophys. Acta, 516, 1-25.

Vaheri, A., Alitalo, K., Hedman, K., Kurkinen, M., Saksela, O., and Vartio, T., 1980, Fibronectin and its loss in malignant transformation, in "Biochemistry of Normal and Pathological Connective Tissues". Robert, A.M. and Robert, L. eds., CNRS, Paris, N° 287, Vol. II, pp 249-254.

Vuento, M., and Vaheri, A., 1979, Purification of fibronectin from human plasma by affinity chromatography under non-denaturing conditions. Biochem. J., 183, 331-337.

Yamada, K.M., and Olden, K., 1978, Fibronectin-adhesive
    glycoproteins of cell surface and blood. Nature
    (Lond), 275, 179-184.
Yamada, K.M., Yamada, S.S., and Pastan, I., 1976, Cell
    surface-protein partially restores morphology
    adhesiveness and contact inhibition of movement
    to transformed fibroblasts. Proc. Nat. Acad. Sci.
    USA, 73, 1217-1221.
Yamada, K.M., Olden, K., and Pastan, I., 1978, Transfor-
    mation sensitive cell surface protein : isolation,
    characterization and role in cellular morphology
    and adhesion. Ann. N.Y. Acad. Sci., 312, 256-277.

IMMUNOTHERAPY OF SPONTANEOUSLY ARISING RAT MAMMARY TUMOURS

R.W. Baldwin, M.V. Pimm and N. Willmott

Cancer Research Campaign Laboratories
University of Nottingham
Nottingham, England

Numerous studies with experimentally-induced animal tumours have demonstrated the potential of introducing immunotherapy as a component in the treatment of human malignant disease (Baldwin and Pimm, 1978 ; Baldwin and Byers, 1979 ; Milas and Scott, 1977) and many clinical trials are currently in progress (Goodnight and Morton, 1978). But many of the experimental tumours used in designing immunotherapy protocols, e.g. carcinogen-induced tumours have been criticized as not being appropriate models for human malignant disease since they frequently express neoantigens which elicit strong rejection responses, whereas the clinical evidence for host immunity to human cancer is not fully substantiated (Castro, 1978). The studies presented here were designed to investigate whether naturally arising (spontaneous) rat mammary carcinomas can be controlled by immunotherapy. Several approaches were evaluated for this purpose including active specific immunotherapy involving treatment with vaccines containing tumour cells together with an immunological adjuvant, since this approach is effective with carcinogen-induced tumours (Pimm and Baldwin, 1978 ; Baldwin and Byers, 1979). Regional immunotherapy, in which immunostimulating agents are administered so as to localize in tumour deposits, was also evaluated since there is a growing evidence to indicate that non-specific immunity mediated by macrophages and/or natural killer cells can be effective against animal and human tumours (Baldwin and Byers, 1979 ; Herberman and Holden, 1979).

The mammary adenocarcinomas used in these studies all arose without deliberate induction in syngeneic WAB/Not rats maintained in the Department (Baldwin et al, 1979a). These were maintained by routine subcutaneous trocar passage in syngeneic female rats. In some studies tumour cells were implanted into the mammary pad in order to evaluate therapy of local mammary growths and metastatic deposits (Greager and Baldwin, 1978 ; Willmott et al, 1979a).

Active Specific Immunotherapy

Active specific immunotherapy involves treatment with vaccines containing an appropriate tumour antigen preparation usually with an immunological adjuvant so as to enhance, or even qualitatively alter, immune responses in a tumour-bearing host. It, therefore, follows that the innate immunogenicity of the tumour under treatment will control the effectiveness of the form of treatment. This is exemplified by a series of studies with the spontaneous rat mammary carcinomas since only three of nine tumours studied were shown to express tumour associated rejection antigens (TARA) at least at levels capable of inducing significant levels of immunity (Baldwin et al, 1979a). This was assessed by the capacity of rats immunized by surgical removal of a developing tumour graft or repeated implantation of γ-irradiated tumour cells to reject tumour challenge. For example, two mammary carcinomas Sp4 and Sp15 were immunogenic eliciting resistance to challenge with 2×10^4 and 1×10^3 cells respectively of the autologous tumour compared to the minimum inoculum for growth in untreated rats (1×10^3 cells). Immunization with the other mammary carcinomas provided no immunity to challenge with the autologous tumour even though threshold doses of tumour cells were injected. In the immunotherapy trials, rats receiving a subcutaneous challenge with mammary carcinoma cells were treated contralaterally with vaccines of viable or irradiated tumour cells in admixture with either BCG (Glaxo percutaneous vaccine) or C. parvum (CN 6134 : Wellcome Research Laboratories). This series of experiments summarized in Table 1, illustrates that growth of the moderately immunogenic mammary carcinoma Sp4 could be controlled with this type of therapy using either BCG or C. parvum as the adjuvant. It was also possible to use γ-irradiated Sp4 cells as a source of tumour antigen as well as viable tumour cells whose growth was restricted by injection together with the bacterial adjuvant (Pimm et al, 1978 ; Willmott et al, 1979b). In contrast, these approaches

TABLE 1

ACTIVE IMMUNOTHERAPY OF SPONTANEOUS RAT MAMMARY CARCINOMAS

Mammary carc.	Tumour vaccine		Controlateral challenge		
	No. cells	Adjuvant	No. cells	Tumour test	takes in: control
Sp4	5×10^4	BCG	5×10^3	0/6	5/6
	1×10^4	BCG	1×10^4	0/12	12/12
	2×10^5	C.parvum	1×10^4	0/13	5/6
Sp15	5×10^6-1RR[*]	BCG	1×10^3	7/12	5/12
	2×10^6-1RR	C.parvum	1×10^3	7/7	6/6
Xp22	5×10^6-1RR	BCG	1×10^3	7/12	9/14
	2×10^6-1RR	C.parvum	1×10^3	4/13	8/11
	2×10^6-1RR	C.parvum	1×10^4	6/6	6/6

[*]1RR : cells attenuated with 15,000 R ^{60} γ-irradiation.

Glaxo BCG percutaneous vaccine (200-1000 µg moist weight)
C. Parvum Wellcome CN6134 (200 µg dry weight).

were totally ineffective with mammary carcinoma Sp15 and Sp22 where TARA could not be detected by immunization/challenge tests (Baldwin et al, 1979a).

The conclusion from these studies is that active specific immunotherapy is only effective against a small proportion of the spontaneously arising mammary carcinomas, being restricted to those tumours with significant TARA expressions. Moreover even with the most immunogenic mammary carcinoma tested (Sp4) the amount of tumour suppressed by this type of treatment was only 1×10^4 tumour cells.

Regional Immunotherapy

Previous studies with a range of carcinogen-induced rat tumours, especially 3-methylcholanthrene-induced sarcomas and aminoazo-dye induced hepatocellular carcinomas have demonstrated that bacterial agents administered in contact with tumour cells suppresses tumour growth, the effect being mediated by host responses rather than direct cytotoxicity of the agents (Pimm and Baldwin, 1978 ; Baldwin and Byers, 1979). This "adjuvant contact suppression" or "regional immunotherapy"

suppression of tumour growth does no necessarily require
T lymphocyte responses to tumour associated antigens,
since suppression of tumour growth could be induced
against tumour cells transplanted into athymic (nude)
mice (Pimm and Baldwin, 1975). In this respect the experiments summarized in Table 2 indicate that C. parvum
injected in admixture with cells derived from three
mammary carcinomas (Sp4, Sp15, Sp22) suppressed tumour
growth even though the latter tumour (Sp22) was not de-
monstrably immunogenic. With BCG, however, tumour growth
was inhibited following treatment of mammary carcinoma
Sp4 only.

Treatment of Mammary Tissue Growths and Metastatic Deposits

In order to further evaluate the potential of
regional immunotherapy with BCG or C.parvum preparations,
studies were carried out to evaluate their therapeutic
effect when administered intralesionally into developing

TABLE 2

INHIBITION OF GROWTH OF RAT MAMMARY CARCINOMA CELLS

INJECTED SUBCUTANEOUSLY IN ADMIXTURE

WITH BCG OR C. PARVUM

Mammary Carcinoma	No. Tumour Cells	Tumour Incidence from Cells injected with		
		C. Parvum[1]	BCG	Control
Sp4	1×10^5	0/5	3/5	4/4
	5×10^5	2/11	3/5	11/11
Sp15	2×10^4	2/6	6/6	7/7
	1×10^5	11/12	12/12	13/13
Sp22	2×10^4	0/5	6/6	5/5
	1×10^5	10/12	12/12	11/11

1. 100 µg dry weight bacteria/inoculum
    BCG Glaxo Percutaneous

    C. Parvum Wellcome CN6134

tumours. For this purpose the transplanted tumours
established from the naturally arising rat mammary carcinomas were implanted into mammary tissues of the right
pectoral region (Greager and Baldwin, 1978 ; Willmott
et al, 1979a, 1979b). This transplanted tumour system
was adopted since tumours developing in mammary tissue
show characteristic patterns of metastasis involving the
draining lymph nodes and pulmonary tissue. For example,
mammary carcinoma Sp4 produced widespread metastases
in the draining lymph nodes and pulmonary tissue. In
contrast, all rats implanted with mammary carcinoma
Sp15 in the mammary pad developed lymph node metastases,
but pulmonary metastases were rare (Willmott et al,
1979a).

In the initial studies, multiple doses of BCG
(Glaxo) or C. parvum (Wellcome CN6134) were injected
into mammary carcinoma Sp4 starting 14 days after
mammary pad implantation. As illustrated in Fig. 1, repeated intralesional therapy with BCG was partially

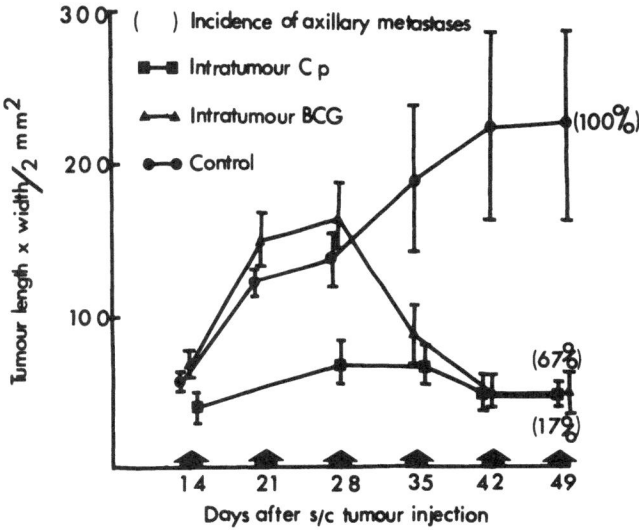

Fig. 1.   Influence of weekly intratumour injection of
          BCG (1.0 mg. Glaxo) or C. parvum (0.7 mg.
          Wellcome CN6134) on growth and spread of mam-
          mary pad implants of mammary carcinoma Sp4.

effective, since this treatment markedly restricted the
growth of the local tumour. But even so, 67 % of the
treated rats still developed regional lymph node metastases. Intralesional injection of Wellcome C. parvum was
markedly more effective since the local tumour was more
effectively controlled and in this case, only 17 % of
treated rats developed regional lymph node metastases.

The Sp4 tumour system has since been developed to
evaluate the efficacy of intratumoral injections of
bacterial agents in the control of mammary tumour growth.
This is illustrated in Fig. 2 which shows the increased
survival of rats bearing mammary pad implants of mammary
carcinoma Sp4 following intratumoral injection of BCG
(Pasteur, Immuno. F.). In this case intralesional BCG
(Pasteur) at a dose of 200µg did not prolong survival
whereas there was a significant response at the higher
dose (1.4 mg). Similar increased survival rates were

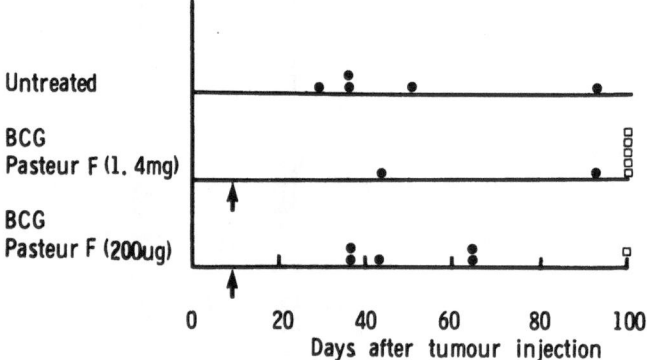

Fig. 2.   Survival of rats with mammary pad implants of
          mammary carcinoma Sp4 receiving a single intra-
          tumoral injection of BCG (BCG Immuno. Pasteur F).
            Rat killed with primary tumour or axillary
          lymph node metastasis 3.5 cm. diameter   -rat
          tumour - free.

obtained following intratumoral treatment with another
BCG preparation (Connaught Multiple Puncture Lyophilized).
But these bacterial agents only produced a significant
prolongation in survival when therapy was initiated at
an early stage of tumour growth. This is illustrated in
Table 3 which compares the response to C.parvum either
as a single or multiple treatment when given early
(9 days) or later (15 and 17 days) after tumour cell
injection. When C. parvum was administered on Day 9
there was a significantly prolonged survival in both
tests. This effect was not obtained when treatment was
delayed, even though in one group repeated doses of
C. parvum was given. In subsequent tests, tumours were
injected with C. parvum (1.4 mg) 15 days after implantation and the mammary tumour growths surgically resected
in day 32 to 35. In this experiment (Fig. 3) intratumoral
injection of C. parvum alone inhibited to some extent
growth of the primary tumour but did not produce any

TABLE 3

INTRALESIONAL THERAPY OF MAMMARY CARCINOMA Sp4

WITH C. PARVUM

Expt.	Treatment[1]	Survival Time[2] (Days)
1	None	20, 20, 27, 27, 27
	C. parvum (1.4 mg) Day 9	27, 55, 5x100+($p<0.01$)[3]
	C. parvum (3x1.4 mg) Days 15, 23, 29	20, 27, 46, 77, 84, 100$^+$ (HS)
2	None	29, 36, 36, 50, 91
	C. parvum (1.4 mg) Day 9	36, 50, 64, 78, 3x100$^+$ ($p<0.05$)
	C. parvum (1.4 mg) Day 17	36, 50, 50, 71, 78, 91, 100 (HS)

1. C. parvum Wellcome CN6134.

2. Mammary carcinoma Sp4 (2×10^4 cells) injected
   into mammary pad Day 0.

3. From Wilcoxon Rank sum test, one tailed.

complete regressions. However, intratumoral C. parvum
combined with surgery was no better than surgery alone,
in this case survival being controlled by the development
of axillary lymph node metastases.

DISCUSSION

     Regional immunotherapy whereby bacterial vaccines
including BCG and C. parvum were injected into tumour
deposits effectively controlled growth of the spontaneously arising rat mammary carcinomas. The clinical
potential of this approach is emphasized by the series
of experiments in which growth of mammary carcinomas
implanted into mammary pad tissue was controlled and in
addition, the development of regional lymph node and
pulmonary metastases was restricted, leading to

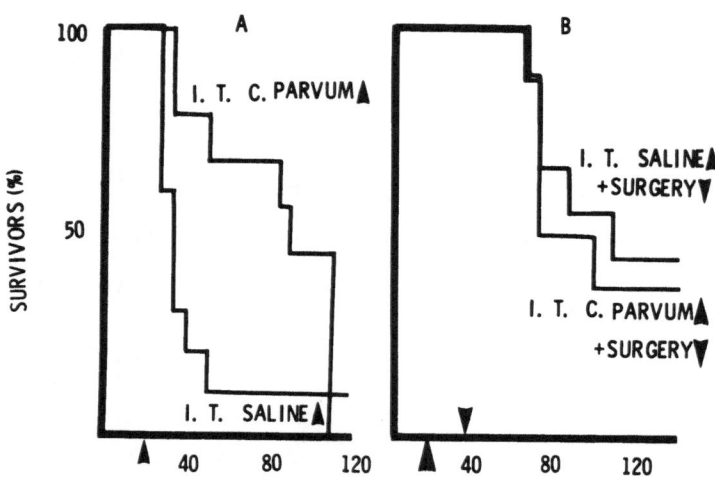

TIME (DAYS) AFTER TUMOR CELL INJECTION

Fig. 3. Effect of Intratumoral (IT) injection and sur-
        gery on survival time of rats bearing Sp4
        tumours. Rats treated with IT injection only
        were killed when their primary tumour or axilla-
        ry lymph node metastases reached 3.5 cm. diame-
        ter. Rats treated by tumour excision were killed
        when distressed due to the growth of metastatic
        tumour (either axillary lymph node or visceral).
        8-10 rats per group. Surviving rats were tumour
        free at the termination of the experiment.

significant prolongation of survival. This effect was
achieved with BCG (Pasteur Immuno. F.) and C. parvum
(Wellcome CN 6134) and in other studies (Willmott
et al, 1980) BCG (Connaught) was found also to be effective. Considering the various parameters of this intratumoral therapy, it is evident that the timing of treatment is most critical. Thus intra-tumoral injection was
most effective when administered early (Day 9) after
mammary pad implantation, and a high dose of C. parvum
or BCG was more effective than a low dose (Fig. 2 ;
Table 3). The therapeutic effect was lost, however,
when treatment was delayed for only 8 days (day 17 after
tumour implantation) and multiple intralesional injections were then not effective. Furthermore, late intratumoral injections of C. parvum combined with surgical
resection of the treated tumour did not signigicantly
prolong survival compared to surgery alone groups.

In further developing intralesional therapy, consideration has to be given to its immunological basis.
Here it must be recognised that the host responses most
likely will be multi-factorial and their combined effectiveness will depend upon the characteristics of individual tumours. The mammary carcinoma Sp4 used in the
present therapeutic studies is moderately immunogenic,
eliciting specifically sensitized lymphocytes which can
effectively suppress growth of the tumour (Baldwin and
Embleton, 1969 ; Baldwin et al, 1979a). The role of these
specifically sensitized lymphocytes is emphasized by
the finding that rejection of tumour Sp4 by active
immunotherapy initiated with tumour cell-BCG vaccines
is abrogated by whole body irradiation (Baldwin et al,
1979b). One pathway leading to tumour rejection, therefore, is through trafficking of specifically sensitized
lymphocytes to the tumour deposit which may then set in
operation a series of cellular interactions. This may
include activation of in situ tumour macrophage and
natural-killer (NK) cells as well as further extrava-
sation of these cells to the tumour deposit (Baldwin
et al, 1979b). Specifically sensitized lymphocytes may,
therefore, have a dual role being "cytotoxic" for tumour
cells and/or providing the "signal" through the release
of soluble factors for influx and activation of other
host cells.

In respect to these concepts, intralesional injection of bacterial vaccines such as BCG or C. parvum will
induce activation of in situ macrophages which either
directly, or indirectly through their effects upon NK
cells (Baldwin and Byers, 1979), will produce an anti-

tumour response. Also macrophage activation will lead
to the release of soluble factors causing further extra-
vasation of host lymphocytes and macrophages to the
tumour bed. This may have particular significance when
considering the therapy of tumours with little or no
immunogenicity since the local delayed type hypersensitivity response elicited by bacterial vaccines may prove
to be important. This is emphasized by experiments
showing that rejection of non-immunogenic mammary carcinomas (Sp15 and Sp22) could be obtained when tumour
cells were injected in admixture with BCG in rats pre-
sensitized to BCG, but not in naive rats (Pimm and
Baldwin, unpublished findings). A controlling factor
may be the degree of host cell infiltration with particular tumours since it has been shown that mammary
carcinomas Sp15 and Sp22 do not provoke a significant
macrophage infiltration (Baldwin et al., 1976). This
correlates with their lack of response to regional immunotherapy (Greager and Baldwin, 1978). In comparison
mammary carcinoma Sp4 produces a greater degree of
macrophage infiltration and as illustrated its growth
can be suppressed by intralesional injection of BCG
or C. parvum.

ACKNOWLEDGEMENTS

        This work was supported by grants from the
Cancer Research Campaign, U.K. and by Public Health
Service contract NO1-CB64042 from the Tumor Immunology
Program, Division of Cancer Biology and Diagnosis,
National Cancer Institute, U.S.A.

REFERENCES

Baldwin, R.W., and Byers, V.S., 1979, Immunoregulation
        by bacterial organisms and their role in the
        immuno-therapy of cancer, Springer Semin.
        Immunopathol., 2, 79-100.
Baldwin, R.W., and Embleton, M.J., 1969, Immunology
        of spontaneously arising rat mammary adenocar-
        cinomas. Int. J. Cancer, 4, 430-439.
Baldwin, R.W., and Pimm, M.V., 1978, BCG in tumor immu-
        notherapy. Adv. Cancer Res., 28, 91-147.
Baldwin, R.W., Embleton, M.J., and Pimm, M.V., 1979a,
        Host responses to spontaneous rat tumors, in :
        "Anti-viral mechanisms in the control of neo-
        plasia", Chandra, P., ed., Plenum Press,

New York, pp. 333-353.

Baldwin, R.W., Hopper, D.G., and Pimm, M.V., 1976, Bacillus Calmette Guérin contact immunotherapy of local and metastatic deposits of rat tumors. Ann. N.Y. Acad. Sci., 277, 124-134.

Baldwin, R.W., Pimm, M.V., and Robins, R.A., 1979b, Active specific immunotherapy : experimental studies, in : Advances in Medical Oncology, Research and Education. 6, 67-75.

Castro, J.E., 1978, Immunological Aspects of Cancer, J.E. Castro ed., p. 1-14, MTP Press Lancaster, U.K.

Goodnight, J.E., and Morton, D.L., 1978, Immunotherapy of malignant disease. Ann. Rev. Med., 29, 231-283.

Greager, J.A., and Baldwin, R.W., 1978, Influence of immunotherapeutic agents on the progression of spontaneously arising, metastasizing rat mammary adenocarcinomas of varying immunogenicities. Cancer Res., 38, 69-73.

Herberman, R.B., and Holden, H.T., 1979, Natural killer cells as antitumor effector cells. J. Natl. Cancer Inst., 62, 441-445.

Milas, L., and Scott, M.T., 1977, Antitumor activity of corynebacterium parvum. Adv. Cancer Res., 26, 257-306.

Pimm, M.V., and Baldwin, R.W., 1975, BCG immunotherapy of rat tumour in athymic nude mice. Nature (Lond.) 254, 77-78.

Pimm, M.V., Cook, A.J., Hopper, D.G., Dickinson, A.M., and Baldwin, R.W., 1978, BCG treatment of transplanted rat tumours of spontaneous origin. Int. J. Cancer, 22, 426-432.

Willmott, N., Austin, E.B., and Baldwin, R.W., 1979a, Comparative studies of the metastatic potential of three transplantable rat mammary carcinomas of spontaneous origin. Br. J. Exp. Path., 60, 499-506.

Willmott, N., Pimm, M.V., and Baldwin, R.W., 1979b, C. parvum treatment of transplanted rat tumours of spontaneous origin. Int. J. Cancer, 24, 323-328.

Willmott, N., Austin, E.B., Pimm, M.V., and Baldwin, R.W., 1980, Evaluation of intratumoral Corynebacterium parvum and BCG in the treatment of a transplanted rat mammary carcinoma of spontaneous origin. Submitted.

MORPHOLOGICAL ASPECTS OF IMMUNOTHERAPY IN BREAST CANCER

J.M. Verley[1], K.H. Hollmann[1], R. Villet[2] and
J. Reynier[2]

1. Hopital Marie-Lannelongue, 133 avenue de la
   Résistance, 92350 Le Plessis Robinson, France
2. Hopital Boucicaut, Service de Chirurgie ,
   78 rue de la Convention, 75730 Paris Cedex 15,
   France

There is evidence to believe that numerous immunostimulating agents of bacterial origin inhibit tumor
growth in a variety of experimental systems and in some
human tumors. The mechanism of this action seems to be
mainly related to stimulation of the reticuloendothelial
system (or mononuclear phagocyte system, Lennert, 1978)
with activation of macrophages (Halpern et al., 1966),
but its morphological basis has not been clearly elucidated.

In another study we examined the tumors and the
draining lymph nodes after local injection of a new
immunostimulating agent P 40, in rats bearing DMBA-
induced mammary carcinoma (Verley et al., 1981). This
report gives more detailed results and deals with the
morphological modifications encountered in the tumors,
the draining lymph nodes and the RES (liver and spleen)
after injection of P 40 by different routes.

MATERIAL AND METHODS

Experimental Model

In this study Sprague-Dawley female rats were used
and mammary tumors were induced by administering a single

intragastric dose of 9-10-dimethyl 1-2 benzanthracen
(DMBA) diluted in sesame oil as described by Huggins et
al. (1961).

In animals so treated, multifocal mammary tumors
developed in the different mammary glands, a high percentage of which (80-85 %) between the 7th and 17th week
following instillation of the carcinogen. At the time
immunostimulating treatment was given, the mean number
of tumors per animal was 2.8, and tumor size varied from
0.3 to 3 cm in diameter. Histologically, almost all the
tumors were adenocarcinomas of regular structure, generally surrounded by fibrous tissue. Their differentiation
varied from rat to rat, from tumor to tumor and within
the same tumor. Mitotic activity was always moderate, and
distant metastases were not observed.

This model is interesting in that it provides primary mammary tumors attached to their normal draining
lymph and blood vessels. Moreover, such tumors are histologically classified as adenocarcinomas of the ducts,
which are close to human breast cancer. They are assumed
to be immunogenic and they develop in an intact, presumed immunologically competent host.

The disadvantages of the model are 1. the multifocal
development of the mammary tumors simultaneously involving several mammary glands, 2. the possible immunosuppres-
sive effect of the carcinogen, and 3. the absence of
distant metastases. But in spite of its disadvantages,
we found the above model particularly close to human
breast cancer.

Immunostimulating agent

P 40 was used as the immunostimulating agent. It is
a fraction from the bacterial wall of Corynebacterium
granulosum, isolated at the Pasteur Institute of Paris
by Bizzini et al. (1978). It resists chemical and enzymatic degradation as well as autoclave sterilization for
20 minutes at 120°C. It can be preserved without forma-
lization, which avoids the toxicity related to the use
of formaldehyde and formaldehyde's own immunostimulating
effect (Fauve, 1975), which could otherwise interfere
with the bacterial extract's effect.

Experimental Procedure

The rats were divided into three main groups
(Table 1) :

TABLE 1

		Animals sacrified	Animals kept under observation
DMBA treated animals	120		
Surviving DMBA treated animals	85		
Mammary tumors bearing rats			
P 40 intra-tu.	40	30	10
P 40 peri-tu.	7	7	
P 40 i.v.	18	8	10
Control mammary tu. bearing rats			
untreated	16	6	10
saline intra-tu.	4	4	
Control non tu. bearing rats			
untreated	7	7	
P 40 in the foot pad	5	5	

TABLE 2

IMMUNOTHERAPEUTIC REGIMEN ADMINISTERED FOR THREE CONSECUTIVE DAYS

	Number of rats treated	Dosis per tumor (µg) and per day	Dosis per animal (µg) and per day
- Mammary tumors bearing rats			
P 40 i.tu.	6	17-100	100
	6	71-500	500
	6	333-2.000	2.000
	22	1.500-2.000	1.500-4.000
P 40 peri-tu.	7	1.500-2.000	1.500-4.000
P 40 i.v.	18	-	2.000
- Controls (fresh animals)			
P 40 in the foot pad	5	-	1.000

1. Mammary tumor bearing rats treated with P 40, either
    -· by local administration, intra- or peritumorally, or
    - by systemic i.v. injection ;
2. Mammary tumor bearing rats either
    - untreated or
    - treated by injection of physiologic saline ;
3. Non tumor bearing rats, either
    - untreated or
    - treated with injection of P 40 in the foot pad of
      the front limb.

Table II indicates the doses of P 40 given. In all cases, the immunostimulating agent was administered for three consecutive days.

In the animals treated by local injection (intra or peritumoral), the dose per injection varied from 100 to 4,000 μg in each rat. The dose injected into a given tumor was calculated according to the size and the number of tumors per rat and varied from 17 to 2,000 μg.

The rats treated by intravenous injection received 2,000 μg of P 40 at each injection.

The non mammary tumor bearing control rats treated with P 40 injection in the foot pad received 1,000 μg at each injection.

Nine to fifteen days following the last injection, all the rats were killed, with the exception of : 10 intratumorally treated rats ; 10 having received i.v. treatment ; and 10 untreated mammary tumor bearing control rats, which were all kept under observation. Tissue samples from the tumors, the draining and controlateral lymph nodes, the liver and the spleen were removed from the killed rats and fixed for histological and fine structure examination.

RESULTS

Untreated control rats

In the non mammary tumor bearing control animals not receiving any immunostimulating agent, all the organs examined were structurally normal. The lymph nodes were rather small and atrophic with small follicles.

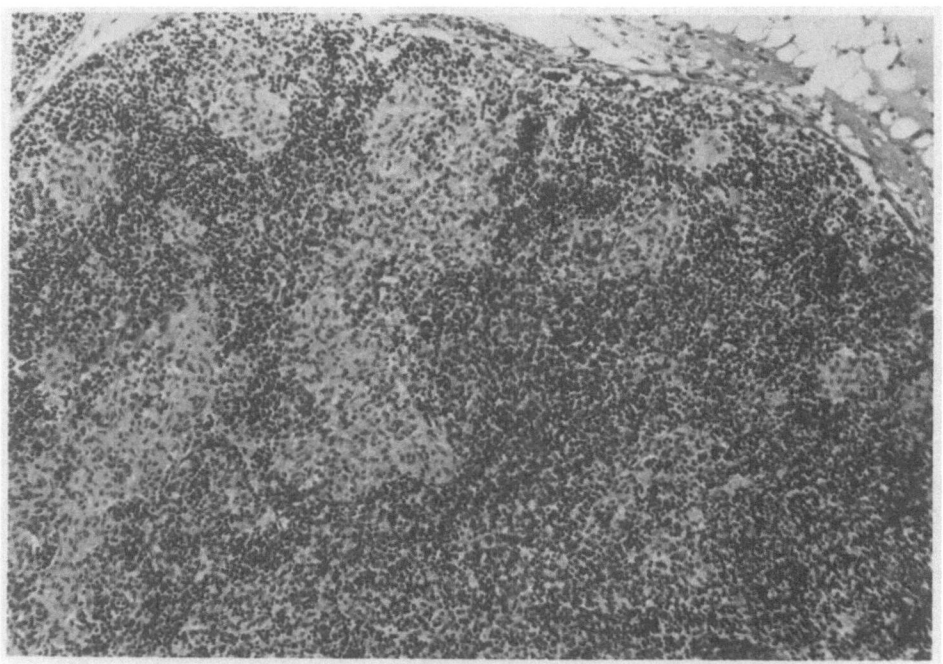

Fig. 1. Draining lymph node of P 40 injected foot pad
        in non-tumor bearing rat (Paraffin section,
        hematein and eosin x135).

Non mammary tumor bearing rats treated by P 40 injection in the foot pad

In this group, the draining lymph nodes of the treated limb were slightly enlarged. Upon histopathological
study, the lymph follicles were found to be somewhat
hyperplastic, with reduced germinal centers. A significant feature was the presence of a multifocal granulomatous reaction, predominant in the cortical area, in
the periphery of the lymph follicles (Fig. 1). The granulomas consisted of large macrophage histiocytes containing abundant, eosinophilic cytoplasm and irregularly
outlined nuclei with prominent nucleoli. The controlateral lymph nodes were unchanged. The structure of the
spleen and liver was normal.

Untreated tumor bearing rats

The structure of the untreated tumors and of those
treated with physiologic saline remained unchanged (Fig 2).

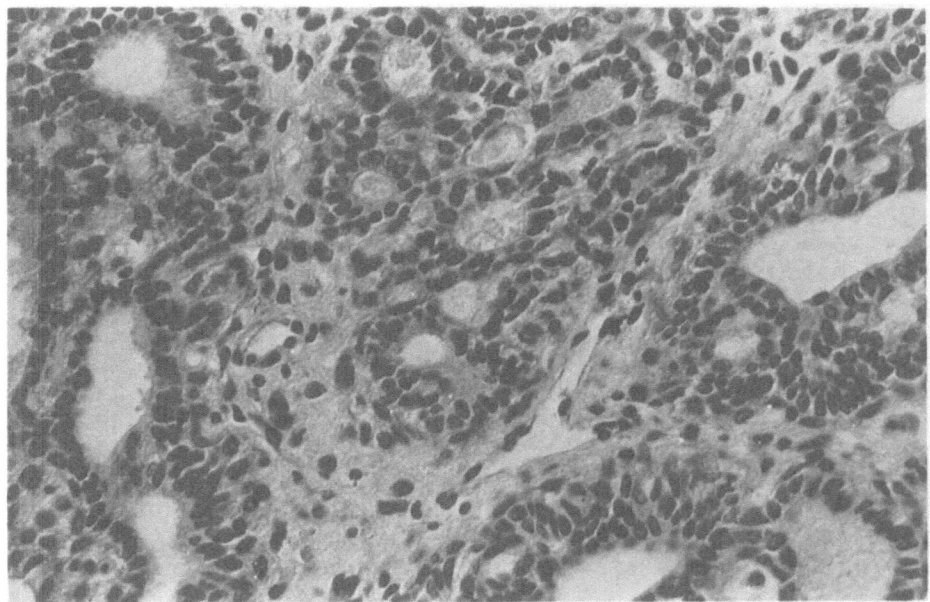

Fig. 2. Untreated DMBA-induced mammary adenocarcinoma
of the rat. (Paraffin section, hematein and
eosin).   x 350

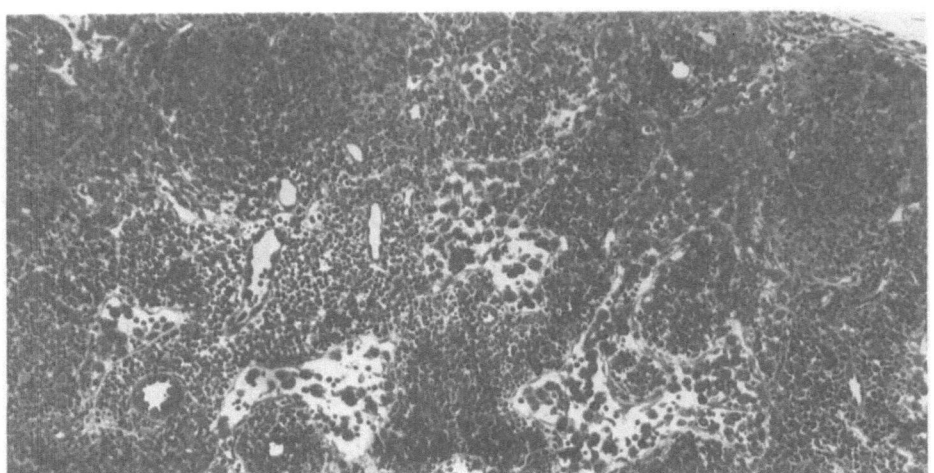

Fig. 3. Draining lymph node of untreated mammary carcinoma. Hyperplasia of the thymus-dependent paracortical region and of the medullary cords
with plasmocytosis, and sinus histiocytosis.
(Araldite embedded, 0.5μm section, Toluidine
blue, x115).

A few necrotic foci were present in the voluminous tumors,
but no significant inflammatory infiltration was observed,
in particular, few, if any, macrophages.

The draining lymph nodes had slightly increased in
volume. Histologically, their general structure was preserved with numerous light germinal centers in the cortex.
The thymus dependent paracortical region and the medullary cords were hyperplastic and contained many plasmocytes.
The lymphatic sinuses, particularly in the paracortical
and medullary area, were full of histiocytes intermingled with a few mastocytes (Fig. 3).

Examined on half-thin araldite sections, the histiocytes resembled large free cells in the lumina of
the sinuses, either isolated or in clusters. They had
abundant cytoplasm rich in vacuoles and dense bodies.
Their cytoplasmic contour was well defined and uneven,
with numerous tousled surface projections. The nuclei
were voluminous and notched, with small but well defined
nucleoli (Fig. 4). This is the characteristic feature
of sinus histiocytosis, as described by classic histo-
logists.

Furthermore, the half-thin araldite sections indicate that the histiocytes originate either from the
cells lining the sinus walls or from submarginal histiocytic reticular cells which invade the sinus lumen between the bordering sinus cells (Fig. 5).

Electron microscope study confirmed and completed
the above observations. The histiocytes were clearly
separated from one another, and not syncytial. They
were large-sized cells containing uneven nuclei and more
or less well defined nucleoli. Their cytoplasm was
abundant with numerous peripheral projections. They
contained a few endoplasmic reticulum, generally medium-
sized Golgi apparatus and large, smooth vacuoles. But
the most characteristic feature was the existence of
large amount of small lysosomes, of slightly variable
density and shape, corresponding to so-called "primary"
lysosomes (Fig. 6).

In these non immunostimulated mammary tumor bearing
rats no changes occurred in the liver or spleen.

P 40 treated mammary tumor bearing rats

The structural alterations observed in this group
differed in extent and intensity according to the

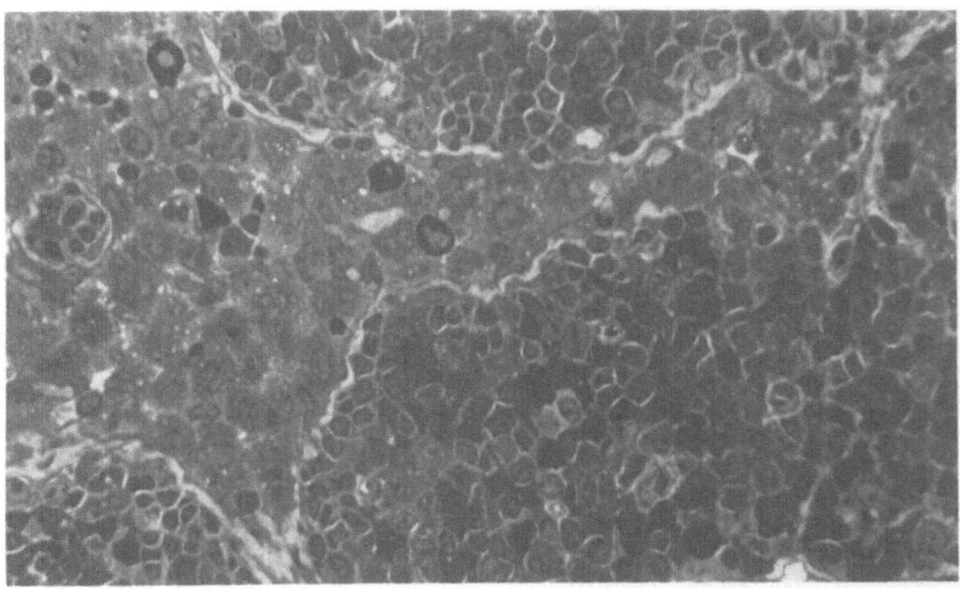

Fig. 4. Draining lymph node of untreated mammary carcinoma. Sinus histiocytosis. (Araldite embedded,
0.5 µm section, Toluidine blue. x 560).

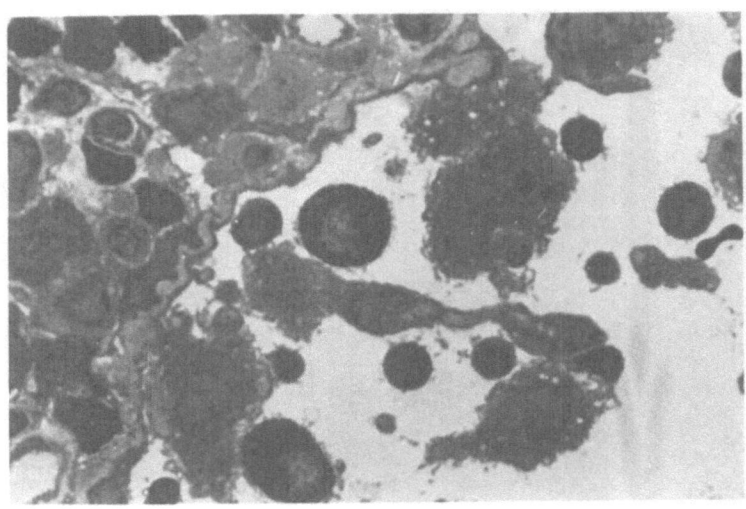

Fig. 5. Draining lymph node of untreated mammary carcinoma. Sinus histiocytosis : the histiocytes
arise from the cells lining the sinus wall and
from underlining so-called submarginal reticulum cells. (Araldite embedded, 0.5 µm section,
Toluidine blue, x 1,150).

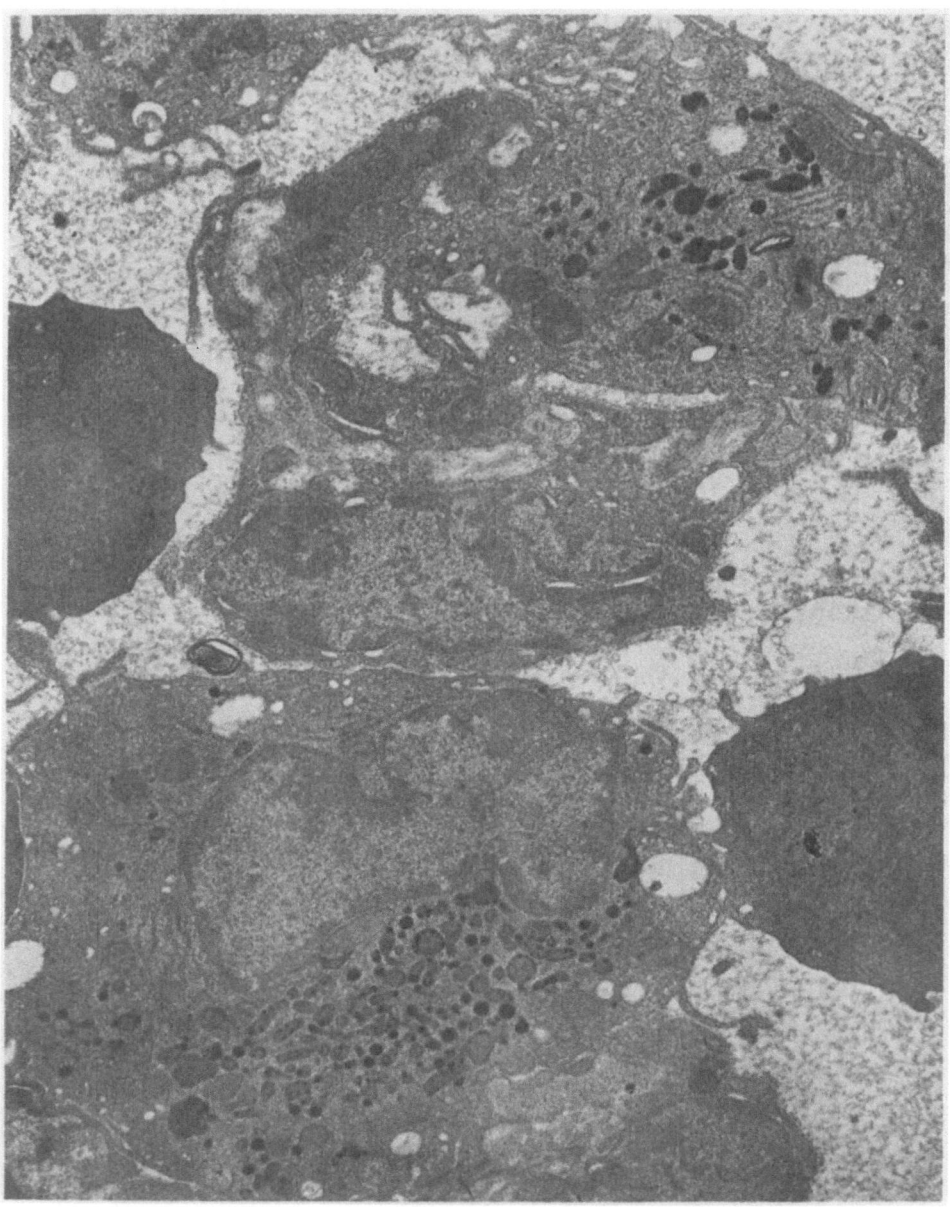

Fig. 6. Draining lymph node of untreated mammary carci-
        noma. Sinus histiocytosis : the histiocytes are
        covered with filiform cytoplasmic projections
        and contain numerous small lysosomes of the
        primary type. (Electron micrograph, Lead
        citrate,x10.000).

administration route and dose of the immunostimulating
agent.

  Intravenous administration of P 40 induced structural modifications in the liver and spleen, mainly the
appearance of many histiocytic granulomas.

  In the liver, the granulomas were usually located
in the portal spaces, but were also found along the
sinusoids. Each granuloma consisted of a cluster of
macrophage histiocytes sometimes surrounded by a few
lymphocytes (Fig. 7).

  In the spleen, the granulomas developed in the
peripheral part of the germinal centers. Their structure
was similar to the histiocytic granulomas observed in
the liver, but here they were particularly numerous.
The proliferation of histiocytic granulomas was associated with considerable erythroblastosis and a megakaryocyte reaction (Fig. 8).

  In the i.v. P 40 treated rats, no structural modifications were observed in the tumors, which showed no
signs of necrosis, inflammatory infiltration or regression. In addition, the draining lymph nodes of the
tumors and the distant lymph nodes remained unchanged.

  Local injection of P 40, whether intra or peritumoral, induced dramatic structural modifications which
were much greater and more extensive than following
systemic i.v. injection. The changes concerned not only
the liver and spleen, but also the injected tumors and
their draining lymph nodes.

  The tumors were destroyed to various degrees and
invaded by a large amount of mononuclear cells (Fig. 9).
This mononuclear infiltration, consisting mainly of histiocytes and also lymphocytes, was either diffuse or
granulomatous. A strong sclerotic reaction also occurred
and developed among the tumor remnants.

  Under the electron microscope (Fig. 10), the histiocytes were characterized by a very uneven outline of
the cytoplasm with numerous thin filiform projections
frequently in contact with those of the neighboring
cells. The cytoplasm contained numerous mitochondria, well
developed Golgi bodies, some endoplasmic reticulum and
numerous large-sized lysosomes, with a homogeneous electron dense matrix and an even countour.

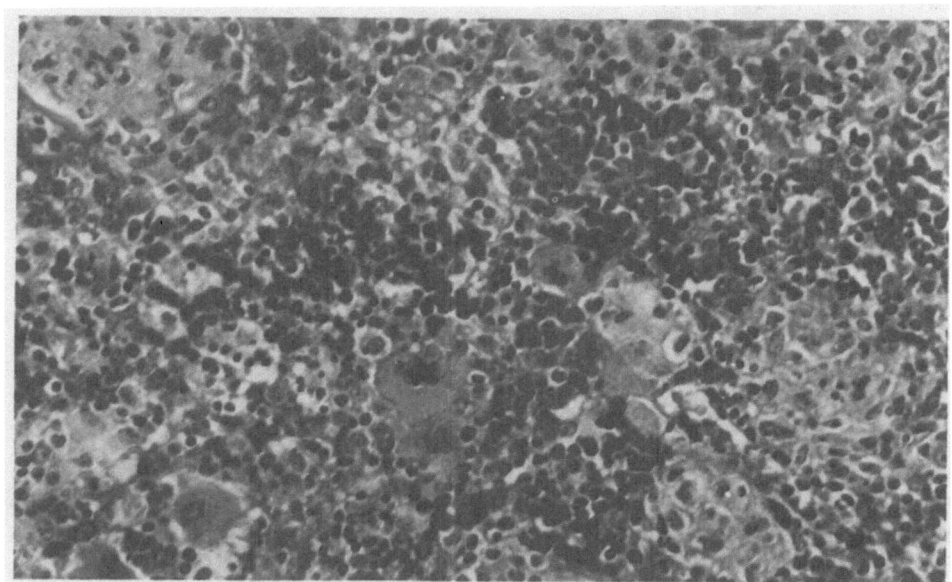

Fig. 7. Liver of P 40 i.v. injected mammary tumor bear-
        ing rat. (Paraffin section, hematein and eosin,
        x 350).

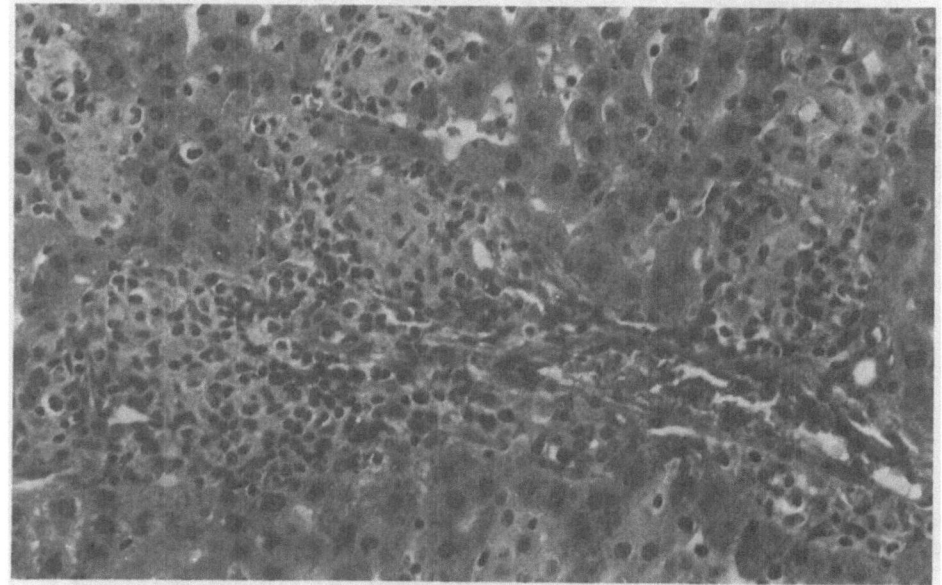

Fig. 8. Spleen of P 40 i.v. injected mammary tumor
        bearing rat. (Paraffin section, hematein and
        eosin. x 350).

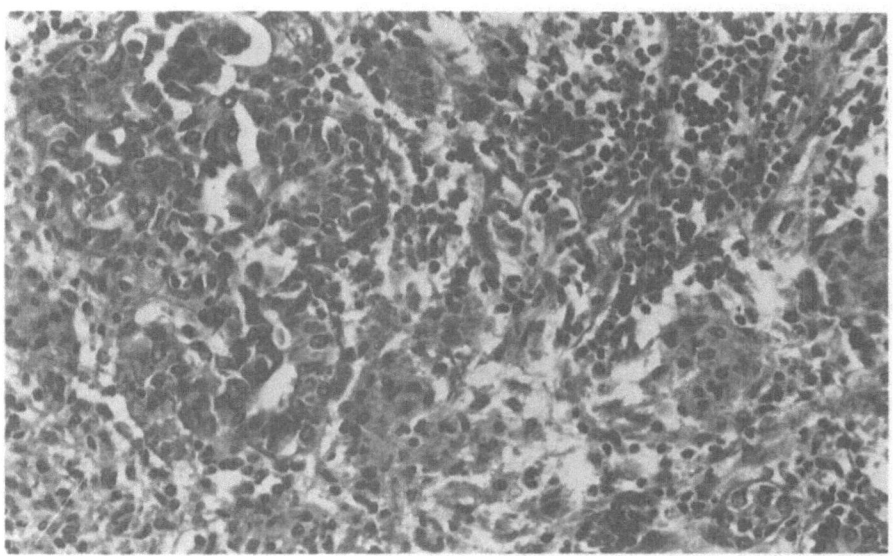

Fig. 9. Locally P 40 treated mammary carcinoma. The tumor is destroyed and invaded by a large amount of mononuclear cells. (Paraffin section, hematein and eosin, x350).

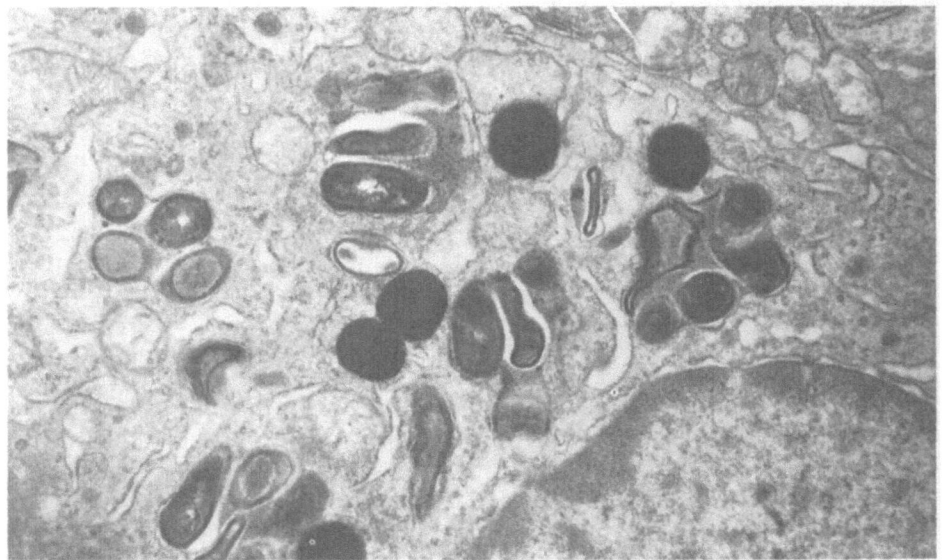

Fig. 10. Locally P 40 treated mammary carcinoma. The histiocytes contain numerous remnants of bacteria and large lysosomes. (Electron micrograph, Lead citrate, x20.500).

Aside from these organelles, there were other structures of rounded or oval shape and of about 1 μm in
size. They had a less electron dense matrix and a more
uneven contour than the lysosomes and were surrounded
by a thick, dense membrane. These structures were obviously phagocytized remnants of disintegrated bacteria.

The draining lymph nodes had undergone profound
changes. On paraffin sections, their general structure
had become denser, with the disappearance of the germinal centers and rarefaction of the medullary cords in
the paracortical region. Plasmocytosis and mastocytosis
were less pronounced and sinus histiocytosis had almost
disappeared.

The most remarkable alteration was the presence of
numerous granulomas (Fig. 11). The reaction was analogous
to that observed in the draining lymph nodes of the non
mammary tumor bearing rats treated by P 40 injection in
the foot pad, but more intense. It developed in the cortical area in the periphery of the lymph follicles, then
in the paracortical region and in the medullary cords.

In cases of weak reaction, the granulomas were
compact, well defined, isolated from one another and
located exclusively in the cortex. They showed no signs
of degeneration. The cells had homogeneous eosinophilic
cytoplasm with undistinguishable cytoplasmic borders
(Fig. 12).

In cases of stronger reaction, the granulomas
coalesced and occupied practically the lymph node as
a whole. They were loosely grouped, with their cells
separated from each other, and had numerous cytoplasmic
projections sometimes intermingling with those of neighboring cells. The nuclei had become small and pyknotic.

Half-thin araldite sections showed that the granulomas were situated in the paracortical and medullary
regions of the node parenchyma in close neighbourship
to the sinuses. They were generally in contact with
the sinus wall and apparently developed from the here
situated submarginal reticulum cells, (Fig. 13).

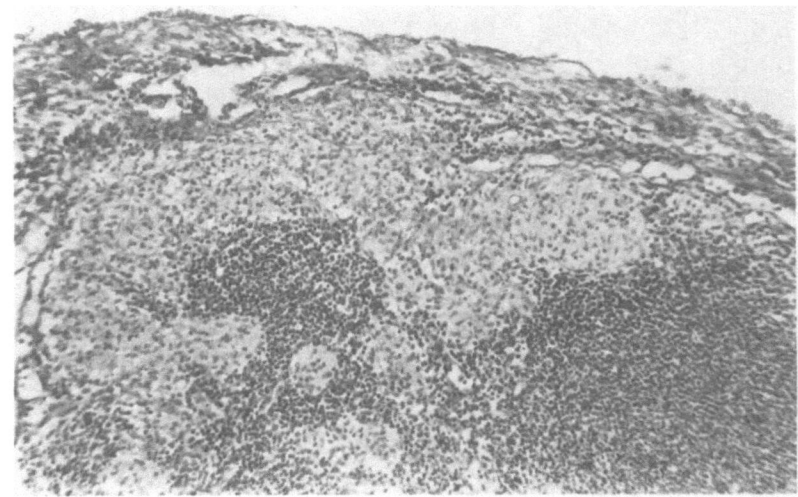

Fig. 11. Draining lymph node of locally P 40 treated mammary carcinoma. Coalescent granulomas in the cortical region. (Paraffin section, hematein and eosin, x120).

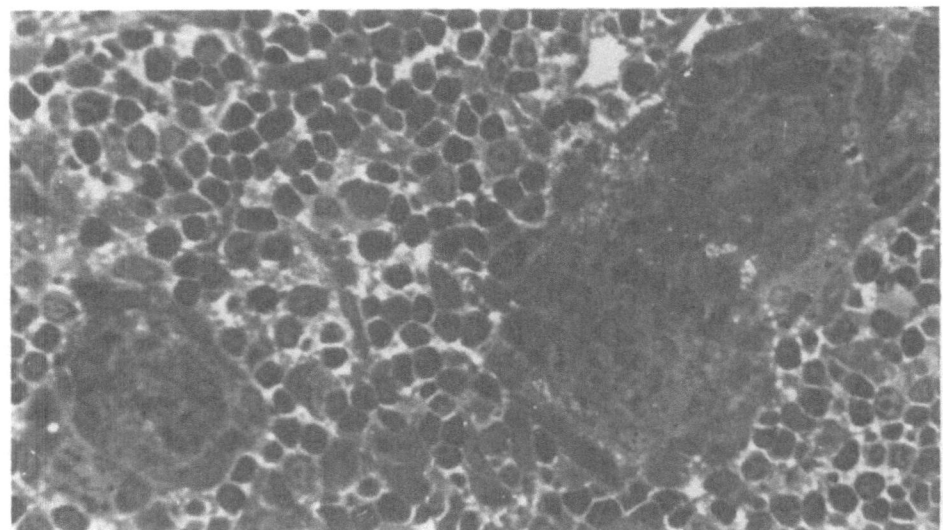

Fig. 12. Draining lymph node of locally P 40 treated mammary carcinoma. Two focal granulomas in the paracortical region consisting of large histiocytes. (Araldite embedded, 0.5 μm section, Toluidine blue, x 750).

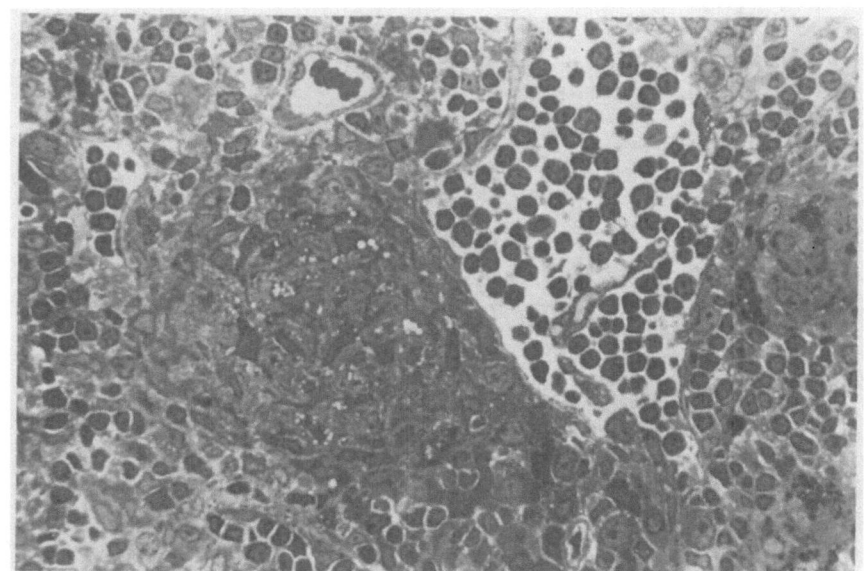

Fig. 13. Draining lymph node of locally treated mammary
carcinoma. The granulomas develop inside the
lymph cords from the cells of the reticular
network. Sinuses are not invaded by the proces-
sus. (Araldite-embedded, 0.5 μm section,
Toluidine blue, x560).

Under the electron microscope (Figs. 14 and 15) the
histiocytes of the granuloma closely resembled those of
sinus histiocytosis. However, the nucleoli were more
prominent and well defined, the lysosomes appeared larger
and either dense and homogeneous or light and dotted with
dense spots. They resembled so-called secondary lysosomes.

The liver contained numerous histiocytic granulomas,
the aspect and distribution of which was analogous to
that of the ones observed after i.v. P 40 injection.

The spleen also had many histiocytic granulomas,
erythroblastosis and a megakaryocyte reaction.

The intensity of the histiocytic reaction was closely related to the doses of P 40 injected. Doses below
100 g were almost ineffective. Doses of 500 μg sometimes
produced large tumor necrosis and considerable cellular
reactions. But the most consistent and intense reactions

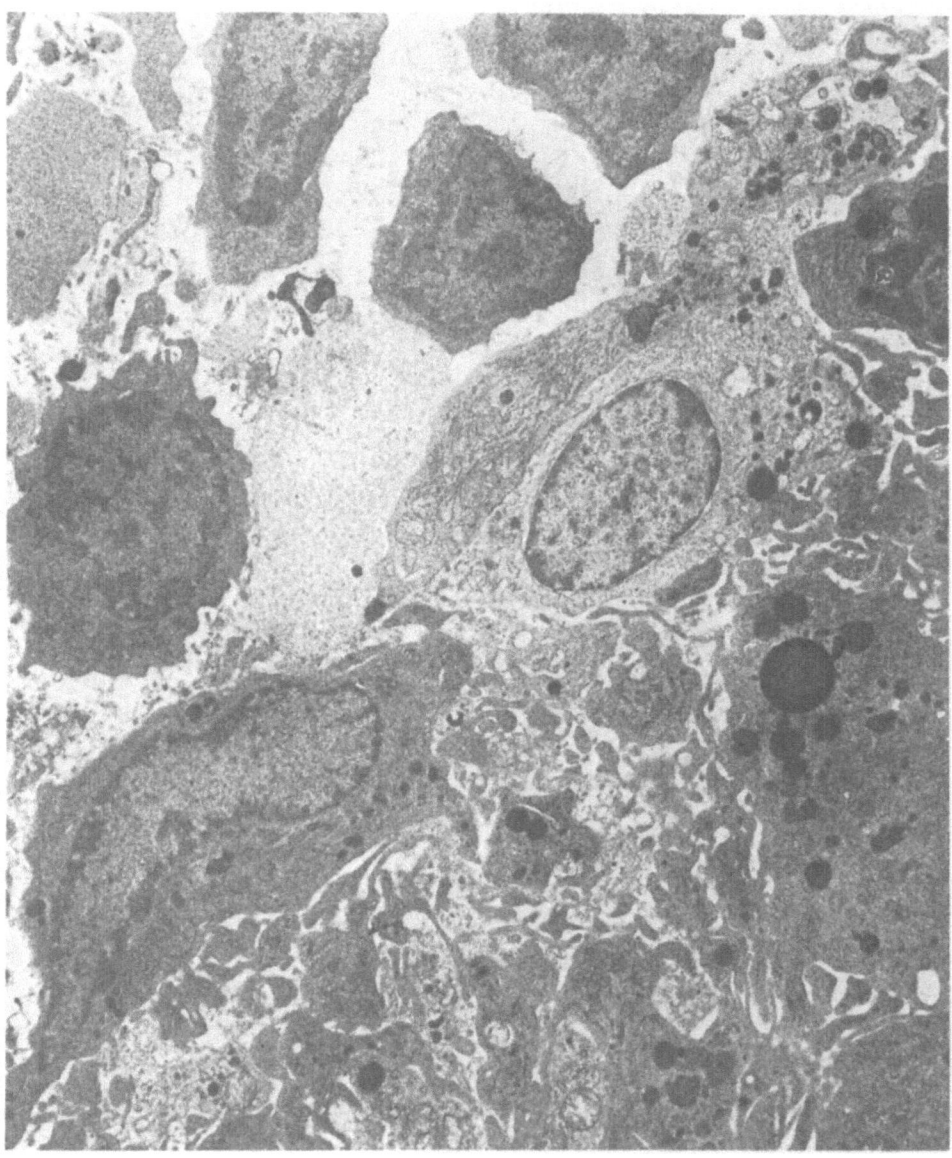

Fig. 14. Draining lymph node of locally treated mammary carcinoma. At the lower right, a granuloma composed of histiocytes with long interdigitating cytoplasmic projections and numerous big lysosomes. At the upper left, a portion of a sinus containing lymphocytes. There is a sharp limit between the granuloma and the sinus wall. (Electron micrograph, Lead citrate, x8.100).

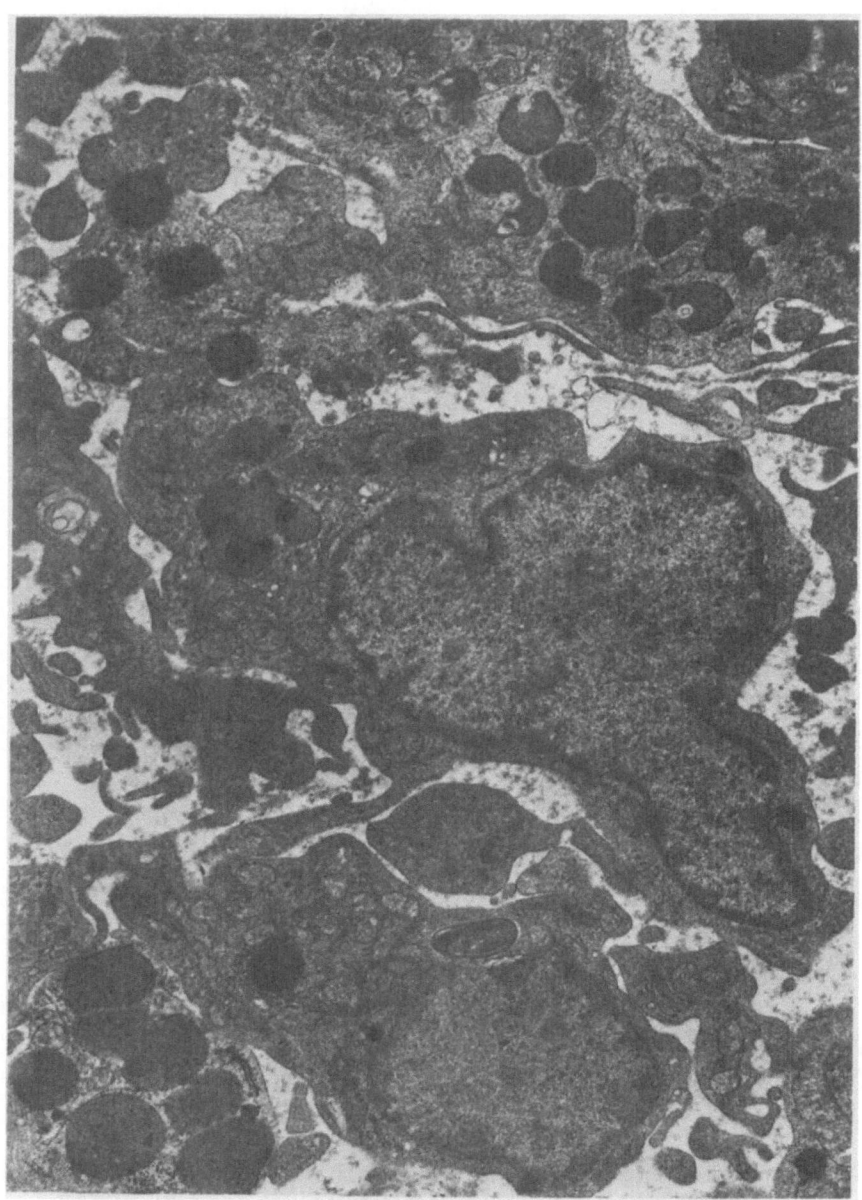

Fig. 15. Draining lymph node of locally treated mammary
         carcinoma. The histiocytes of the granuloma
         contain numerous large pale lysosomes of se-
         condary type. (Electron micrograph, Lead
         citrate, x10.800).

were obtained with doses of 2,000 μg per tumor. Intra or
peritumoral injection of the immunostimulating agent gave
identical results in both the type and intensity of the
reaction.

DISCUSSION

     The present observations can be summarized as
follows (Table III) :

     1. In untreated mammary tumor bearing rats, the
draining lymph nodes show a reaction associating sinus
histiocytosis and plasmocytosis of the lymph cords. The
mammary tumors are unchanged and the liver and spleen
remain normal.
     2. In non mammary tumor bearing rats, P 40 injection
in the foot pad induces histiocytic granulomas only in
the lymph nodes draining the treated limb. At the time
of our observations (7-15 days following injection of
the immunostimulating agent), the liver and spleen
appeared histologically normal.
     3. In mammary tumor bearing rats killed 7-15 days
following 3 i.v. injections of P 40, histiocytic granulomas are noted in the liver and spleen. The tumors
remain intact and their draining lymph nodes show sinus
histiocytosis analogous to the cases observed in mammary
tumor bearing rats not treated by an immunostimulating
agent.
     4. In mammary tumor bearing rats treated locally and
killed as above, alterations are much more extensive :
the tumors are necrotic, sometimes completely ; the
draining lymph nodes are infiltrated by histiocytic granulomas sometimes in clusters ; and the liver and spleen
also contain numerous histiocytic granulomas.

     As for the immunologic significance of these results,
the modifications observed in the draining lymph nodes of
untreated DMBA-induced mammary tumors closely resemble
those seen in cellular immunity, as described for example
in graft rejection. In cellular immune response, lymphoproliferative reaction in the paracortical and medullary
cord regions with an increase in plasmocytes is associated with the appearance of numerous macrophages in the
paracortical sinus, in other words sinus histiocytosis
(Simar, 1973). This suggests that in our experimental
model, the DMBA-induced mammary tumors are immunogenic,
as in other chemically induced animal tumors (Prehn,
1975 ; Baldwin, 1976).

TABLE 3
HISTOLOGICAL MODIFICATIONS AFTER P 40

ANIMALS	SITE OF REACTION			
			SYSTEMIC	
	TUMOR	DRAINING LYMPH NODES	LIVER	SPLEEN
Tu. bearing untreated	-	• Sinus histiocytosis • Plasmocytosis in the lymph cords	-	-
Tu. bearing treated P 40 intra- or peritu.	• Necrotic changes • Infiltration of histiocyte-macrophage	• Histiocytic granulomas • Sinus histiocytosis	HISTIOCYTIC GRANULOMAS	• Megakaryocytosis • Erythroblastosis
Tu. bearing treated P 40 i.v.	-	• Sinus histiocytosis • Plasmocytosis in the lymph cords	HISTIOCYTIC GRANULOMAS	• Megakaryocytosis • Erythroblastosis
Control, non tu. bearing P 40 in the foot-pad	-	• Histiocytic granulomas	-	-

Furthermore, it is well known that human breast cancer, in favorable cases, is associated with sinus histiocytosis and lymphoproliferative reaction in the draining lymph nodes, as observed by many authors (Cutler et al., 1966; Silverberg et al., 1970; Black et al., 1975 ; Hunter et al., 1975 ; Kozlowski and Hrabowska, 1978). This suggests that in such favorable cases, the cancer is immunogenic and the host immunocompetent.

The reaction induced by the immunostimulating agent is somewhat different from sinus histiocytosis and seems to have another significance.

Here the basic reaction is the formation of a granuloma consisting of macrophage histiocytes corresponding to reticuloendothelial cell clusters stimulated by the bacterial extract. In the lymph nodes, immunostimulated cells differ from the histiocytes in sinus histiocytosis in that they are located in the lymph cords and not within the sinus lumina. In the liver, stimulated cells correspond to Kupffer cells.

Such a granulomatous reaction is a specific immune reaction induced by various microorganisms (Bartlett et al., 1972 ; Hanna et al., 1973). For instance, Hanna and coworkers (Hanna et al., 1972 ; Zbar et al., 1972) describe modifications similar to ours in draining lymph nodes injected with BCG. This so-called histiocytic reaction is interpreted by Lennert (1979) as of preepithelioid cell nature. It is important to emphasize that this specific immune reaction induced by microorganisms implies immunocompetence of the host, since it disappears in immuno-suppressed hosts, as shown by Scott (1974), Baldwin (1973) and others.

The granulomatous reaction reflecting stimulation of the reticuloendothelial system is observed in tumor bearing hosts as well as in non tumor bearing hosts. The same observations as ours have also been made by other authors describing non tumor bearing animals treated with subcutaneous injection of immunostimulating agents (Khalil et al., 1975), i.v. injection (Halpern et al., 1963a; Moore et al., 1963 ; Khalil et al., 1975) or i.p. injection (Halpern et al., 1963b ; Meyer et Grundmann, 1980). The study of Halpern et al. (1963b) concerns non tumor bearing mice receiving i.p. injection of Coryne-

bacterium phlei : the resulting modifications in the
liver and spleen are identical to those found in this
study.

The importance of the administration route of the
immunostimulating agent should also be stressed. In non
tumor bearing mice, Khalil et al. (1975) showed that
systemic i.v. injection of BCG induces a very pronounced
reaction, which is more diffuse than following subcutaneous injection of the immunostimulating agent. Fourteen
to eighteen days after i.v. injection, a granulomatous
reaction develops in the liver, spleen, lymph nodes and
lungs of the mice, whereas in those treated by subcutaneous injection, the histiocytic granulomas are only
observed locally at the site of injection and in the
draining lymph nodes.

Our study, however, shows that in tumor-bearing
animals, local injection (intra or peritumoral) of the
immunostimulating agent is more efficient than i.v. injection, and induces a granulomatous reaction, not only
in the liver and spleen, but also in the tumors, more or
less completely destroying them, and in the draining lymph
nodes. As in the study of Khalil et al. (1975), the non
tumor bearing control animals receiving P 40 injection
in the foot pad, only showed a localized granulomatous
reaction not extending beyond the draining lymph nodes
of the site of injection.

These results emphasize the importance of direct
contact between the immunostimulating agent and tumoral
antigens, illustrating the three main conditions for
effective immunotherapy : 1. antigenicity of the tumor ;
2. immunological competence of the host ; and 3. local
administration of the immunostimulating agent.

These morphologic results are in accord with the
experimental studies by Fisher et al. (1978), Greager
and Baldwin (1978) and others, who showed that in tumor-
bearing animals local injection of an immunostimulating
agent is more effective than systemic injection. Clinical
results have also been obtained in the treatment of malignant melanomas by immunostimulating agents : Rosenberg
and Rapp (1976) stressed that the efficiency of BCG immunotherapy is greater if the host is immunocompetent and
that intralesional injection is more efficient than
intradermal injection distant from the tumors.

These results should be taken into account for clinical application of immunotherapy in human breast cancer.

ACKNOWLEDGMENTS

     This work was partly supported by a contract from
CHU Necker Enfants Malades (Pr. J. Reynier), with the
help of the Ligue Nationale Française contre le Cancer,
the FEGEFLUC and the International Society against
Breast Cancer.

     We thank also the Ecole de Chirurgie, Paris (Direc-
teur scientifique : Pr. C. Cabrol) and Dr. Bizzini (Pasteur Institute) which kindly provided the immunostimulating agent P 40.

     The skillfull collaboration of Melle G. Amichot
and Mme J. Garaudel is gratefully acknowledged.

REFERENCES

Baldwin, R.W., 1973, Immunological aspects of carcino-
          genesis. Adv. Cancer Res., 16, 1-75.
Baldwin, R.W., 1976, Relevant animal models for tumor
          immunotherapy. Cancer Immunol. Immunother., 1,
          197-198.
Bartlett, G.L., Zbar, B., and Rapp, H.J., 1972, Suppression
          of murine tumor growth by immune reaction to the
          Bacillus Calmette Guerin strain of Mycobacterium
          bovis. J. Natl. Cancer Inst., 48, 245-257.
Bizzini, B., Maro, B., and Lallouette, P., 1978, Isolement
          et caractérisation d'une fraction (P 40) isolée
          de Corynebacterium Granulosum. Médecine et Mala-
          dies infectieuses, 8, 408-414.
Black, M.M., Zachrau, R.E., Shore, B., Moore, D.H., and
          Leis, H.P., 1975, Prognostically favorable immu-
          nogens of human breast cancer tissue : Antigenic
          similarity to murine mammary tumor virus. Cancer,
          35, 121-128.
Cutler, S.J., Black, M.M., Friedell, G.H., Vidone, R.A.,
          and Goldenberg, I.S., 1966, Prognostic factors
          in cancer of the female breast. Cancer, 19,
          75-82.
Fauve, R.M., 1975, Stimulating effect of Corynebacterium
          parvum and Corynebacterium extract on the macro-
          phage activities against Salmonella typhimurum
          and Listeria monocytogenes. In : B. Halpern (ed.),
          Corynebacterium parvum. Application in experimental
          and clinical oncology. pp 77-83. New York : Plenum
          Press.
Fisher, B., Gebhardt, M., Linta, J., and Saffer, E., 1978,
          Comparison of the inhibition of tumor growth fol-

lowing local or systemic administration of Corynebacterium parvum or other immunostimulating
agents with or without cyclophosphamide. Cancer
Res., 38, 2679-2687.

Greager, J.A., and Baldwin, M.W., 1978, Influence of
immunotherapic agents on the progression of spontaneous arising metastazing rat mammary adenocarcinomas of varying immunogenicities. Cancer Res.,
38, 69-73.

Halpern, B., Prevot, A.R., Biozzi, G., Stiffel, C.,
Mouton, D., Morard, J.C., Bouthillier, Y., and
Decreusefond, C., 1963a, Stimulation de l'activité
du système réticuloendothélial provoquée par Corynebacterium parvum. J. Réticuloendothél. Soc.,
1, 77-96.

Halpern, B.N., Haguenau, F., and Hollmann, K.H., 1963b.
Modifications ultrastructurales observées dans
le foie et dans la rate de souris après injection
d'extraits bactériens. In : Rôle du système ré-
ticulo-endothélial dans l'immunité antibactérienne
et anti-tumorale. B.N. Halpern ed., Centre National
de la Recherche Scientifique, Paris, pp 249-259.

Halpern, B., Biozzi, G., Stiffel, C., and Mouton, D.,
1966, Inhibition of tumor growth by administration
of killed Corynebacterium parvum. Nature, 212,
853-854.

Hanna, M.G., Jr., Zbar, B., and Rapp, H.J., 1972, Histo-
pathology of tumor regression after intralesional
injection of Mycobacterium bovis. I. Tumor growth
and metastasis. J. Natl. Cancer Inst., 48, 1441-
1455.

Hanna, M.G., Jr., Snodgrass, M.J., Zbar, B., and Rapp,
H.J., 1973, Histopathology of tumor regression
after intralesional injection of Mycobacterium
bovis. IV. Development of immunity to tumor cells
and BCG. J. Natl. Cancer Inst., 51, 1897-1908.

Huggins, C., Grand, L.G., and Brillantes, F.P., 1961,
Mammary cancer induced by a single feeding of po-
lynuclear carbons and its suppression. Nature, 189,
204-207.

Hunter, R., Ferguson, D., and Coplleson, W., 1975, Survival with mammary cancer related to the interaction of germinal center hyperplasia and sinus
histiocytosis in axillary and internal mammary
lymph nodes. Cancer, 36, 526-539.

Khalil, A., Bourut, Ch., Halle-Pannenko, O., Mathe, G.,
and Rappaport, H., 1975, Histologic reactions of
the thymus, spleen, liver and lymph nodes to
intravenous and subcutaneous BCG injections.
Biomedicine, 22, 112-121.

Kozlowski, H., and Hrabowska, M., 1978, Stages of the
    development of immunologic response in regional
    lymph nodes draining breast cancer. Neoplasma,
    25, 445-452.
Lennert, K., 1978, Malignant lymphomas. Springer, Berlin,
    Heidelberg, New York.
Lennert, K., 1979, Introductory remarks. In : Function
    and structure of the immune system. W. Müller-
    Ruchholtz and H.K. Müller-Hermelink eds., Plenum
    Press, New York. pp.1-9.
Meyer, E.M., and Grundmann, E., 1980, BCG-induced changes
    in size of thymic cortex and thymus-dependent
    areas in spleen and lymph nodes of mice. Clin.
    Exp. Immunol., 39, 60-65.
Moore, R.D., Lamm, M.E., Lockman, L.A., and Schoenberg,
    M.D., 1963, Cellular aspects of the action of
    Freund's adjuvant in the spleen and lymph nodes.
    Brit. J. Exp. Path., 44, 300-311.
Prehn, R.T., 1975, Relation-ship of tumor immunogenicity
    to concentration of the oncogen. J. Natl. Cancer
    Inst., 55, 189-190.
Rosenberg, S.A., and Rapp, H.J., 1976, Intralesional
    immunotherapy of melanoma with BCG. Med. Clin.
    North Am., 60, 419-430.
Scott, M.T., 1974, Corynebacterium parvum as a therapeutic
    antitumor agent in mice. II. Local injection.
    J. Natl. Cancer Inst., 53, 861-865.
Silverberg, I., Chitale, A., Hind, A., Frozier, A., and
    Kevitt, S., 1970, Sinus histiocytosis and mammary
    carcinoma. Cancer, 26, 1177-1185.
Simar, L.J., 1973, Modifications structurales des gan-
    glions drainant un greffon allogénique. Relation
    avec la réaction inflammatoire du greffon. Arch.
    Anat. Path., 21, 13-28.
Verley, J.M., Hollmann, K.H., Villet, R., and Reynier, J.,
    Immunostimulation of rats bearing DMBA induced
    mammary carcinoma. Histopathology and ultrastruc-
    ture of the tumors and regional lymph nodes after
    local injection of P 40. In press.
Zbar, B., Bernstein, I.D., Bartlett, G.L., Hanna, M.G.,
    and Rapp, H.J., 1972, Immunotherapy of cancer :
    Regression of intradermal tumor and prevention of
    growth of lymph node metastases after intralesional
    injection of living mycobacterium bovis. J. Natl.
    Cancer Inst., 49, 119-130.

REGRESSION IN NORMAL AND PATHOLOGICAL MAMMARY TISSUES

J. de BRUX

Institut de Pathologie
53 rue des Belles Feuilles
75116 Paris, France

The mammary gland is a labile organ capable of acti-
vely developing and becoming functional, then regressing
and involuting when the stimuli are suppressed. Regression
occurs at the end of lactation. Involution takes place
in old age by supression of pituitary and ovarian stimuli.
Moreover, in some pathological conditions, regressive
phenomena may be observed in some benign lesions or even
in carcinoma.

REGRESSION OF THE MAMMARY GLAND AT THE END OF LACTATION

With the end of lactation a regression takes place
in the mammary gland (Fig. 1). The process begins in the
distal part of the gland and progresses towards the
large ducts (Martinez-Hernandez et al., 1976). It implies
the cessation of the secretory activity with stasis of
previously elaborated secretory material and the reduc-
tion of the glandular structures which return to a resting stage (Verley and Hollmann, 1967 ; Hollmann and
Verley, 1967 ; Hollmann, 1974). The secretion remaining
in the gland is absorbed by digestion in the cytoplasm
of the glandular cells, transported through the enlarged
intercellular spaces, and sucked up by the well developed
capillaries of the stroma.

The glandular tissue is reduced by degeneration of
secretory cells and by decrease of cytoplasmic volume in
surviving cells. This process involves the participation
of lysosomes. Under electron microscope (Hollmann and

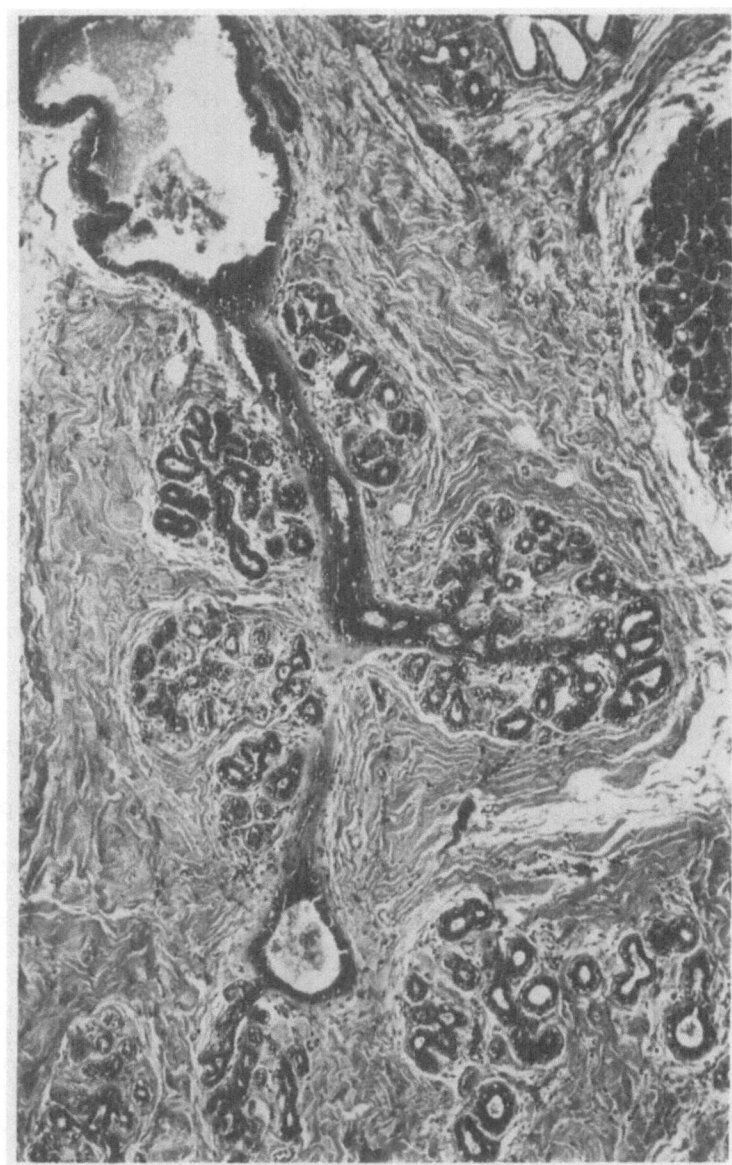

Fig. 1.   Regression of the mammary gland at the end of
          lactation. Cystic dilatation of the terminal
          ducts. H & E, x 125.

Verley, 1967) the amount of ergastoplasm and Golgi elements rapidly decreases whereas free ribosomes appear.
In surviving cells the autolytic process is limited to
small areas of cytoplasm. Dying cells become vacuolated
and are either eliminated as colostrum bodies in the
acinar lumen or lysed and eliminated in the interstitium.
During this process the junctional complexes appear well
preserved. The myoepithelial cells do not undergo degeneration and apparently play an important role in main-
taining the surviving cells together (Verley and Hollmann,
1967 ; Hollmann and Verley, 1967). In the beginning of
regression the basal membrane undergoes modifications :
it is larger and looser, more irregular and sinuous.
When regression is complete the myoepithelial cells
secrete a ground substance which reconstitute the basal
membrane of the remaining ducts. Sometimes pseudolactating
lobules persist (residual lactation acini ; McFarland,
1922).

INVOLUTION OF THE MAMMARY GLAND AT MENOPAUSE

Involution of the mammary gland at menopause is
multicentric and lasts approximately 3-5 years. Clinically it is often confused with cystic disease. During
that period, part of the gland remains normal, and part
hyperplastic.

Involution involves the glandular structures, ducts
and acini, and the intra- and interlobular connective
tissue.

The first step of the involution is characterized
by a thickening of the intralobular connective tissue,
the fibrillary and edematous nature of which disappears
and is replaced by collagen fibers secreted by fibroblasts. The myoepithelial cells, which are normally flat,
become rounder and their cytoplasm vacuolized. They
degenerate, due to progressive disappearance of transfer
phenomena between the epithelium and the interstitial
connective tissue.

In certain cases, the myoepithelial cells secrete
glycoaminoglycans and the glandular structures become
surrounded by a hyaline basal membrane, following increase
and thickening of the reticular fibers. In times, the
basal membranes fuse with the densified interstitial
connective tissue. It should be noted that elastic fibers
are never found.

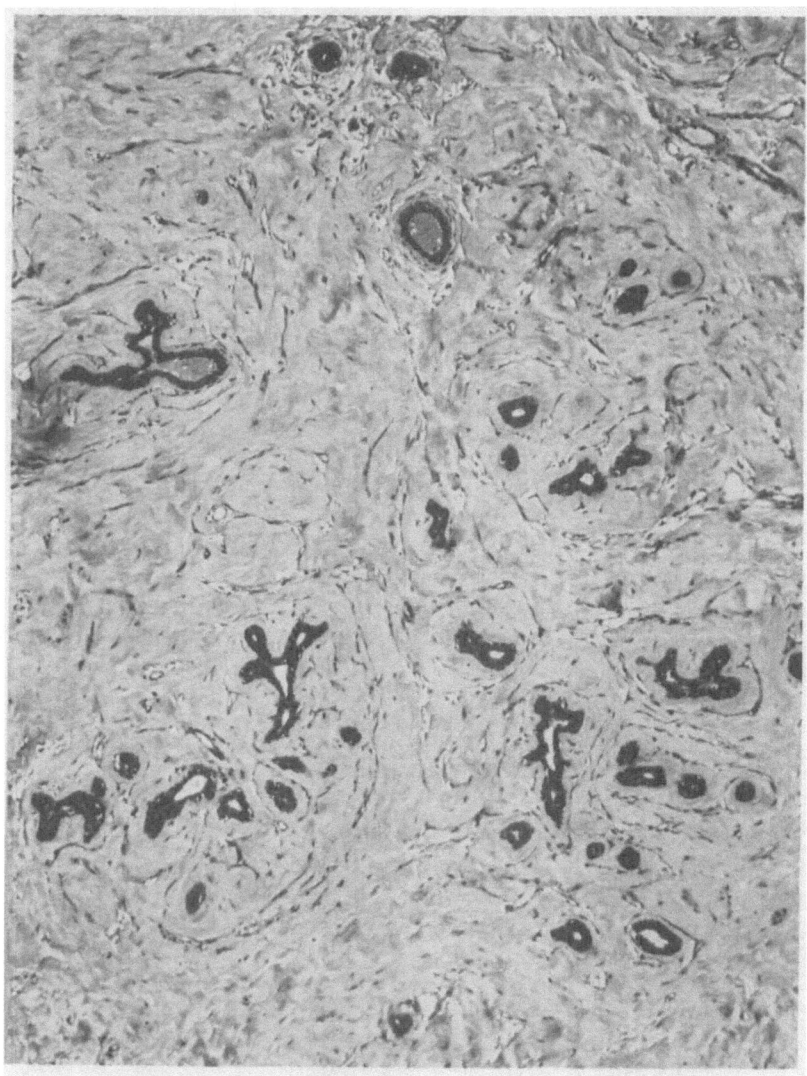

Fig. 2.   Involution at menopause. Sclerosis induced by
          the myoepithelial cells. Disappearance of the
          alveolar structures and persistence of small
          ducts. H & E, x 125.

At the end of the process, the mammary tissue has disappeared and is replaced by homogeneous, more or less hyalinized stroma surrounding a few persisting ducts. (Fig. 2). Occasionally, the sclerosis occurs focally. The thickening of the stroma around the extralobular terminal ducts induces the distal cystic dilatation of small lobules, besides other flattened ducts in the process of disappearing, as described by Bonser et al. (1961) as cystic lobular involution.

REGRESSION PHENOMENA IN MAMMARY CARCINOMA

It may seem unusual to discuss regression in as malignant a process as mammary carcinoma, but particular images appear in precancerous lesions and in beginning cancers, the significance of which should be discussed. Two factors are involved in tumor regression : immune processes and processes occuring in the ground substance. The latter are still controversial.

Tumor regression of Immune Origine

The concept of immune-induced regression is based on the observation of medullary carcinoma. The prognosis of this lesion, according to certain authors (Richardson, 1956), seems to be better than that of other cancers of no special type, particularly if its cellular structure and generally severe nuclear grade are taken into account.

In medullary carcinoma, the cancerous masses are surrounded by dense sheets of lymphocytes which dissociate the tumoral strands and isolate small groups of cells. Thus, tumoral cells undergo cytoplasmic and nuclear lysis, and then disappear (Fig. 3).

In the center and on the margin of these areas, fibroblasts appear and secrete collagen fibers which gradually form a stroma rich in mucopolysaccharides that tends to strangle persisting cancerous trabecles.

The massive lymphoid infiltrates, consisting mainly of T lymphocytes, that destroy the carcinomatous cells and thus secondarily induce the onset of sclerosis, are the expression of an immune reaction of the host to its tumor.

In 1976, Cantor and Weissmann subdivided T cells according to the functions :

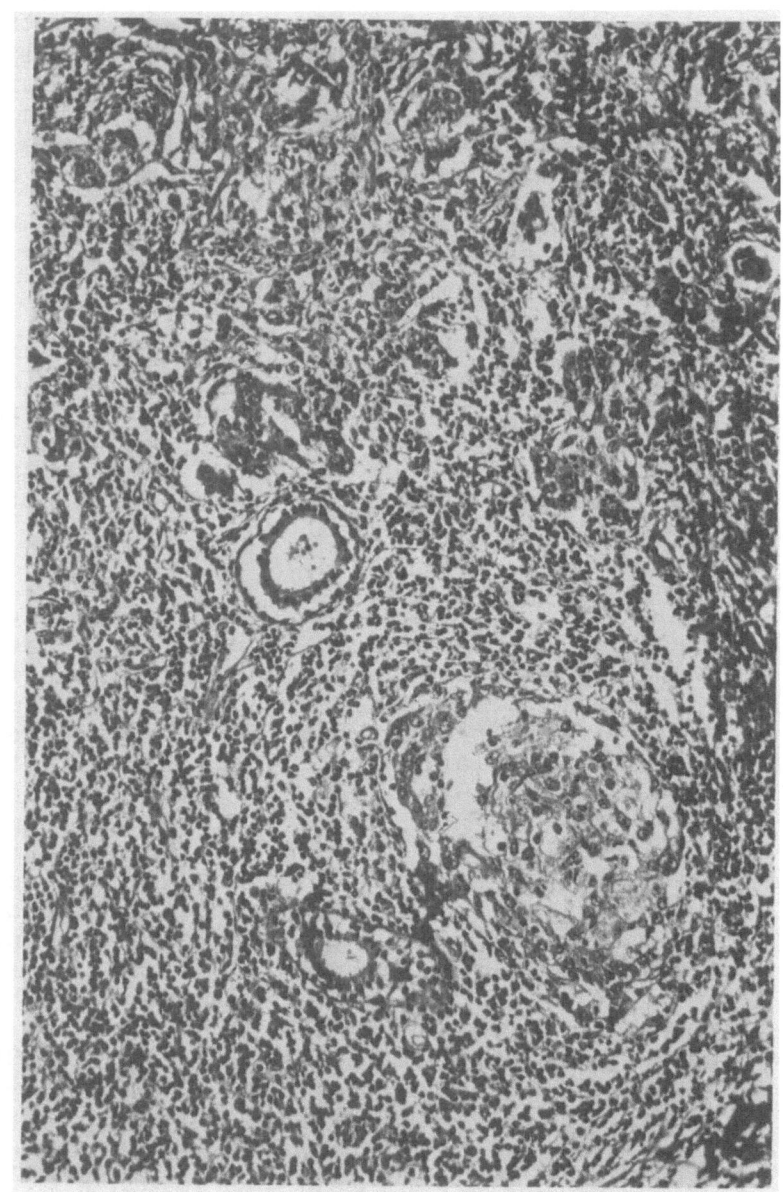

Fig. 3. Medullary carcinoma : progressive disappearance
        of the carcinomatous cells and infiltration
        of lymphocytes. H & E, x 160.

T_h recognize the antigen obtained by macrophage action on the cancer cell and intensifies T_c and B cell activity, determining their specificity for that antigen.

T_c of high cytotoxic activity, recognize the antigens on the surface of abnormal cells or foreign bodies and lyse them by direct contact.

T_d transfer specific activities (lymphokines) of T_h cells to the macrophages. They have no lytic power on target cells.

T_s suppresse the immune reaction by acting on T_h and B cells.

T_c lymphocytes lyse cancer cells by direct contact of gammaglobuline receptors of the lymphocyte membrane with tumor cell antigens (Cottier et al., 1972). This action involves an enzymatic activity.

But lysis also depends on a complement which binds antibody molecules. The latter must be evenly aligned on the surface of the cancer cells. The antibody/complement bind occurs according to the following ratio : 2 molecules of IgG for one complement molecule ; or one IgM molecule for one complement molecule.

In addition to the direct action of T lymphocytes, macrophages sensitized by MAF (Macrophage Activating Factor) also induce cellular immunity.

Such cellular immunity appears also in precancerous lesions and in carcinomas in situ, before the development of metastases. In these cases, the recognition of tumoral antigens does not necessarily coincide with the onset of malignant transformation. Thus, lymphocyte infiltration surrounding carcinoma in situ is less a sign of early tumoral antigen recognition than its consequence.

In cancers of no special type, the dense lymphocyte infiltrate within or surrounding the cancerous mass (Fig. 4), associated with periductal and perivenous lymphoid sheets, is interpreted as the expression of strong cellular immunity, especially in beginning cancer and according to Black (1973) is an indication of a good prognosis.

Furthermore, if the lymphocyte infiltration around and within the tumor is accompanied by follicular hyper-plasia of the lymph nodes, with or without association of sinus histiocytosis, the prognosis should be consi-

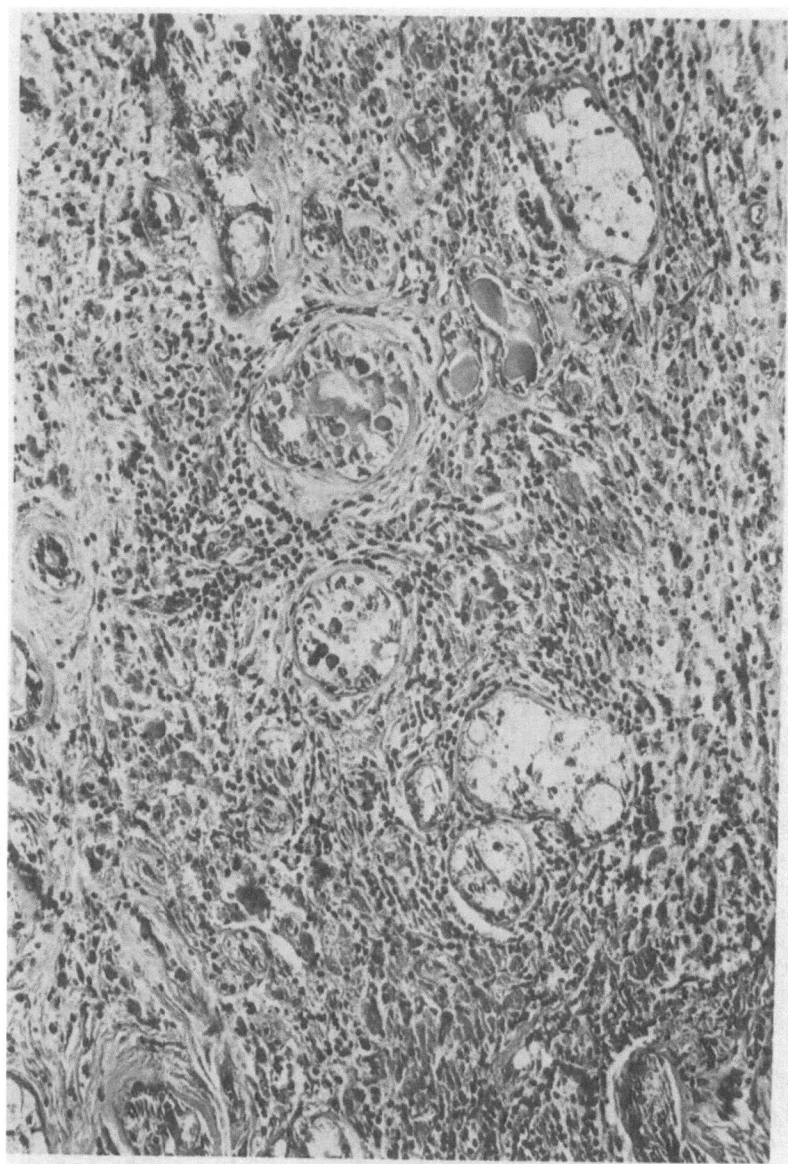

Fig. 4. Regression in a ductal carcinoma. Lymphocytic
         infiltration and sclerosis with disappearance
         of the carcinomatous cells. H & E, x 125.

dered as better, according to Hamlin (1968), Black and
Leis (1971) and Di Paola et al. (1974).

Tumor regression by modification of the ground substance

Apart from the role of the immune cells, other
factors, the mechanisms of which are unclear, may inter-
vene in the destruction of cancer cells. A number of beginning mammary carcinomas seem to have partially and
even totally healed spontaneously. Such a process depends
on necrosis of the stroma around precancerous lesions or
intraductal carcinoma, either in situ or with a beginning
infiltration. Askanazy (1931) estimated that the presence
of sclerosis around duct ectasia indicated a precancerous
state. In 1958, Orr suggested the same hypothesis concerning collagenosis and subepithelial elastosis. Azzopardi
and Laurini (1974), however, feel that there is no correlation between elastosis and malignancy, because such
phenomena occur in carcinoma as well as in certain benign
lesions such as sclerosing adenosis and certain types of
dysplasia, for instance dysplasia with epithelial infiltration.

It is therefore likely that those modifications are
related to the activity of the ductal cells which secrete
enzymes inducing metamorphism of the stroma with variable
secondary connective reconstruction.

The ground substance shows alterations corresponding
to "fibrinoid necrosis", a rather vague term but that
helps distinguish this metamorphism from amyloidosis,
which differs in its histochemical and immunofluorescent
reactions (Tremblay, 1974, 1976 ; Tobon and Salazar,
1977). The fibrinoid necrosis consistently appears around
the ducts, the flattened lumina of which disappear secondarily. The latter are sometimes lined with a cuboidal
epithelium with hyperchromatic nuclei (Fig. 5, 6 and 7).
Carcinomatous cells may fill the lumina. Elastic fibers,
after Weigert's stain, appear in the stroma, thick, wavy,
tangled or parallel, particularly in the central portion
of dense hyaline sclerosis. They also develop in the
venous walls and increase in the arteries.

The significance of the above described connective
tissue metamorphisms raise two questions :

1. Which cells direct the transformation of the
stroma and the differentiation of the elastic fibers ?
2. Should this transformation be considered to
favor cancer cell invasion, or on the contrary cancer
regression ?

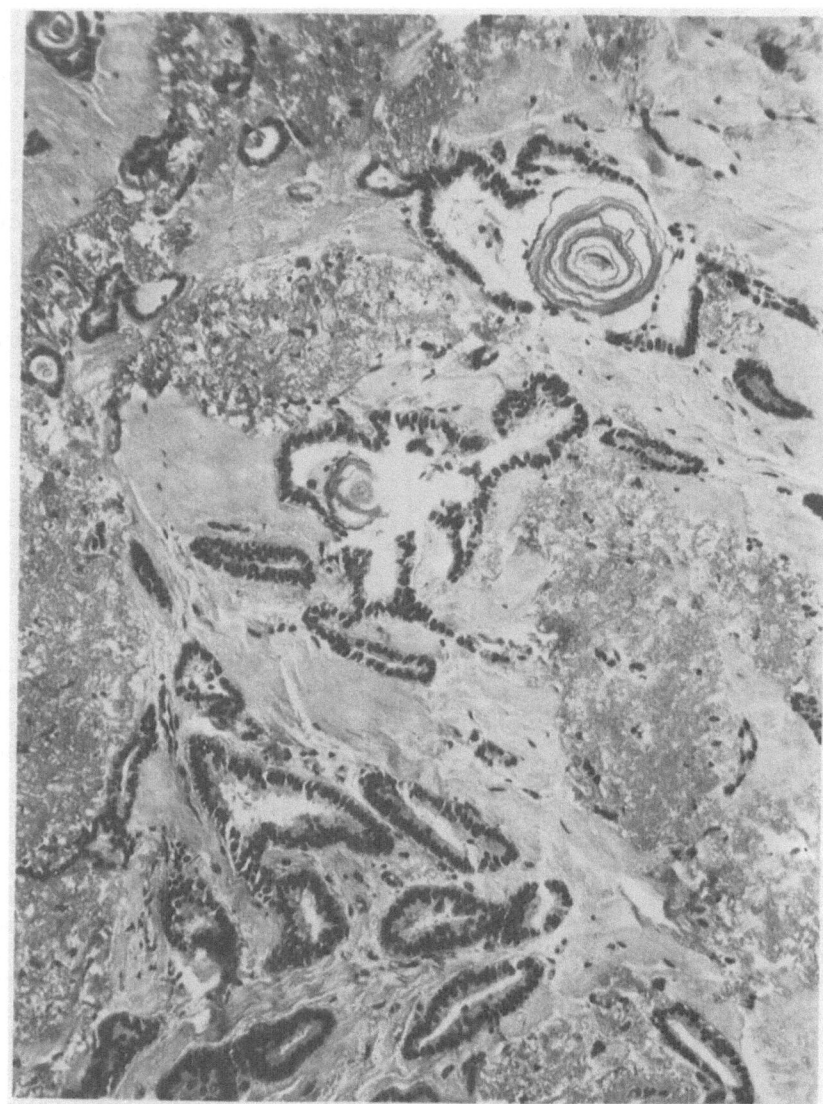

Fig. 5.   Well differentiated carcinoma.
          Elastogenesis in the stroma.
          H & E, x 160.

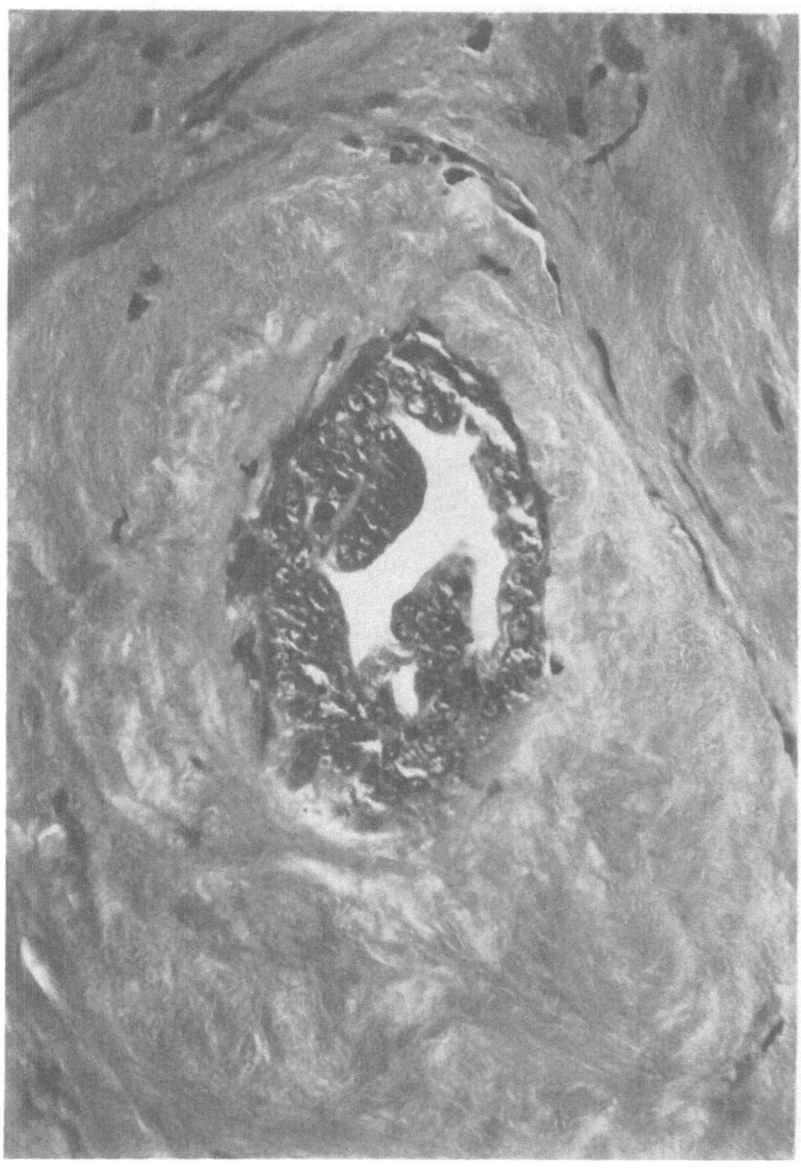

Fig. 6. Large sclerosis around a small duct carcinoma.
H & E, x 350.

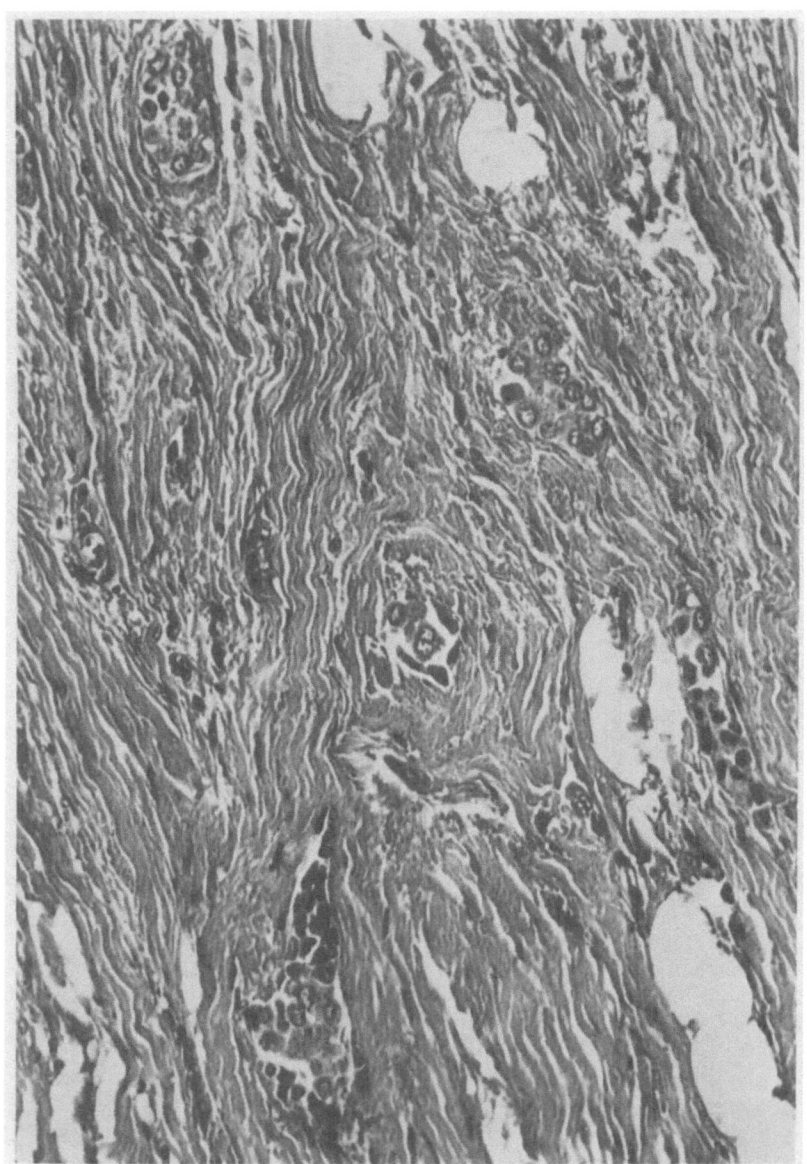

Fig. 7. Sclerosis in the adipose tissue after
         carcinomatous infiltration.
         H & E, x 250.

Tremblay (1976), studying the structure of the elastic fibers under electron microscope, showed that the central part is made of an amorphous substance and that, in the periphery, microfibrils can be distinguished. The variations between the two constituents, according to Tremblay, depend upon their degree of maturity, that is, the polymerization rate of the ground substance.

Hay (1970), studying embryonic tissue by radio-autography, and Ozzello (1959, 1970), studying in situ ductal carcinoma by electron microscopy, were able to demonstrate that the basal membrane was permeable and even favored the migration of embryonic cells and cancer cells, respectively, even when the basal membrane appears intact. As shown by Bossmann and Hall (1974), cancer cells secrete collagenosis enzymatic systems (sialyl transfe-rase, glycosyltransferase, neuraminidase) which are measured in the blood serum and which play a part in the functioning and regulation of the proteoglycoaminoglycans. These enzymatic secretions may be hormone-dependent, probably on estrogens, since Masters et al. (1976) dis-covered estrogen receptors in the cells of carcinoma with elastosis. The glycoproteins of microfibrillary structure will secondarily differentiate and become elas-tic fibers insoluble in water or in alkalyne solutions.

The cells inducing elastin synthesis are probably fibroblasts and/or myoepithelial cells (Azzopardi and Laurini, 1974 ; Tremblay, 1976), but according to Douglas and Shivas (1974), the cancer cells themselves could be directly involved in this mechanism. However, the fact that elastogenesis occurs in some benign lesions seems to indicate that it involves particular enzymatic capa-cities of mammary epithelial cells.

Such a hypothesis would answer the second question : the focal regression found in some carcinomas therefore depend on the ductal cell itself. These cells secreting proteolytic enzyme would determine the depolymerization of the connective tissue and would favor stromal inva-sion. As the cancer cells disperse, they induce the collagen metamorphism. Subsequently, elastogenic scle-rosis will be able to break down the carcinomatous cells.

REFERENCES

Askanazy, M., 1931, Die Beziehungen der gutartigen
     Erkrankungen der Brustdrüse zum Mamma Karzinom.

Beiträge zur pathologischen Anatomie und zur allgemeinen Pathologie ; 87, 396-424.

Azzopardi, J.G., and Laurini, R.N., 1974, Elastosis in breast cancer. Cancer, 33, 174-183.

Black, M.M., and Leis, H.P., 1971, Cellular response to autologous breast cancer tissue. Cancer, 28, 263-273.

Black, M.M., 1973, Human breast cancer ; a model for cancer immunology. Inst. J. Med. Sci., 9, 284-299.

Bonser, G.M., Dosset, J.A., and Jull, J.W., 1961, Human and experimental breast cancer, Pitman Medical, London.

Bossman, H.B., and Hall, T.C., 1974, Enzyme activity in invasive tumors of breast and colon. Proc. Nat. Acad. Sci. U.S.A., 71, 1833-1835.

Cantor, H., and Weissmann, J., 1976, Development and functions of subpopulation of thymocytes and T lymphocytes. Prog. Allergy, 20, 1-6.

Cottier, H., Turk, J., and Sobin, L., 1972, A proposal standardized system of reporting human lymph node morphology in relation to immunological function. Bull. W.H.O., 47, 375-379.

Di Paola, M., Angelini, L., Bertolotti, A., and Colizza, S., 1974, Host resistance in relation of survival in breast cancer. Brit. Med. J., 4, 266-271.

Douglas, J.G. and Shivas, A.A., 1974, The origins of elastica in breast carcinoma. J. Royal Coll. Surg. Edimburgh, 19, 89-93.

Hamlin, I.M.E., 1968, Possible host resistance in carcinoma of the breast. A histological study. Brit. J. Cancer, 22, 383-387.

Hay, E., 1978, Role of basement membrane in development and differentiation. In : Biology and chemistry of basement membranes, Kefalides, N.A. (ed), Academic Press, New York and London, pp 119-136.

Hollmann, K.H., 1974, Cytology and fine structure of the mammary gland. In : Lactation I, Larson B.L. and Smith V.R. eds, Academic Press, New York, 3-95.

Hollmann, K.H., and Verley, J.M., 1967, La régression de la glande mammaire à l'arrêt de la lactation. II. Etude au microscope électronique. Z. Zellforsch., 82, 222-238.

McFarland, J., 1922, Residual lactation acini in female breast : their relation to chronic cystic mastitis and malignant disease. Arch. Surg., 5, 1-6.

Martinez-Hernandez, Fink, L.M., and Pierce, B., 1976, Removal of basement membrane in the involving breast. Lab. Investig., 34, 455-462.

Masters, J.R.W., Sangster, K., Hawkins, R.A., and Shivas, A.A., 1976, Elastosis and oestrogen receptors in human breast cancer. Brit. J. Cancer, 33, 342-343.

Orr, J.W., 1958, The significance of connective tissue changes within the ducts in relation to mammary carcinoma. In : International Symposium on Mammary Cancer, Severi L. ed., p. 209, Perugia, Italy.

Ozzello, L., 1959, the behavior of basement membranes in intraductal carcinoma of the breast. Am. J. Pathol., 35, 887-895.

Ozzello, L., 1970, Epithelial-stroma junction of normal and dysplastic mammary glands. Cancer, 25, 586-600.

Richardson, W.W., 1956, Medullary carcinoma of the breast: a distinctive tumor type with a relatively good prognosis following radial mastectomy. Brit. J. Cancer, 10, 415-418.

Tobon, H., and Salazar, H., 1977, Tubular carcinoma of the breast. Clinical, histological and ultrastructural observations. Arch. Path. Lab. Med., 101, 310-316.

Tremblay, G., 1974, Elastosis in tubular carcinoma of the breast. Arch. Path., 98, 302-307.

Tremblay, G., 1976, Ultrastructure of elastosis in scirrhous carcinoma of the breast. Cancer, 37, 307-316.

Verley, J.M., and Hollmann, K.H., 1967, La régression de la glande mammaire à l'arrêt de la lactation. I. Etude au microscope optique. Z. Zellforsch., 82, 212-221.

THE NATURAL HISTORY OF HUMAN BREAST CANCER

M. Tubiana, A.J. Valleron and E. Malaise

Institut Gustave Roussy
94800 Villejuif, France

Breast carcinoma stands out for its broad spectrum of clinical behaviour, ranging from that of a highly aggressive neoplasm which disseminates shortly after diagnosis and causes death rapidly to that of a virtually chronic disease, compatible with many decades of survival even when initial therapy has failed to eradicate the cancer.

During this last decade, there have been many studies of the kinetics of tumor cell proliferation (Steel, 1977 ; Tubiana and Malaise, 1976) as well as the growth rates of human cancers (Sommers, 1973) and in particular of breast carcinomas (Gioanni et al., 1979; Meyer et al., 1978 ; Meyer and Hixon, 1979 ; Tubiana et al., 1975). Therefore it is of interest to consider to what extent this large amount of data can help in understanding the natural history of breast cancer (Berg and Robbins, 1966 ; Brinkley and Haybittle, 1975 ; Cutler et al., 1969). For the clinician, two questions are of paramount importance. Firstly, could an earlier detection of the primary tumor reduce the incidence of metastasis and what gain in complete cure rates can be expected from progress in the diagnostic process ? In order to answer this question we must establish the time at which the metastases were initiated and what percentage of them originated during the 3 to 6 months preceding clinical diagnosis. Secondly, do cell kinetics provide valuable prognostic information ? Adjuvant chemotherapy is for some patients a useful tool for the treatment of occult metastases, but this treatment is long,

toxic and not always well tolerated. Moreover its side-
effects are far from being negligible. Any prognostic
indicator which can help one to select the patients who
might benefit from adjuvant therapy is therefore of great
value. Let us consider these two points after a brief
review of our current knowledge about the growth rate of
human tumors.

CELL POPULATION KINETICS IN MALIGNANT TISSUES

        Malignant tumors are distinguished functionally
from normal tissues by a number of characteristics, notably continuous growth and distant metastasis.

        From a dynamic point of view, the basic difference
between a normal renewal tissue and a cancerous one is
that in the normal tissue there is an effective balance
between cell production and cell loss whereas in tumors,
cell production exceeds cell loss. If the net production
rate of cells were to remain constant a tumor would grow
exponentially. An exponential growth is fully characterized by its doubling time, that is the time interval
during which the volume of the tumor (or the number of
neoplastic cells) doubles. In practice the net production
rate of neoplastic cells varies greatly among different
cancer types as shown by the wide range of volume doubling times (DT). For human tumors the doubling times
vary from about one week to many years (Charbit et al.,
1971 ; Steel, 1977 ; Tubiana and Malaise, 1976). Indeed
rapid growth is not a characteristic of human cancers
and in general the cell proliferations in human tumors
are far less than those of normal human fetal tissues or
of many normal tissues stimulated to divide, for example
in the course of regeneration.

        In considering problems of the kinetics of cell
proliferation in human tumors it is important to define
the main parameters which are used in such studies. The
cell cycle time is equal to the time interval between
2 mitoses in the dividing cells of a cell population.
In human tumors the cell cycle time ranges from about
2 to 5 days and is therefore far less variable than the
doubling time (Tubiana and Malaise, 1976). The main
event which occurs during the cell cycle is the duplication of DNA. The phase of the cycle during which the
cell synthetizes the DNA is called the S-phase, the
duration of which is about one third that of the cell
cycle (Tubiana and Malaise, 1976). Cells in the S-phase,

and only them, incorporate thymidine, a specific pre-
cursor of DNA. After administration of radioactive thymidine, cells in the S-phase can be identified by autoradiography and the percentage of labelled cells is
called the labelling index (L.I.). (Chavaudra et al.,
1979).

The whole population of tumor cells does not divide :
a large proportion of the cells do not proliferate and
are quiescent. The ratio $\frac{P}{P + Q}$ (where P is the number
of proliferating cells and Q the number of quiescent
cells) is called the "Growth Fraction". Knowing the LI
and the relative durations of the S-phase and of the
cell cycle, one can calculate the growth fraction (G.F.).
Its numerical value ranges in human tumors from less
than 1 % to nearly 100 % (Malaise et al., 1973). The
G.F. is correlated with the histologic type of the tumors but can also vary greatly within a given type of
tumor. This variation is particularly wide for breast
cancers (Tubiana et al., 1975).

The potential doubling time is defined as the
doubling time which would be observed in the absence of
any cell loss, and is easy to calculate if one knows
the growth fraction and the duration of the cell cycle ;
it would be equal to the cell cycle time if all the
tumor cells were dividing (Growth Fraction equal to
unity). The comparison between the rate of production
of new cells with the observed growth rate of the tumor,
that is between the potential doubling time and the
actual doubling time, enables one to evaluate cell loss.
With many human tumors the extent of the cell loss is
very high and the cell loss factor, representing the
ratio of rate of cell loss to rate of new cell production, is sometimes more than 90 %. Growth fraction and
cell loss are the two major factors which determine the
growth rates of tumors (Steel, 1977 ; Tubiana and Malaise,
1976).

OCCURENCE OF METASTASES IN BREAST CANCERS

The various studies which have been carried out
show that metastases of breast cancers can become clinically detectable as late as 20 years (Berg and Robbins,
1966) after treatment of the primary tumor ; however
about half of them are detected during the 2.5 years
following surgical treatment (Cutler et al., 1969).

The growth rates of breast cancer have been measured by a few authors. The volume of the tumor is measured with X-Rays (mammography for the primary tumors, chest X-Ray for the lung metastases) and the time course change in volume is assessed by sequential X-Rays. We have previously reviewed our own data as well as the other published data (Tubiana et al., 1975). For most of the cases the growth of the tumor or of the metastases is exponential during the observation time and can be characterized by its doubling time (DT) ; however in some patients, and in particular for some of those who have been observed over a long period of time, a departure from exponential growth has been observed (Rambert et al., 1968 ; Steel, 1977).

The geometric mean DT of primary breast tumors has been found to be about 3.5 months but the spread of individual values is wider than in most other human cancers (Tubiana et al., 1975). The mean DT of lung metastases of breast carcinomas appears to be significantly shorter and is equal to 2.2 months (Tubiana et al., 1975). This is consistent with the observation made in other types of cancers in which the DT of the metastases has also been found to be shorter than the DT of the primary tumor (Malaise et al., 1973). The interpretation of this finding is not obvious. A simple explanation is that there is some clonal selection and that the metastases originate preferentially from relatively rapidly proliferating cells.

The data of Cutler et al. (1969) on a series of patients with breast cancers show a correlation in each patient between the duration of the first complete remission after treatment of the primary tumor and survival after first relapse suggesting that both are linked with the growth rate of the metastases. In fact we have shown previously the existence of a statistically significant correlation between the mean doubling time of the metastases of different histologic types of tumors and the mean survival after dissemination. It was clearly shown that the longer the mean doubling time the longer was the mean survival (Malaise et al., 1974). However, the relationship between the two parameters was not linear. Besides Kusama et al. (1972) have measured retrospectively the doubling times of a series of breast cancers on mammographies and have compared them with the outcome of the patients. In this series it was calculated that there is a correlation between the DT and the duration of survival.

We have recently performed a prospective study in which the labelling indices (LI) of breast carcinoma were measured consecutively in 128 patients and compared with the course of the disease (Tubiana et al., in press).

Samples of breast carcinomas were obtained in patients subjected to radical mastectomy. For patients initially treated by pre-operative radiotherapy cancer specimens were obtained by drill biopsies carried out before the initiation of radiotherapy. The fraction of neoplastic cells in the DNA synthetic phase of the cell cycle (S-phase) was measured by incubation of small specimens, less than 1 mm thick, with tritiated thymidine (^{3}H-TdR) and subsequent autoradiography. The length of follow-up was longer than six years for all patients. A significant correlation has been observed between on the one hand the LI of the primary tumor and on the other hand the time intervals between initial treatment and relapse or between the first relapse and death : the higher the LI, the shorter these time intervals. Thus our data extend and confirm the previous data. It was known that the LI of a tumor and its doubling time are highly correlated (Malaise et al., 1973) and it was suspected although not definitely proved that the DT of a primary tumor was correlated with the DT of its metastases (Charbit et al., 1971). Our data strongly suggest a correlation between the LI of the primary tumor and the DT of the metastases.

All these data stress that the natural history of a cancer depends upon the kinetics of cell proliferation. It is therefore legitimate to use available data on growth rates of lung metastases from breast cancers to calculate how long before their detection they originated ; in other words at what age did they become clinically detectable ?

Two types of models can be used for this estimation. The first is the so-called <u>exponential model</u> ; it assumes that the growth remains exponential during the life history of the metastases, from the seeding and mitosis of the few clonogenic cells which initiated the metastasis until clinical detection. This means that the DT remains constant during the entire history of the metastasis. This model is the simplest and most commonly used for human cancers because it has generally been observed that the growth rate of human tumors is exponential for the whole of the period during which their volume can be measured, that is in fact during a relatively short time interval corresponding to only 3 or 4 DT.

The second model which can be used is <u>Gompertz's</u> <u>model</u>. In this model the DT lengthens progressively as the tumor grows. Gompertz's model fits well the growth of the experimental tumors which it is possible to follow from the onset of the tumor, when only a few tens of cells are present, until the death of the animal when the tumor comprises 10^9 to 10^{10} cells, i.e. for about 30 DT. The only human tumor for which a Gompertzian growth has been demonstrated is multiple myeloma (Salmon and Durie, 1975) because the existence of an immunological marker enables to follow the growth over many logs, from about 10^6 cells until 10^9 or 10^{10} cells. However a progressively retarded growth is observed in some other human tumors and this suggests that for these tumors a Gompertzian model would be better than an exponential one (Rambert et al., 1968 ; Steel, 1977).

In 1975 we used the exponential model for the study of the natural history of breast cancer (Tubiana et al., 1975). Fig. 1 summarizes our findings. Extrapolation of the exponential growth curve suggests that the average age of the metastases when they are detected is about 4.5 years. As half of the metastases are detected during the first 2.5 years after treatment of the primary tumor, this means that half of the metastases start their growth two years or more before the time at which the primary tumor reached a clinically detectable size. If this model is correct a progress in diagnostic techniques which would permit the detection of breast cancer on an average six months earlier would result only in a relatively small decrease in the incidence of metastases.

Let us consider now the predictions of Gompertz's model. With this model the determination of the growth function requires 4 parameters : the DT and the size of the tumor at the time it was detected, the initial number of cells at seeding and the maximum volume reached by the tumor at the plateau of the curve. As compared to the exponential model, the only new parameter which has to be assumed is the volume of the tumor at plateau. In a preliminary computation we have assumed, at detection, a mean doubling time of 3.5 months and a size of 10^9 cells (1g). Fig. 2 illustrates the results obtained assuming a plateau value of 5 kgs and an initial

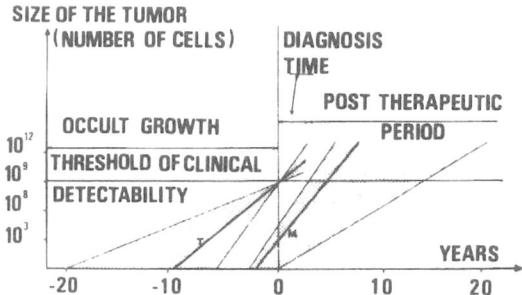

Fig. 1.   Natural history of breast carcinoma as predic-
           ted by the exponential model. The left side
           corresponds to the hidden history of the cancer,
           that is before it becomes clinically detecta-
           ble. T is for the primary tumor, M for metas-
           tases. Knowing the doubling time (D.T.) at
           diagnosis period and assuming that the D.T.
           remains constant throughout the whole history
           of the primary tumor or of the metastasis, it
           is easy to estimate how long before their cli-
           nical detection the primary tumor or the me-
           tastasis originated.
           The grey area corresponds to the range of D.T.,
           from tumors with a slow growth rate to tumor
           with a rapid growth rate. In only relatively
           few patients metastases start their growth
           during the few months preceding the treatment
           of the primary tumor.

number of cells equal to 1. Under these assumptions the
hidden history of the tumor is 4.5 years, instead of
9 years with corresponding exponential model. It is
worthwhile noting that these results are not significantly modified if one assumes plateau values ranging from
1 to 5 kgs and an initial number of cells varying between
1 and 1 000 (the range of the occult period is 38-53
months). The occult period for metastases, with a D.T.
at discovery of 2.2 months, ranges from 20 to 30 months
for a plateau value ranging from 0.1 to 0.5 kg. This
suggests that many of the metastases originated only a
few months or weeks before the diagnosis of the primary

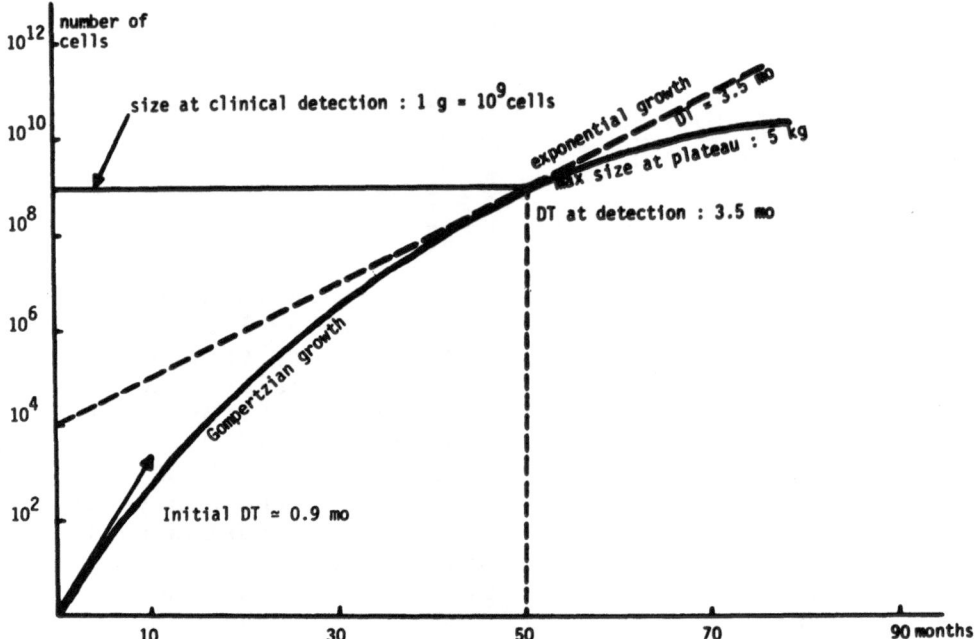

Fig. 2.   Natural history of breast cancer as predicted
          by Gompertz's model. In this model the doubling
          time lengthens progressively as the tumor grows.
          The left side corresponds to the hidden his-
          tory of the primary tumor.
          Assuming a same D.T. at the time of clinical
          detection of the primary tumor (3.5 months)
          this model predicts a shorter duration of the
          hidden history than the exponential model :
          50 months instead of 9 years.

tumor and that a small progress towards earlier diagnosis
would result in a notable decrease in the frequency of
patients with occult metastases. Preliminary data
showing an improvement of about 30 % in survival caused
by a screening program involving systematic mammography
(Strax, 1978) are consistent with the prediction of
such a model.

It is also noteworthy that the Gompertzian model's
predictions are consistent with the data of Philippe
and Le Gal (1968). These authors studied the time interval between surgical procedure and the detection of
recurrencies in the cutaneous scar of mammectomies.

Assuming an exponential growth they found that this time
interval corresponded to an average D.T. of 40 days which
is notably shorter than the D.T. of 2.2 months observed
for lung metastases. This discrepancy might be explained
by Gompertz's model. As shown on fig. 2, Gompertz's model
predicts for a tumor with a volume of 1 gram at detection
and with a D.T. of 2.2 months, a time interval between
birth and detection which is equal to that predicted by
the exponential model assuming a constant D.T. equal to
40 days.

KINETIC PARAMETERS OF CELL PROLIFERATION AND COURSE OF
THE DISEASE

     The detachment of cells from a tumor is certainly
not synonymous with metastasis formation, nonetheless
it represents the initial step of the process leading
to metastases (Poste and Fider, 1980). The occurrence
of metastases is therefore dependent on the characteristics of the detachment of cancer cells from primary
tumors as well as on the arrest of these cells in a
suitable tissue and the capability and opportunity for
some of the arrested cells to develop into metastases.
It is therefore plausible that the rate of cell detachment influences the incidence of metastases. Of all the
factors which affect the complex process of cell detachment and cell release, the proliferative activity of
the tumor might be one of the most important. In fact
it has been shown in vitro that increasing growth rate
facilitates detachment from glass and plastic surfaces
(Weiss, 1977). In addition, other factors generally
associated with proliferation also enhance cell detachment, such as activation of lysosomes, increased endo-
cytosis and changes in membrane permeability. Although
it is obvious that some slow growing tumors, such as
prostate, kidney and thyroid carcinomas, often metas-
tasize, it is tempting to hypothesize that one of the
factors which contributes to the high incidence of metastases is the rapid growth of the primary tumor
(Glucksmann, 1948 ; Slack et al., 1969 ; Weiss, 1977).

     In order to investigate this hypothesis for breast
cancers, we undertook a search for a correlation between
the kinetic parameters of the primary tumor and the
course of the disease after initial treatment prospec-
tively in a series of patients. As mentioned above we
measured the LI in the breast carcinomas of 128 patients
all treated by the same techniques (simple mastectomy
and axillary dissection, followed for the patients with

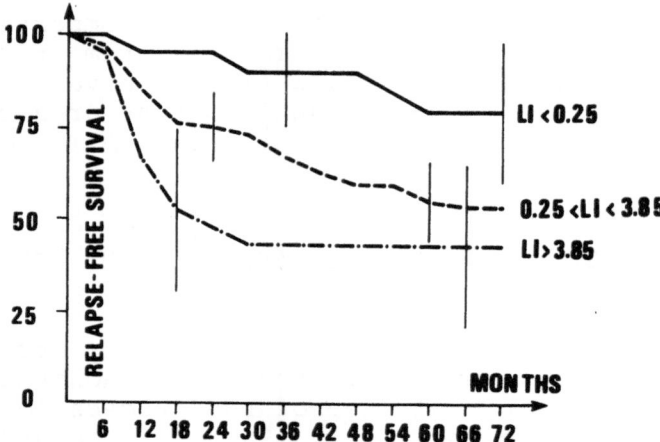

Fig. 3. Proportion of surviving patients free of relapse
at various time intervals after the treatment
of the primary tumor, in group of patients
with a high, median or low labelling index
(LI) (from Tubiana et al., in press).

metastasis bearing lymph nodes by post-operative radiotherapy). The follow-up period for all the patients is
now greater than 6 years (Tubiana et al., in press).

As can be seen on Figs. 3 and 4 for the group with
a high LI the survival and relapse-free curves decreased
abruptly during the first 2 years and then reached a
plateau. For the subgroup with a medium LI the decrease
was slower but at the sixth year no plateau is reached
and the trend suggests that despite the less rapid
evolution after primary therapy, the relapse-free survival and survival rates in this group will ultimately
be similar to those of the high LI subgroup. However the
subgroup with the low LI has a different trend. The
proportion of relapse is small, about 20 % by the 6th
year, and the shape of the curve suggests that the

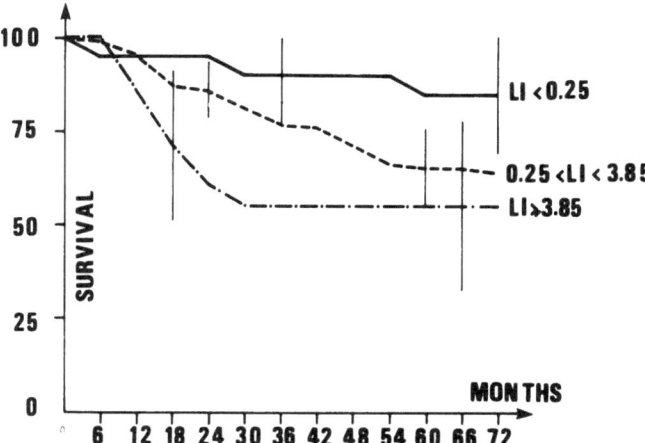

Fig. 4.   Proportion of surviving patients after treat-
          ment of the primary tumor in the 3 LI sub-
          groups (from Tubiana et al., in press).

outcome in this subgroup will definitely be better than
in the other two subgroups.

     Thus there is a clear association between the LI
and the incidence of relapse. However this correlation
might have been due to a coincidental correlation between the LI and other prognostic indicators. In order
to answer this question we studied the correlations
between the LI and various prognostic indicators. This
investigation was for the most part negative. No statistical correlation was found between the LI and UICC
staging, the existence or absence of an inflammatory
reaction, the age of the patients, their hormonal status,
or the histologic type of the tumor. It is well known
that the incidence of metastases is influenced by the
size of the mammary tumor at the time of initial treatment and this might be explained by a correlation between
the amount of cell release and the number of cells present in the tumor. Another interpretation has been
discussed previously : it has been suggested that the
growth rate of the primary tumor and its volume at

diagnosis were not independent factors, the larger tumors being on average the tumors with the higher growth rate (Berg and Robbins, 1966 ; Kusama et al., 1972). However this interpretation is not confirmed by our study as we did not find a correlation between the size of the tumor and the LI.

Another prominent prognostic indicator is the number of metastasis bearing axillary lymph nodes. Previous studies have shown that this number has a prognostic significance independent of the size of the tumor , (Contesso et al., 1977). Our study shows that it is also independent from the LI. This is in accordance with previous data which indicate that the mean survival time after initial treatment is not influenced by the number of involved axillary nodes (Tubiana et al., 1975).

Therefore in summary it seems that the LI gives a significant independent indication of prognosis. This is confirmed by statistical analysis showing that the LI prognostic value remains significant after adjustment for other parameters : size of the tumor, involvement of axillary nodes, age, hormonal status, existence of an inflammatory reaction.

The only statistically significant correlation that we found is between the LI and the histologic grading (Bloom and Richardson, 1957). Further analysis has shown that there was no correlation between the LI and the nuclear or the differentiation components of the histologic grading whereas a significant correlation existed between the mitotic component of the histologic grading and the LI ; this correlation is not surprising because both reflect the proliferative activity of the tumor. Thus this activity assessed either by the LI or the mitotic index, provides significant prognostic information. This is in accordance with some clinical studies performed twenty years ago in which the growth rate of the tumor was assessed by questioning the patients and which showed a lower survival for patients with a rapid growth rate (Lalanne, 1963 ; Richards, 1948 ; Rigby-Jones, 1963).

A striking feature of our data is that they show a remarkably good prognosis for the low LI group of patients despite the presence in this group of many patients with poor prognostic indicators. This finding is consistent with the data of Kusama et al.,(1972). These authors studied the survival of patients after surgical treatment

for breast cancer of various growth rates. They found
that the long term survival was significantly better
only in the subgroup with a doubling time longer than
6 months. In all the other subgroups despite considerable
spread of the DT and of the proportion of survival after
short-term follow-up, the long-term survival was the same.
This suggested a lower probability of cell dissemination
in this subgroup with a long DT.

REFERENCES

Berg, J.W., and Robbins, G.F., 1966, Factors influencing
        short and long term survival of breast cancer.
        Surg. Gynec. Obstet., 122, 1311-1316.
Bloom, H.J.G., and Richardson, W.W., 1957, Histological
        grading and prognosis in breast cancer. A study
        of 1 409 cases of which 359 have been followed
        15 years. Brit. J. Cancer, 11, 359-377.
Brinkley, D., and Haybittle, J.L., 1975, The curability
        of breast cancer. Lancet, 2, 95-97.
Charbit, A., Malaise, E., and Tubiana, M., 1971, Relation
        between the pathological nature and the growth
        rate of human tumors. Europ. J. Cancer, 7, 307-
        315.
Chavaudra, N., Richard, J.M., and Malaise, E.P., 1977,
        Labelling index of human squamous cell carcinomas.
        Comparison of in vivo and in vitro labelling
        methods. Cell Tissue Kinet., 12, 145-152.
Contesso, G., Rouesse, J., Petit, J.Y., and Mouriesse,
        H., 1977, Les facteurs anatomo-pathologiques du
        pronostic des cancers du sein. Bull. Cancer (Paris),
        64, 525-536.
Cutler, S.J., Asire, J.A., and Taylor, S.G., 1969, Classi-
        fication of patients with disseminated cancer of
        the breast. Cancer, 24, 861-869.
Gioanni, J., Farges, M.F., Asin, Ch., and Lalanne, C.M.,
        1979, L'index de marquage dans les cancers du sein
        et des voies aéro-digestives supérieures. Bull.
        Cancer (Paris), 66, 479-484.
Glucksmann, A., 1948, The relation of radiosensitivity
        and radiocurability to the histology of tumor
        tissue. Br. J. Radiol., 21, 559-566.
Kusama, S., Spratt, J.S., Donegan, W.L., Watson, F.R.,
        and Cunningham, C., 1972, The gross rates of
        growth of human mammary carcinoma. Cancer (Philad.),
        30, 594-599.
Lalanne, C.M., 1963, Taux d'accroissement et pronostic
        des tumeurs malignes du sein. In "Symposium on

the Prognosis of Malignant Tumours of the Breast",
    p. 16, Karger, Bâle.
Malaise, E.P., Chavaudra, N., and Tubiana, M., 1973,
    The relationship between growth rate, labelling
    index and histological type of human solid tumours.
    Europ. J. Cancer, 9, 305-312.
Malaise, E.P., Chavaudra, N., Charbit, A., and Tubiana,
    M., 1974, Relationship between the growth rate of
    human metastases, survival and pathological type.
    Europ. J. Cancer, 10, 451-459.
Meyer, J.S., Bauer, W.C., and Rao, B.R., 1978, Subpopu-
    lations of breast carcinoma defined by S-phase
    fraction, morphology, and estrogen receptor con-
    tent. Lab. Invest., 39, 225-235.
Meyer, J.S., and Hixon, B., 1979, Advanced stage and
    early relapse of breast carcinomas associated with
    high Thymidine labelling indices. Cancer Research,
    39, 4042-4047.
Philippe, E., and Le Gal, Y., 1968, Growth of 78 recurrent
    mammary cancers. Quantitative study. Cancer
    (Philad.), 21, 461-467.
Poste, G., and Fider, I.J., 1980, The pathogenesis of
    cancer metastasis. Nature, 283, 139-146.
Rambert, P., Malaise, E., Laugier, A., Schlienger, M.,
    and Tubiana, M., 1968, Données sur la vitesse de
    croissance des tumeurs humaines. Bull. Cancer
    (Paris), 55, 323-342.
Richards, G.E., 1948, Mammary cancer, Part I. Brit. J.
    Radiol., 21; 109-127.
Rigby-Jones, P., 1963, Prognosis of malignant tumours
    of the breast in relation to rate of growth and
    axillary lymph node involvement as observed cli-
    nically. In "Symposium on the Prognosis of Mali-
    gnant Tumours of the Breast", p. 24, Karger, Bâle.
Salmon, S.E., and Durie, B.G.M., 1975, Cellular kinetics
    in multiple myeloma. A new approach to staging
    and treatment. Arch. Intern. Med., 135, 131-138.
Slack, N.H., Blumenson, L.E., and Bross, I.D.J., 1969,
    Therapeutic implications from a mathematical model
    characterizing the course of breast cancer. Cancer
    (Philad.), 24, 960-971.
Sommers, S.C., 1973, Growth rates, cell kinetics and
    mathematical models of human cancers. Pathobiology
    Annual, vol. 3, p. 309, Appleton-Century-Croft,
    New York.
Strax, P., 1978, Evaluation of screening programs for
    the early diagnosis of breast cancer. Surgical
    Clinics North-America, 58, 667-679.
Steel, G.G., 1977, Growth kinetics of tumours, Clarendon
    Press. Oxford.

Tubiana, M., Chauvel, P., Renaud, A., and Malaise, E.P.,
    1975, Vitesse de croissance et histoire naturelle
    du cancer du sein. Bull. Cancer (Paris), 62,
    341-358.
Tubiana, M., and Malaise, E.P., 1976, Comparison of cell
    proliferation kinetics in human and experimental
    tumors : response to irradiation. Cancer Treat.
    Rep., 60, 1887-1895.
Tubiana, M., Pejovic, M.J., Renaud, A., Contesso, G.,
    Chavaudra, N., Gioanni, J., and Malaise, E.P.,
    1980, Kinetic parameters and the course of the
    disease in breast cancer. Submitted to Cancer.
Weiss, L., 1977, A pathobiologic overview of metastasis.
    Sem. Onc., 4, 5-17.

TUMOR ASSOCIATED MARKERS IN BREAST CANCER

P. Franchimont[1], P.F. Zangerle[1*], J. Collette[1],
C. Colin[2], P. Osterrieth[3], J.C. Hendrick[1**],
J.R. Van Cauwenberge[2], and J. Hustin[2]

Institute of Medicine,
Radioimmunoassay Laboratory[1], Obstetrics and
Gynecology Department[2], Bacteriology and Viro-
logy Department[3],
University of Liège, Belgium

Several tumor markers have been assayed in serum
of patients suffering from breast diseases in order to
improve the early detection of cancer, to contribute to
its diagnosis, to evaluate the local and metastatic extension of the neoplasia, to monitor the follow-up of
previously diagnosed cancer and to provide useful prognosis information. In this article, the potential interest of some tumor markers will be stressed as the limits
of some others.

RESULTS OF INDIVIDUAL TUMOR MARKERS

Oncofoetal antigens.

Two oncofoetal antigens were assayed : alpha foeto
protein (α-FP) (Franchimont et al., 1975) and carcino
embryonic antigen (CEA) extracted from liver metastasis
(Franchimont et al., 1974).

1. As described previously (Franchimont et al., 1977)
α-FP is never positive whatever the stage of the breast

* Aspirant Chercheur du F.N.R.S.
** Chargé de Recherches du F.N.R.S.

cancer (T), the extension of the neoplasm (N,M) and the mode of treatment. Thus,α-FP measurement has no clinical interest in breast cancer.

2. CEA determination is an useful criterion in the diagnosis, follow-up and prognosis of breast cancer. In the serum of 935 blood donors, the detectable levels never exceed 10 ng/ml. The results obtained in a population of women with breast diseases (Franchimont et al., 1977) are illustrated in table 1. CEA is discriminating between benign and malignant breast diseases and the incidence of positivity as the absolute concentration of CEA increases when metastases exist. Furthermore, abnormal postoperative CEA levels are associated with lymph node extension (table 1).

Placental antigens

HCG and its α-and β-subunits were assayed using specific radioimmunoassays (Franchimont et al., 1978). In the normal population native HCG, α-and β-subunit levels never exceeded 1 ng/ml, 3,5 ng/ml and 1,5 ng/ml respectively. The incidence of pathological values of α-(> 3,5 ng/ml) and β (> 1,5 ng/ml) subunits is lower in breast cancer population than in non benign breast diseases. Native HCG levels were found elevated in 6 of 39 breast cancer patients (15%) at the onset of clinical symptoms (T_1,T_2,T_3,N_O,M_O) in absence of matastasis (N_O) and before any treatment. Surprisingly, none of 25 patients with metastatic disease had elevation of HCG and its α-and β-subunits. Thus, there is a weak incidence of abnormal HCG levels in breast cancer and no discrimination between benign disorders and malignant breast diseases for α-and β-HCG subunits.

Milk Proteins

Amongst milk proteins, two were extensively investigated in our laboratory : casein (Hendrick et al., 1976; Franchimont et al., 1979) and Gross Cystic Disease Fluid Protein (G.C.D.F.P.) (Haagensen et al., 1976) ; Zangerle et al., 1979).

Kappa casein. Casein may be considered as a good marker for the functional activity of the normal mammary gland (Franchimont et al., 1979). Thus, serum K casein levels increased during pregnancy and reached very high values when milk is produced during the first days of lactation.

TABLE 1

NATURE OF THE DISEASE	TOTAL n	CEA > 10 ng/ml		CASEIN > 25 ng/ml	
		n	%	n	%
Benign breast diseases	55	0	0	1	1.7
Breast cancer :					
– Onset of the disease (T_1, T_2, T_3, N_0, N_1, M_0)	39	20	51	6	15
– With metastases (M+)	25	14	56	11	44
– After surgical removal :					
N–	30	0	0	1	1.7
M+	.39	15	39	7	19

In breast cancer, immunoreactive kappa casein is detected at higher concentration than in normal population (i.e. >25 ng/ml) as illustrated in table 1. The metastatic extension increases both the incidence of positive casein values and the absolute levels (Franchimont et al., 1977).

Lung, digestive and urinary tract cancers can also release casein like materials in the blood which demonstrates the existence of an ectopic exocrine secretion (Franchimont et al., 1979).

As it will be demonstrated later on, casein level may provide a criterion of prognosis when assayed with CEA.

Gross Cystic Disease Fluid Protein (G.C.D.F.P.). Haagensen et al. (1976) recently described a glycoprotein isolated from breast gross cyst disease fluid with a molecular weight of 15.000. This G.C.D.F.P. is believed to be an epithelial cell secretory product, is present in milk and saliva and is expressed in very high concentrations in the fluid of breast cysts.

With the radioimmunoassay carried out in our laboratory (Zangerle et al., 1979), G.C.D.F.P. levels were most often undetectable in the serum of 277 normal subjects. Only in three subjects of the normal population, G.C.D.F.P. levels were higher than 5 ng/ml (1 %). In 1 of 30 (3 %) lactating women, levels were higher than 5 ng/ml whereas no value as high as 5 ng/ml were detected in the serum of 17 pregnant women. In contrast with casein, G.C.D.F.P. does not appear as functional index of normal mammary gland.

G.C.D.F.P. levels were higher than 5 ng/ml only in 1,5 % of patients with non benign breast diseases (251 cases).

In breast diseases, the incidence of G.C.D.F.P. levels higher than 5 ng/ml and the mean levels are elevated in benign cystic disease and in breast cancer whatever the stage (table II) compared with the values observed in non cystic breast benign diseases.

When metastasis exists, the incidence and the absolute levels of G.C.D.F.P. increase (Zangerle et al., 1979).

TABLE II

BREAST DISEASES	n	INCIDENCE OF G.C.D.F.P. LEVELS higher than 5 ng/ml		MEAN LEVELS ng/ml $\pm$ SEM
		n	%	
Non cystic breast diseases	85	3	3.5	2 ± 1.04
Cystic breast diseases	53	30	58	12 ± 3.2
Breast carcinoma	98	64	66	44 ± 8.3

G.C.D.F.P. appears to be specific for breast diseases
as it is very rarely detected in serum in patients with
benign diseases or cancers of lung, digestive and other
origins.

Hormones

Levels of calcitonin, parathormone, prolactin were
always detected in the normal range when assayed with
our radioimmunological methods in serum of patients with
benign and malignant breast diseases (Heynen, 1976).

Viral peptides from MuMTV

Some publications have described that antigens extracted from human breast cancer cross reacted with pep-
tides contained in MuMTV. Thus, Black et al.(1976) described an antigen GP50 in breast cancer cross reacting
with GP47 from MuMTV. Furthermore, a protein with a
molecular weight of 27.000 was described in "virus core"
prepared from human milk (Furmanski et al., 1976) and
antibodies to antigens related to the core antigens of
MuMTV were detected in the serum of breast cancer patients
(Muller et al., 1976).

On that basis, we initiated a work on RIA of all the
constituants of MuMTV and of antibodies against them.

Presently, two specific radioimmunoassays were
carried out, one for GP47, the main envelope glycoprotein
of MuMTV (Zangerle et al., 1977) and the other for P28
the main core protein of MuMTV (Hendriek et al., 1978).

Although GP47 and P28 were measured in several organs
and serum of infected and tumor bearing mice, no substance immunologically related to GP47 and P28 were detected
either in sera from 107 normal subjects, 65 women with
benign mastopathy (9 fibroadenoma, 36 polycystic diseases,
20 considered to be a risk of developing breast cancer),
89 from women with breast cancer at different stages of
clinical evolution, or in 15 cystic fluids or in 12 milks
or in 50 breast cancer extracts. Furthermore, no antibody
against GP47 and P28 was detected in the same media.

More than ten different antisera for each antigen
were used to exclude the possible selection of antibody
only directed against antigenic groups specific for MuMTV.

Sporadic positive results could be interpreted by
the fact GP47 and P28 are damaged by proteases present

either in the serum or in organ extracts. Thus, RIA may give false positive results.

Before concluding to the absence of cross reaction between constituants of MuMTV and human breast cancer, this work should be extended to the other components of MuMTV and to the whole virus. Some works seem to indicate that antibodies detected in serum of women with breast cancer are directed against the whole virus (Day, 1979) and that antiserum against whole virus gives positive results by immunofluorescence when reacting with some breast cancer tissues (Loisillier et al., 1979).

CLINICAL INTEREST OF ASSAYING MARKERS

On the basis of our work the assay of tumor markers may be interesting in the following areas.

Factor of risk

Till now, assays of tumor markers do not provide any indication on the risk for a women to develop a breast cancer. But G.C.D.F.P. could be useful for that purpose as it is a specific breast marker and its incidence of positivity is high in gross cystic disease. A long term evaluation of more than 2.000 patients with gross cyst disease has revealed that breast carcinoma developed at more than four times the frequency in normal women (Haagensen et al., 1976).

An epidemiological and histological study of women with breast cyst disease and positive G.C.D.F.P. in blood is needed to accept or refute this epithelial protein as a biological index of risk.

Tumor markers and diagnosis

As previously stated (Franchimont et al., 1976), measurement of tumor markers is an useful diagnostic procedure which, however, is neither absolute nor specific.

Simultaneous assays of several tumor markers decrease the incidence of "false negative" cancer. In breast cancer, CEA is abnormally high in 51 % of cases at the onset of clinical symptoms whereas abnormally high CEA or casein levels are detected in 65 % of these cases.

Furthermore, the detection of abnormal levels of specific marker such as G.C.D.F.P. leads to the diagnosis of a breast disease.

Extension of the tumor

As many authors and our group have already demonstrated (Franchimont et al., 1977), the incidence of positivity as the absolute levels of CEA, kappa casein and G.C.D.F.P. increase with the local and metastatic extension of breast cancer (Franchimont et al., 1977).

Tumor markers and prognosis

Two retrospective studies were done and confirm the main interest of cancer markers as an index of prognosis.

Breast tumors were removed from 69 patients in 1966. Compared with the incidence before surgery the incidence of positivity of at least one of the two cancer antigens assayed (CEA and kappa casein) dropped from 65 % to 33 %. Thirty patients had no evidence of lymph node involvement or of distant metastases ($N-, M_o$). Casein was found only in one case. The incidence of positivity of at least one antigen was therefore 1 out of 30. In contrast, 39 patients who had been treated surgically had at least one lymph node metastasis in the draining gland (N+). The frequency of appearance of casein and CEA was 7 and 15 on 39 cases respectively (table 1). One case was positive for CEA and casein and, then, 21/39 were tumor marker positive (56 %).

Two years later, local recurrence and/or metastases have appeared in 4 of 30 cases N-,CEA- (one of the 4 patients was casein positive), in 10 of 24 cases N+CEA- (5 of them were casein positive) and in 10 of 15 patients N+CEA+. Local and distant recurrence was observed in 16/22 (72 %) with abnormal high levels of casein or CEA and in only 8/47 (17 %) in absence of these tumor markers.

Extension may be predicted when CEA or casein is detected in abnormally high levels in absence or in presence of lymph node invasion.

As casein and CEA, Gross Cyst Disease Fluid Protein is not detected in serum of women after removal of breast tumor when lymph nodes are not invaded (0/9) whereas 9/13 patients with lymph node metastasis are G.C.D.F.P. positive.

In a retrospective study, Colin (1979) correlated the evolution of small breast cancer (T_1, T_2) after surgical removal with several parameters : number of invaded lymph nodes, invasion of mammary chain nodes, histological grade, thermographical and radiological stages and increased levels of CEA or casein.

No patient with a good prognosis i.e. alife without local or distant recurrence two years after removal of the tumor had high CEA or kappa casein levels. No invasion of lymph nodes and weakly evolutive aspects of histological, radiological and thermographical investigations were observed in these cases. In contrast, high CEA and/or casein levels were measured in 11 of 16 patients with bad prognosis and who died within two years following the operation. Lymph nodes of these patients were invaded, and/or radiological, thermographical and histological investigations gave highly evolutive results. Nine patients with recurrence and/or metastasis but still alife two years after breast cancer removal were classified in the category of poor prognosis. CEA or casein were detected in the serum of three of them.

Thus, increased levels of CEA and casein are always measured in patients with poor or bad prognosis whereas absence of CEA and casein are observed in patients of the three groups, the incidence decreasing with aggravation of the prognosis.

ACKNOWLEDGEMENTS

Supported by Grant n° 20305 from National Foundation for Medical Research (F.R.S.M.) and by C.G.E.R. Foundation for Cancer Research.

REFERENCES

Black, M.M., Zachrau, R.E., Dion, A.S., Shore, B., Fine, D.L., Leis, H.P. Jr., and Williams, C.J., 1976, Cellular hypersensitivity to GP55 of RIII Murine Mammary Tumor Virus and GP55-like protein of human breast cancers. Cancer Res., 36, 4137-4142.

Colin, C., Submitted for publication (1979).

Day, N.K., 1979, Communication at the XXVII Annual Colloquium on : "Protides of the biological fluids", Brussels.

Franchimont, P., Debruche, M.L., Zangerle, P.F., and
      Proyard, J., 1974, Carcinoembryonic antigen (CEA).
      In : "Radioimmunoassay and Related Procedures in
      Medicine", Vol. II, International Atomic Energy
      Agency, Vienne, 267-274.
Franchimont, P., Zangerle, P.F., Debruche, M.L., Proyard,
      J., Simon, P., and Gaspard, U., 1975, Dosage
      radioimmunologique de l'alpha foeto proteine dans
      les différentes conditions normales et patholo-
      giques. Ann. Biol. Clin., 33, 139-148.
Franchimont, P., Zangerle, P.F., Nogarede, J., Bury, J.,
      Molter, F., Reuter, A., Hendrick, J.C., and
      Collette, J., 1976, Simultaneous assays of cancer-
      associated antigens in various neoplastic disor-
      ders. Cancer, 38, 2287-2295.
Franchimont, P., Zangerle, P.F., Hendrick, J.C., Reuter,
      A., and Colin, C., 1977, Simultaneous assays of
      cancer associated antigens in benign and malignant
      breast diseases. Cancer, 39, 2806-2812.
Franchimont, P., Reuter, A., and Gaspard, U., 1978, Ecto-
      pic production of human chorionic gonadotropin
      and its α-and β-subunits. In : "Current Topics in
      Experimental Endocrinology", L. Martini and
      V.H.T. James, Eds., Academic Press, New York,
      London, Vol. 3, 204-216.
Franchimont, P., Hendrick, J.C., Thirion, A., and
      Zangerle, P.F., 1979, Kappa casein : an index of
      normal mammary function and tumor associated
      antigen. In : "Immunodiagnosis of Cancer", R.B.
      Herberman and K.R. McIntire, Eds., M. Dekker,
      Inc., New York, Basel, Part I, 499-512.
Furmanski, P., Loeckner, C.P., Longley, C., Larson, L.J.,
      and Rick, M.A., 1976, Identification and isolation
      of the major core protein from the oncornavirus-
      like particle in human milk. Cancer Res., 36,
      4001-4007.
Haagensen, D.E. Jr., Mazoujian, G., Holder, W. Jr.,
      Kister, S.J., and Wells, S.A. Jr., 1976, Evalua-
      tion of a breast cyst fluid protein detectable
      in the plasma of breast carcinoma patients.
      Ann. Surg., 3, 277-289.
Hendrick, J.C., Thirion, A., and Franchimont, P., 1976,
      Radioimmunoassay of casein. In : "Cancer Related
      Antigens", P. Franchimont, Ed., North-Holland,
      Amsterdam, 51-59.
Hendrick, J.C., François, C., Calberg-Bacq, C.M., Colin,
      C., Franchimont, P., Gosselin, L., Kozma, S.,
      and Osterrieth, P.M., 1978, Radioimmunoassay for
      protein p28 of murine mammary tumor virus in
      organs and serum of mice and search for related

antigens in human sera and breast cancer extracts.
Cancer Res., 38, 1826-1830.

Heynen, G., 1976, Discussion in "Cancer Related Antigens",
P. Franchimont, Ed., North-Holland, Amsterdam,
New York, 160-162.

Loisillier, F., Saracino, J., Metivier, D., and Burtin,
P., 1979, Characterisation of an antigen associated
to human mammary carcinoma. In : "Protides of the
biological fluids", XXVII Annual Colloquium,
Brussels, Abstr. n° 65.

Muller, M., Zotter, S., and Kemmer, C., 1976, Specificity
of human antibodies to intracytoplasmic type A
particles of the murine mammary tumor virus.
J. Natl. Cancer Inst., 56, 295-303.

Zangerle, P.F., Calberg-Bacq, C.M., Colin, C., Franchimont, P., François, C., Gosselin, L., Kozma, S.,
and Osterrieth, P.M., 1977, Radioimmunoassay for
glycoprotein GP47 of murine mammary tumor virus
in organs and serum of mice and search for related
antigens in human sera. Cancer Res., 37, 4326-4331.

Zangerle, P.F., Collette, J., and Franchimont, P., 1979,
Specific radioimmunoassay for gross cystic disease
fluid protein (G.C.D.F.P.). Submitted for publication.

CONTRIBUTION OF ESTROGEN RECEPTORS TO THE STRATEGY
OF BREAST CANCER TREATMENT

J.C. Heuson[1], R. Paridaens[1], E. Ferrazzi[2],
N. Legros[1], G. Leclercq[1], and R.J. Sylvester[3]

Institut J. Bordet,
Centre des tumeurs de l'université libre de
Bruxelles,
1000 Bruxelles - Belgium

INTRODUCTION

Polychemotherapy and hormonal therapy are currently the major therapeutic modalities in advanced breast cancer. The former is the most effective ($\geqslant 50$ percent response rate) but the second is less toxic, with a response rate of about 30 %. The recent development of estrogen receptor determination in breast cancer tissue samples has improved the clinician's ability to use these modalities either separately or together in an optimum manner.

Estrogen receptors are soluble proteins present in the cytoplasm of various normal and neoplastic tissues. They seem to play a key role in the mechanisms of action of the estrogens in these tissues. Estrogens such as the

1.Service de Médecine et Laboratoire d'Investigation Clinique H.J. Tagnon. Clinique et Laboratoire de Cancérologie Mammaire.
2.E.O.R.T.C. fellow sponsored by the Swiss Leage against Cancer
3.Statistician of the E.O.R.T.C. Data Center.
These institutions are affiliated with the European Organization for Research on Treatment of Cancer (E.O.R.T.C.). The Data Center is part of this Organization.

natural hormone 17 β-estradiol bind to the receptors in
the target tissues and form high-affinity complexes that
are translocated into the cell nuclei. The complexes then
affect the transcriptional activity of DNA and thereby
act as regulators of cell growth or differentiation.

Since the pioneer work of Jensen et al. (1971),
numerous studies have confirmed the clinical usefulness
of estrogen receptor determination in metastases from
breast cancer. Thus, estrogen receptor-positive (ER+)
tumors have a 55 percent chance to respond to endocrine
treatments while receptor-negative (ER-) tumors have
a response rate of about 10 % (McGuire et al., 1975).
We have suggested in a previous work on a small number
of cases that the distinction ER+/ER- was largely artificial at least in terms of clinical prediction of
hormone-responsiveness (Heuson et al., 1977). Rather, the
probability of response to endocrine treatments was a
function of ER concentration, along a continuous gradient
of hormone dependency. The study presented here completes
and extends the former work, and confirms the validity
of the concept proposed. Furthermore, it indicates that
this concept leads to a revision of the traditional
approach to breast cancer treatment and favors the combined use of endocrine and cytotoxic therapies. The
results of clinical trials conducted along this line
by the E.O.R.T.C.[1] Breast Cancer Cooperative Group will
be reported.

RELATIONSHIP BETWEEN ESTROGEN RECEPTOR CONCENTRATION
AND THE PROBABILITY OF A RESPONSE TO ENDOCRINE TREATMENTS

The study reported here includes all patients with
inoperable, recurrent or metastatic carcinoma of the
breast whose response to an endocrine treatment could be
assessed and who had a biopsy taken for estrogen receptor
determination and histology prior to initiation of the
treatment. Any patient with a second cancer (including
second breast) or with CNS or massive liver involvement
was excluded. Any patient having received hormones or
cytotoxic chemotherapy within two weeks of the biopsy
(two months in the case of antiestrogens or depot preparations) or between biopsy and initiation of the
treatment to be evaluated was also excluded.

1. E.O.R.T.C. : European Organization for Research on
   Treatment of Cancer.

The criteria for assessment of patients' response
to treatment were basically those of the E.O.R.T.C.
Breast Cancer Cooperative Group (Heuson et al., 1975).
In brief, the size of each measurable lesion should decrease by at least 50 %. For evaluable but non-measurable
lesions, an objective document (picture, X-ray) establishing tumor regression is required. All cases not
fulfilling the criteria of remission after 3 months of
therapy were considered as therapeutic failures. Premature
interruption of treatment because of drug intolerance,
or patients loss to follow-up were interpreted as causes
of ineligibility instead of therapeutic failures, because
the purpose of the present study was to analyse response
to treatments that were actually administered for a long
enough period of time. The medical records of the patients
added here in complement to the original series (Heuson
et al., 1977) were presented in detail by one of the
authors (E.F.) and assessed for response by two others
(J.C.H. and R.P.) who did ignore the results of the
receptor assays.

The estrogen receptor assays were carried out by
a classical dextrancoated charcoal method based on the
measurement of the binding capacity of cytosol to
^{3}H -17 μ-estradiol (Leclercq et al., 1973). The results
were expressed as femtomoles (10^{-15} moles) per mg of
tissue protein (E.O.R.T.C., 1973). All samples were
verified histologically for the presence of tumor tissue.
Except in two patients, all receptor assays were performed within 6 months of commencement of therapy.

Forty-eight patients were available for assessment
of response to endocrine treatment. One patient had
been assessed twice. A total of forty-nine evaluable
courses of therapy is therefore available. Twelve patients were premenopausal or within less than one year
of their last menstrual period. The other patients were
at least one year after their natural or surgical menopause. Various endocrine treatments were given : surgical
oophorectomy (10), surgical adrenalectomy (9), administration of ethinyl-estradiol (6), antiestrogens (20), androgens (1) and aminoglutethimide (3). Fourteen remissions
were recorded which represents a proportion of success
of 29 percent in the whole group.

Thirty-eight biopsies from 37 patients contained
estrogen receptors (ER+), whereas 11 were negative (ER-).
This proportion of 78 percent ER+ cases is of the same
order as is usually found in the laboratory for unse-
lected cases (Leclercq et al., 1975). ER concentrations

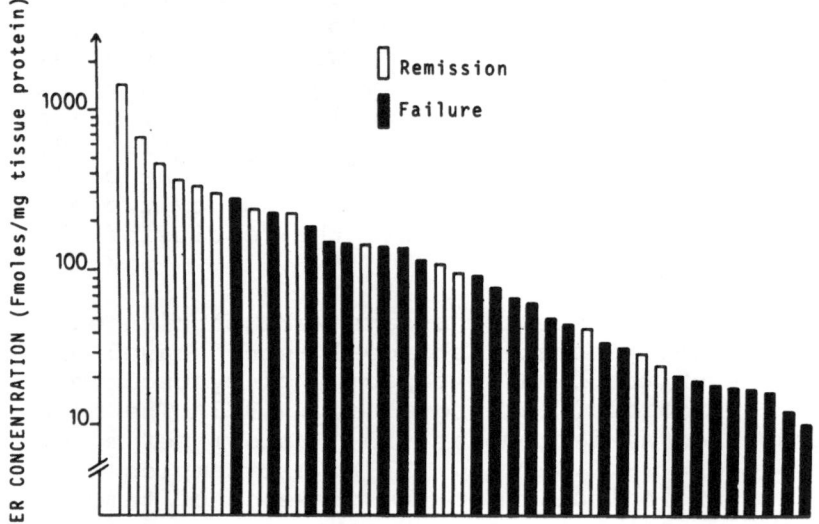

Fig. 1. Estrogen receptor concentrations in individual
        patients who responded (white column) or
        failed to respond (dark column) to endocrine
        treatments.

Table 1 : SIGNIFICANCE OF ESTROGEN RECEPTOR USED AS QUALITATIVE VARIABLE FOR PREDICTION OF RESPONSE TO ENDOCRINE THERAPY

CUT-OFF LEVEL OF ER fmoles/mg tissue protein	PATIENTS WITH ER ABOVE CUT-OFF LEVEL Remissions/total (%)	PATIENTS WITH ER BELOW CUT-OFF LEVEL Remissions/total (%)	STATISTICAL ANALYSIS (x^2) P
0 (ER+/ER-)	14/38 (36,8%)	0/11 (0%)	.045
20	14/31 (45,2%)	0/18 (0%)	.002
80	11/20 (55,0%)	3/29 (10,3%)	.002
200	8/10 (80,0%)	6/39 (15,4%)	.0003

ranged from 0 to 1450 femtomoles per mg of tissue protein.
Therapeutic successes and failures are shown in Fig. 1
as a function of ER concentration. No success was obtained
in the ER- cases. In Table 1, four cut-off points were
tested for their ability to separate responders from non-
responders. It is seen that each cut-off point gives a
significant separation of response rates and that the
most effective one is at the level of 200 femtomoles.
in the ER- poor tumors, the response rate was low : no
remission occurred below the critical level of 20 femtomoles. In contrast, above 200 femtomoles, the response
rate reached 80 percent. Six successes, representing
43 percent of all responses, occurred between these two
levels. The rate of success in the corresponding patients
was 29 percent which is identical to that observed in
the whole series of forty-nine patients.

Statistical analysis was carried further by using
the linear logistic regression model (Cox, 1970). This
model is suitable for studying the relationship between
the probability of a therapeutic response and one or
several potentially related variables. By including as
the only predictive variable the level of ER with reference to the most discriminating cut-off point (Table 1,
ER = 200 femtomoles), the model is highly significant
(P = .00003). It can however be significantly improved
(P = .026) by including a second variable, i.e. ER
concentration taken as a continuous variable. This
indicates that the quantitative variable (concentration)
is more informative than the qualitative variable (cut-
off point). In fact, ER concentration used as the only
variable in the model yields the most significant relationship (P = .000016). The curve of Fig. 2 illustrates
this relationship and shows that the probability of
a response is a continuous function of ER concentration.

This relationship being established, we wondered
whether inclusion of clinical variables of putative
predictive value would further improve the model. The
following 12 clinical variables were analysed in this
regard : age, menopausal status, disease-free interval,
Karnofsky index, prior treatment, soft tissue involvement, lung involvement, liver involvement, dominant
site of disease, number of invaded sites, sites of
biopsy and nature of treatment. After sorting these
variables by conventional statistical methods (chi-
square), the five most significant variables were age,
menopausal status, bone involvement, prior treatment
and present treatment. These variables were then tested
by being added one by one in the model constructed with

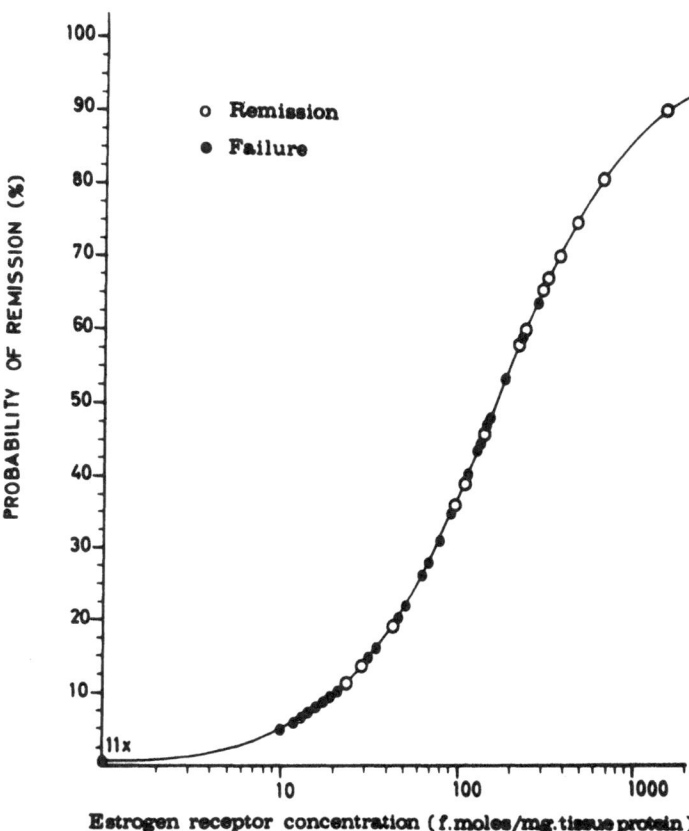

Fig. 2.   Relationship between estrogen receptor concen-
           tration and probability of response to endo-
           crine therapy. The experimental data were
           analized by using the linear logistic regres-
           sion model. The model that best fits the data
           is ln $\frac{P}{1-P}$ = -5.504 + 2.488 X, where P is the

           probability of response and X the logarithm of
           receptor concentration. The figure is a gra-
           phical representation of this formula.
           Using the linear logistic regression model,
           the symbols on the curve give the expected
           probabilities of response calculated for each
           of the 49 patients from their receptor concen-
           tration. The open circles (o) refer to the
           cases of remission, the filled circles (●) to
           those of failure.

ER concentration as the first variable (Fig. 2). It was
found that only age and menopausal status significantly
improved the predictive value of the model. This is
explained, at least in part, by the fact that ER concentration increases with age and interval after the
menopause (McGuire et al., 1975 ; Leclercq et Heuson,
1976). Details concerning the improved model will be
discussed elsewhere.

Analysis of the relationship between ER concentration
and probability of response to endocrine treatments
lends itself both to practical applications and to
biological considerations. For practical purposes, the
curve of Fig. 2 is used for therapeutic decisions. For
a given patient, ER concentration is located on the
abscissa and the corresponding probability of response
is read on the ordinate. This however cannot be done
when tumor tissue is not available for biopsy. The
question then arises as to whether ER assay performed
earlier on the primary tumor can be used in the prediction of response at this later stage. This question
will be studied in the next paragraph.

On the other hand, analysis of the data by the
linear logistic model suggests that breast cancers are
distributed along a continuous gradient of hormone
dependency which is measured by the ER content. ER-
poor tumors rarely respond to endocrine treatments.
The higher the level of ER, the higher is the likelihood
of obtaining a clear-cut success. It should be stressed
however that the criteria used to define a clear-cut
success (remission) are very stringent. It is likely
that an actual response is often below detectability
and passes unrecognized. Such subclinical successes
occuring along the whole assay of ER concentrations
are of great potential value to the patient provided
that they are complemented by chemotherapy. This concept of a possible synergism between endocrine therapy
and chemotherapy was explored in two clinical trials
conducted by the E.O.R.T.C. Breast Cancer Cooperative
Group. These trials will be summarized in the last
paragraph of this communication.

SIGNIFICANCE OF ER ASSAY IN PRIMARY BREAST CANCER AS
PREDICTOR OF HORMONE DEPENDENCY AT A LATER STAGE

The potential usefulness of assaying ER in the
primary tumor at the time of mastectomy for the

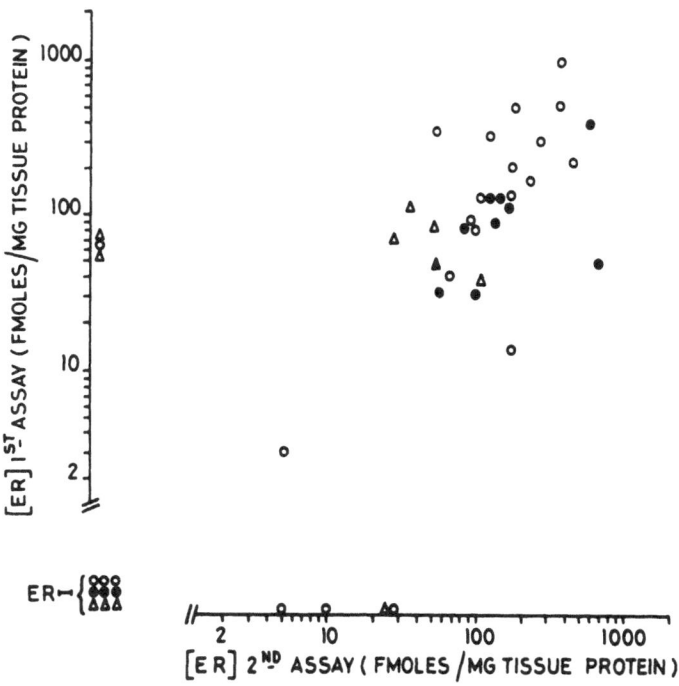

Fig. 3. Estrogen receptor (ER) variations in neo-
         plastic tissue during the course of disease.
         On the graph, individual patients are repre-
         sented in function of the ER concentrations
         found in two consecutive biopsies. The
         following symbols have been used, according
         to the menopausal status of the patients and
         to the site of the first biopsy :
         premenopausal patients, first assay performed
                 on the primary (△)
                 or on a soft tissue metastasis (▲).
         postmenopausal patients, first assay performed
                 on the primary (○).
                 or on a soft tissue metastasis (●).

assessment of hormone dependency at a later stage was
studied in forty-four patients. In forty-two of them,
there were two sequential assays, and in two others,
there were three. A total of 46 pairs of consecutive

assays is thus available. Thirty-three consisted of a
primary lesion and a subsequent metastasis, and 13 of
two consecutive metastases. None of the patients had
received any systemic treatment prior to or between
tissue sampling.

The results are depicted in Fig. 3. The mean duration
of time separating consecutive assays was 16 months
(range : 15 days to 63 months). Thirty patients had
two receptor-positive assays and nine had two negative
assays. In this regard, consecutive assays were thus
concordant in 39 patients (85 %).

In the set of 92 samples, receptor concentration
ranged from 0 to 1140 femtomoles per mg of tissue protein. In the group of premenopausal patients, however,
the range was smaller (0 to 123 femtomoles). Wilcoxon's
Rank Sum Test showed that this difference between pre-
and postmenopausal women is significant (P = .01 for
primary tumors ; P = .001 for metastases). Similar
data have already been reported (McGuire et al., 1975 ;
Leclercq and Heuson, 1976).

The variations of receptor concentration during
the course of disease were analysed. This analysis required the logarithmic transformation of the data to
insure a near-normal distribution. Patients were then
divided into two groups, according to the initial receptor status, positive or negative. Grouping all receptor-
positive (ER+) patients together (33), the correlation
between the two consecutive assays was significant at
P = .013 (r = .4286 ; d.f. = 31). In addition, the
change in ER concentrations according to the duration
of time between the consecutive assays (data not shown)
was studied and no correlation was found. When ER+ cases
were broken down according to the menopausal status, it
was found that the correlation in the postmenopausal
patients was significant at P = .018 (r = .4619 ;
d.f. = 24), but the correlation in the premenopausal
patients was not significant (r = .003 ; d.f. = 5).
It should be noted however that there were only 7 premenopausal ER+ patients so that one cannot determine
with any certainty whether or not a correlation exists.

Since the assumption of normality is not satisfied
for the receptor-negative cases, these patients could
not be analysed using the same statistical techniques.
It was found that 4 out of 5 premenopausal patients,
and 5 out of 8 postmenopausal patients remained receptor-

negative at the second assay. Thus, a total of 9 out of
13 patients (69 %) remained receptor-negative at the
second assay, with a 95 % confidence interval of
(38.6 %, 90.9 %) calculated for this proportion. Although
the confidence interval is quite wide, the 4 patients
who became receptor-positive presented very low levels
of receptor concentration (< 30 femtomoles per mg of
tissue protein). The variations in these cases would
thus not significantly affect the assessment of hormone
responsiveness as measured by the linear logistic
regression model.

These data indicate that a generally good correlation exists, except for premenopausal women in whom
insufficient data are available,between consecutive
assays at least when no intercurrent treatment has been
given. Under such circumstances and with the provision
that more data are needed in premenopausal patients,
it is concluded that hormone dependency can be assessed
from a previous assay and that therefore performing
routine receptor assays on the primary tumor is most
useful. On the other hand,in the presence of intercurrent treatment, a biopsy of metastatic tissue should
probably be assayed immediately before any therapeutic
decision is taken.

COMBINATION OF ENDOCRINE AND CYTOTOXIC TREATMENTS :
E.O.R.T.C. CLINICAL TRIALS

As discussed in a previous paragraph, the analysis
of estrogen receptors-clinical correlations suggests
that breast cancers are distributed along a continuous
gradient of hormone dependency and provides evidence for
a possible synergism between endocrine therapy and
cytotoxic chemotherapy. Two recent clinical trials conducted by the E.O.R.T.C. Breast Cancer Cooperative
Group are exploring such a possible synergism.

Alternated cyclical chemo-hormonal therapy

This treatment involved the concomittant use of the
antiestrogen Tamoxifen and of two monthly-alternated
cyclical cytotoxic combination (Heuson et al., 1980).
The given purpose of this alternation was to avoid or
delay the occurrence of drug resistance and the development of cumulative toxicity of certain drugs (adriamycin,
vincristine). This therapeutic strategy proved successful in Hogdkin's disease (Case et al., 1976) and undifferentiated small-cell bronchial carcinoma (Cohen et al.,

Table 2

TREATMENT AND DOSE SCHEDULES OF ALTERNATED CYCLICAL
CHEMO-HORMONAL THERAPY

THERAPY[a]	DRUG	DOSE[b]	SCHEDULE	ROUTE
A	Adriamycin	75 mg/m2	day 1	IV
	Vincristine	1.4 mg/m2	days 1& 8	IV
	Tamoxifen	20 mg	twice/day	PO
B	Cyclophosphamide	100 mg/m2	days 1 to 14	PO
	Methotrexate	60 mg/m2	days 1 & 8	IV
	Fluorouracil	600 mg/m2	days 1 & 8	IV
	Tamoxifen	20 mg	twice/day	PO

a : Treatments A and B are alternated monthly.

b : The doses of cytotoxic drugs are reduced in
the case of excessive hematologic toxicity.

Table 3 : THERAPEUTIC RESULTS OBTAINED WITH ALTERNATED CYCLICAL CHEMO-HORMONAL THERAPY

DOMINANT SITE OF LESIONS	EVALUABLE CASES			ALL CASES	
	Number of patients	CR[a] N° (%)	CR + PR[b] N° (%)	Number of patients	CR + PR N° (%)
Soft tissue	15	9 (60%)	11 (73%)	18	11 (61%)
Bone	10	1 (10%)	6 (60%)	18	6 (33%)
Viscera	49	6 (12%)	36 (73%)	59	36 (61%)
Total	74	16 (22%)	53 (72%)	95	53 (56%)

a : CR = complete response   b : PR = partial response

1979). The two drug combinations used here were selected
because Brambilla et al., (1976) demonstrated their therapeutic efficacy and lack of major cross-resistance in
advanced breast cancer. Drug doses and schedule of administration are described in Table 2.

Ninety-five postmenopausal patients with advanced
breast cancer were treated according to this protocol
in 10 different institutions. Seventy-four were evaluable
by the UICC criteria (Hayward et al., 1977) and were
assessed each by two extramural reviewers. The therapeutic
results are shown in Table 3. Complete or partial
remission was obtained in fifty-three patients (72 %),
with a median duration of 16 months. The median survival
in remitters lasted 29 months and, in non-remitters,
10 months.

Table 4 compares these data with those of five large
historical series of endocrine therapy and of cytotoxic
chemotherapy. The results of the present trial are by
far superior to those of endocrine therapy alone for
which the remission rate was only about 30 percent. The
combined endocrine-cytotoxic therapy thus provided an
additional quota of long survivors that amounted either
to 26 or 42 percent depending upon whether all cases or
only assessable cases are taken into consideration. One
should indeed emphasize the fact that these comparisons
are performed on non-randomized series and should
therefore be interpreted with caution.

Randomized trial of CMF ± Tamoxifen

In view of the foregoing encouraging results, it
was decided to determine the part played by the endocrine
therapy in association with chemotherapy. Therefore,
the E.O.R.T.C. Group compared the efficacy of a classical
chemotherapy regimen alone or complemented with Tamoxifen.

Patients were randomized into two groups : group A
was treated with CMF (cyclophosphamide, 100 mg_2per m^2
p.o., days 1 to 14 ; methotrexate, 40 mg per m^2 i.v.,
days 1 and 8 ; 5-fluouracil, 600 mg per m^2 i.v., days 1
and 8), repeated every 28 days ; group B received the
same treatment plus continuous Tamoxifen, 20 mg p.o.
twice daily.

Two hundred-sixty-three postmenopausal patients with
advanced breast cancer were treated in 9 institutions
according to this protocol. Partial preliminary results

Table 4

DURATION OF RESPONSE AND SURVIVAL IN THIS TRIAL
AS COMPARED TO OTHER TREATMENT MODALITIES

TREATMENT	NUMBER OF PATIENTS	RESPONDERS			NON-RESPONDERS
		%	Median duration (months)	Median survival (months)	Median survival (months)
Androgens[a]	521	21%	10	26	6
Estrogens[b]	357	37%		21	7
Adrenalectomy[c]	583	36%		25	8
CMF/AV sequential[d]	105	54%	9	23	10-14
CMF/AV alternating[e]	110	56%	12		
This trial[f] evaluable cases	74	72%	16	29	10
all cases	95	56%	16	29	7

a : Goldenberg et al.(1964).
b : AMA (1960).
c : Silverstein et al. (1975).
d : Brambilla et al. (1976).
e : Brambilla et al. (1978).
f : Heuson et al. (1980).

Table 5

E.O.R.T.C. RANDOMIZED CLINICAL TRIAL COMPARING CMF AND CMF + TAMOXIFEN

PARTIAL PRELIMINARY RESULTS - H.T. MOURIDSEN - COPENHAGEN 1979

THERAPEUTIC RESPONSE	C M F		CMF + TAMOXIFEN	
	Number of patients	Percent of total	Number of patients	Percent of total
Failure	21	29%	10	13%
No change	19	26%	13	17%
Partial response (PR)	26	36%	38	49%
Complete response (CR)	7	9%	16	21%
CR + PR	33	45%	54	70% P = .003
Total	73	100%	77	100%

of this study were presented by H.T. Mouridsen at the
Second E.O.R.T.C. Breast Cancer Working Conference
(Copenhagen, May 31 -June 2, 1979). They are presented
in Table 5 and clearly demonstrate the therapeutic supe-
riority, in terms of remission rate, of the association
CMF + Tamoxifen.

In conclusion, the concept of complementarity
between endocrine therapy and cytotoxic chemotherapy is
substantiated in the light of these preliminary clinical
trials. Endocrine therapy alone should be restricted
to patients selected according to precise criteria. For
the majority of patients however, hormonochemotherapy
should be considered a first-line treatment for which
the most effective modalities remain to be established.
Finally, it should be emphasized that the appreciable
gain in survival due to chemotherapy justifies its
energistic use early in the treatment of advanced breast
cancer.

ACKNOWLEDGEMENTS

This investigation was supported by a grant from the
Fond Cancérologique de la Caisse Générale d'Epargne et
de Retraite de Belgique and by Grant number 5R1OCA
11488-10 awarded by the National Cancer Institute DHEW.

We are indebted to Dr. H.T. Mouridsen who allowed
us to reproduce his data.

REFERENCES

AMA Council on drugs,1960, Androgens and estrogens in
        the treatment of disseminated mammary carcinoma.
        Retrospective study on nine-hundred forty-four
        patients. JAMA, 172,1271.
Brambilla, C., De Lena, M., Rossi, A., Valagussa, A.,
        and Bonadonna, G., 1976, Response and survival
        in advanced breast cancer after two non cross-
        resistant combinations. Br. Med. J., 1, 801-804.
Brambilla, D., Valagussa, A., and Bonadonna, G., 1978,
        Sequential combination chemotherapy in advanced
        breast cancer. Cancer Chemother. Pharmacol.,
        1, 35.
Case, D.C., Young, C.W., Nisce, L., Lee, B.J. III, and
        Clarckson, B.D.,1976,Eight-drug combination chemo-
        therapy (MOPP and ABVD) and local radiotherapy

for advanced Hodgkin's disease. Cancer Treatment
      Reports, 60, 1217-1223.
Cohen, M.H., Ihde, C.C., Bunn, P.A., Fossieck, B.E.,
      Matthews, M.J., Shackney, S.E., Johnston-Early,
      A., Makuch, R., and Minna, J.D., 1979, Cyclic
      alternating combination chemotherapy for small
      cell bronchogenic carcinoma. Cancer Treatment
      Reports, 63, 163-175.
Cox, D.R., 1970, The analysis of binary data. Methuen
      and Co Ltd., London.
E.O.R.T.C. Breast Cancer Cooperative Group, 1973,
      Standards for the assessment of estrogen receptors
      in human breast cancer. Europ. J. Cancer, 9,
      379-381.
Goldenberg, I.S., 1964, Testosterone propionate therapy
      in breast cancer. JAMA, 188, 1069.
Hayward, J.L., Carbone, P.P., Heuson, J.C., Kumaoka, S.,
      Segaloff, A., and Rubens, R.D., 1977, Assessment
      of response to therapy in advanced breast cancer.
      Europ. J. Cancer, 13, 89-94.
Heuson, J.C., Engelsman, E., Blonk-van der Wijst, J.,
      Maass, H., Drochmans, A., Michel, J., Nowakowski,
      H., and Gorins, A., 1975, Comparative trial of
      Nafoxidine and ethinyloestradiol in advanced
      breast cancer. An E.O.R.T.C. Breast Cancer Coope-
      rative Group Study. Br. Med. J., 2, 711-713.
Heuson, J.C., Longeval, E., Mattheiem, W.H., Deboel, M.C.,
      Sylvester, R.J., and Leclercq, G., 1977, Signi-
      ficance of quantitative assessment of estrogen
      receptors for endocrine therapy in advanced breast
      cancer. Cancer, 39, 1971-1977.
Heuson, J.C., Sylvester, R., and Engelsman, E.,1980,
      Alternating cyclical hormonal cytotoxic combina-
      tion chemotherapy in postmenopausal patients with
      breast cancer. An E.O.R.T.C. Trial. Europ. J.
      Cancer, in press.
Jensen, E.V., Block, G.E., Smith, S., Kyser, K., and
      de Sombre, E.R., 1971, Estrogen receptors and
      breast cancer response to adrenalectomy. Natl.
      Cancer Inst. Monogr., 34, 55-70.
Leclercq, G., Heuson, J.C., Schoenfeld, R., Mattheiem,
      W.H., and Tagnon, H.J., 1973, Estrogen receptors
      in human breast cancer. Europ. J. Cancer,9,
      665-673.
Leclercq, G., Heuson, J.C., Deboel, M.C., and Mattheiem,
      W.H., 1975, Oestrogen receptors in breast cancer :
      a changing concept. Br. Med. J., 1, 185-189.
Leclercq, G., and Heuson, J.C.,1976, Estrogen receptors
      in the spectrum of breast cancer. Current pro-
      blems in Cancer, 1, n° 6, R.C. Hickey ed.,

Year Book Medical Publishers, Inc. Chicago, pp. 1-34.

McGuire, W.L., Carbone, P.P., Sears, M.E., and Escher, G.C., 1975, Estrogen receptors in human breast cancer : an overview, in : Estrogen receptors in human breast cancer. McGuire W.L., Carbone P.P. and Vollmer E.P., eds., Raven Press, New York, pp. 1-7.

Mouridsen, H.T., and Palshof, T., 1980, CMF versus CMF plus Tamoxifen in advanced breast cancer in post-menopausal subjects. Europ. J. Cancer, in press.

Silverstein, M.J., Byron, R.L. Jr., Yonemoto, R.M., Riihimaki, D.U., and Schuster, G., 1975, Bilateral adrenalectomy for advanced breast cancer : a 21 year experience. Surgery, 77, 825-832.

HORMONAL DEPENDENCE OF BENIGN BREAST DISEASE, GYNECOMASTIA AND BREAST CANCER

B. de Lignières and P. Mauvais-Jarvis

C.H.U. Necker-Enfants-Malades
149-161 rue de Sèvres
75730 Paris Cédex 15, France

Until recently, the hormone dependence of the human mammary gland appeared unclear. In 1979, conflicting interpretations were still published on the essential physiological and pathological points (Diamont and Hollander, 1979). These contradictions have several origins : until a short time ago, women with breast diseases were exclusively seen by surgeons, radiologists and cancerologists and there were few possibilities of endocrinological investigation. Only the recent epidemiological enquiries draw attention to certain characteristics of genital life, and, above all, the use of various estro-progestative drugs for contraception or treatment of menopause lead to seeking advice from an endocrinologist.

Moreover, most of the basic knowledge has been obtained from exploration of animal mammary glands which cannot necessarily be used to draw conclusions applicable to the human species. There are considerable hormonal differences among mammals, and women are very peculiar in their mammary hormone dependence (Baldwin and Plucinski, 1977). Physiological doses of estradiol stimulate galactophoric growth in the rat, whereas this effect is obtained in the dog by progesterone, and in the guinea pig by a mixture of both (Table 1). Moreover, a synergistic action between estradiol and prolactin is necessary to produce this effect in the rat (Leung and Sasaki, 1973 ; Vignon and Rochefort, 1974). Synergy between progesterone and STH intervenes in the dog (Gräf and Eletreby, 1979). None of the laboratory animals currently used has the same hormonal situation as women, either during the estral

TABLE 1

SPECIFIC HORMONAL DEPENDANCE OF GALACTOPHORIC GROWTH
IN SEVERAL SPECIES

	Estradiol (+ Prolactin)	Estradiol (+ Progesterone)	Progesterone (+ STH)
Rat Mouse Rabbit Cat	+		
Guinea pig Goat Cow		+	
Dog			+

or menstrual cycle or during gestation (Thibault and
Levasseur, 1979 ; Gräf and Eletreby, 1979).

    The experimentation on the dog imposed by the Food
and Drug Administration in the U.S.A. before application
to humans, has thus undoubtedly been detrimental since
it is irrelevant to the human situation. Contrary to
women, estradiol production decreases in dogs during the
luteal phase and pregnancy (Figures 1 and 2), and progesterone is what induces endometrial and galactophoric
hyperplasia (Vandaele, 1977). All the substances related
to progesterone generally induce benign tumors in the
dog, and increase the frequency of malignant mammary
tumors, particularly since the F.D.A. experimental codi-
fied protocols require prolonged administration (2 years)
of doses 2 to 25 fold higher than those projected for
use in the human species (Gräf and Eletreby, 1979). It
is therefore hardly advisable to use the dog in experiments on human hormone physiopathology, since spontaneous
growth of mammary glands occurs in grossly different
hormonal surroundings. In another tissue, the endometrium,

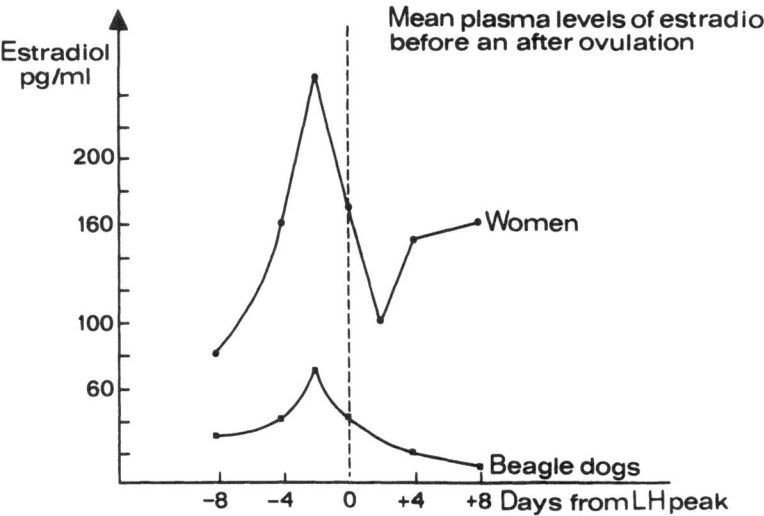

Fig. 1.

it has been well established that progesterone has opposite effects in dogs and women. After numerous years of
discussion, mandatory experimentation on dogs of sexual
steroids destined for human therapeutics, has now been
abandoned by the majority of european countries. It
remains mandatory in the U.S.A..

The rat experimental model, particularly in DMBA
induced mammary cancer, has also been shown to be ina-
dapted to the human species (Pearson and Manni, 1978).
DMBA-induced cancer in the rat is prolactin-dependent
and, even though the tumors contain extradiol receptors,
estrogens have only an indirect effect on its growth,
linked solely to the increase in prolactin secretion
they induce. The experimental variations of estrogeni-
sation do not modify tumoral growth when prolactin impregnation is maintained constant (Nagasawa and Yanaï,
1970). However, all experimentations increasing prolactin production accelerate tumoral growth, and those
which decrease prolactin production induce a decrease
in the tumor, whatever the estrogenic impregnation.

In the human species, however, manipulations of
prolactin secretion have no effect on tumoral growth

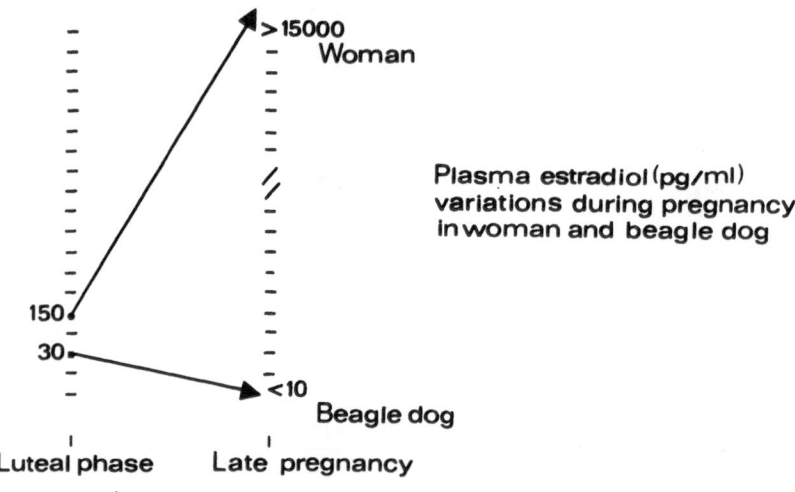

Fig. 2.

(Newsome et al., 1971 ; Turkington et al., 1971 ; Pearson
and Manni, 1978). Generally speaking, in the human, prolactin has almost none of the multiple activities clearly
demonstrated in various animal species (Lancet, editorial,
1979). Information directly concerning the human, should
therefore be clearly separated from that obtained in
other mammals, and animal experimental models accepted
only for those points where precise convergences exist
with the human species (Cardiff et al., 1977).

HORMONAL CONTROL OF THE HUMAN BREAST

The different morphological or histological aspects
which the breast may have, are not irreversibly determined by genetic predestination. On the contrary, endo-
genous perturbation or hormonal therapeutics may disrupt
mammary morphology, whatever the chromosomic sex or age
of the subject may be : an estrogenic treatment in a
male phenotype man of XY chromosomal sex, may develop
mammary glands in the same way as at female puberty, as
is seen with the cancerous of the prostate or in trans-
sexuals. The breasts develop as a whole in a female
manner in XY individuals if they are insensitive to male
hormones and secrete abnormal levels of estradiol
("testicular feminization"). Gynecomastia develops in-
constantly during Klinefelter's XXY syndrome, and estrogenic treatment develops the mammary structures of
subjects with Turner's XO syndrome. Transitory modifications of the mammary gland may be induced by hormonal
manipulations in the infant as well as during childhood
(precocious puberty), in the young male or female adult,
or in the aged (estrogenic treatment for prostate or
breast cancer). The basics of the breast physiology are
therefore not genetically fixed, but correspond to a
daily hormonal balance, of which the essential elements
may be determined.

In women, the breasts (galactophores and connective
stroma) develop with the onset of pubertal estrogenic
secretion (Lee et al., 1976 ; Thorner et al., 1977).
At this time there is no progesterone secretion (Winter
and Faiman, 1973 ; Widholm et al., 1974) and in the
majority of cases, no variation in prolactin levels is
noted (Franks and Brook, 1976). Some authors describe
a minimal increase of prolactin levels (Thorner et al.,
1977) during female puberty. That variation is of such
small amplitude that it remains within the normal range
for children and adults of both sexes, and has no known
biological significance. At the same time, estradiol

levels increase from inactivity to the threshold of
clearly recognized biological activity. The galactophores
and connective tissue of the human breast develop under
the preponderant influence of estradiol. The mammary
gland as a whole acts as a "receptor" tissue to estradiol
since it accumulates, concentrates and retains, for 5 to
6 hours after intravenous injection, the labeled steroid
(Desphande et al., 1967). Estradiol is permanently found
in mammary tissue at concentrations 2 to 20 fold superior to those found in the plasma at the same moment
(Cortes-Gallegos et al., 1975). The cytosolic and nuclear
receptors specific for estradiol have been identified in
human breast samples containing a great density of galactophores (adenomas) (May-Levin et al., 1977 ; Martin
et al., 1978 ; Fournier and Kuttenn, 1980). Galactophores
and connective tissue regress with the disappearance of
estrogenic stimulation (castration, menopause) but the
histological glandular structure may be developed at any
age by administration of estrogens (Huseby and Thomas,
1954).

In men, galactophores and connective tissue remain
atrophied as long as estrogen production is low and
androgen production high. The androgens act as anti-
estrogens and dihydrotestosterone formed by 5 α-reduction
of testosterone appears the strongest of them (Watson
et al., 1977). When the estrogen/androgen ratio is
increased in men, whatever the cause or age of the subject, their mammary glands develop as during the female
puberty.

Gynecomastia appears under the influence of an
increase in estradiol levels. Therefore in neoformed
male mammary tissue, the estradiol concentrations found
are identical to those in the normal female breast
(Cortes-Gallegos et al., 1975).

Gynecomastia may be induced by an anti-androgen
treatment such as with spironolactone (Corvol et al.,
1976) or cimetidine (Winters et al., 1979). Gynecomastia
occurs, roughly and fleetingly, in numerous male ado-
lescents at puberty. This condition evolves as long as
the testicular production of estradiol increases more
rapidly than that of testosterone, then decreases when
this ratio returns to normal (Lee, 1975, Large and
Anderson, 1979).

In addition, local synthesis of estradiol may occur
in the gynecomastia tissue itself (Rajendran et al.,
1975) from steroids circulating in the plasma at normal

levels, as well as from androgens such as testosterone and androstenedione. In such cases only unaromatisable 5 α -dihydrotestosterone would preserve its anti-estrogen effect, but its synthesis depends on the 5 α -reductase activity which undergoes progressive maturation under androgenic influence during puberty. There again, in common gynecomastia situations, plasma or local inbalance between estrogens and androgens appears solely responsible, and there is no proof that other hormones, particularly prolactin, play a direct part (Frantz et al., 1972, Nagel et al., 1973).

HORMONAL DEPENDENCE OF BENIGN BREAST DISEASES

Benign breast diseases which involve connective tissue and galactophores appear to correspond to an excessive estrogenic effect. During spontaneous fibro-cystic disease, mammary tissue contains abnormally high levels of estradiol (Cortes-Gallegos et al., 1975). The concentration of estradiol cytosolic receptor is higher in adenomatous benign tumors with a greater galactophoric hyperplasia. This concentration of estrogenic receptors, is, on the contrary, very low when concerning fibrous non-evolutive tissue (May-Levin et al., 1977 ; Martin et al., 1978 ; Fournier and Kuttenn, 1980). The frequency of benign breast disease decreases after menopause unless estrogenic treatment is administered (Haagensen, 1971). Post-menopausal estrogenic treatment may recreate the radiological and clinical aspects of fibrocystic disease. All these symptoms regress when treatment is suspended (Peck and Lowman, 1978). Benign breast tumors are more frequent in women on estrogenic treatment (without any other hormonal association), than in those of a control population without any treatment (Nomura and Comstock, 1976).

But aside from the iatrogenous pathology, local tissular hyperestrogenesis appears only exceptionally in relation to plasma hyperestrogenesis, and estradiol levels are more often to be found within normal limits (Sitruk-Ware et al., 1977).

However, plasma progesterone levels are frequently low in women with benign breast diseases (Mauvais-Jarvis and Kuttenn, 1975 ; Dargent et al., 1977 ; Gairard, 1979 ; Colin et al., 1978). This progesterone deficiency is almost constant when clinical or thermographical signs of evolutivity of the benign breast disease exist (Sitruk-Ware et al., 1980) and is less pronounced in

the absence of these signs. The progesterone levels may
not be significantly low upon diagnosis of benign breast
disease since purely cystic or fibrous lesions may persist for many months after the hormonal event which
induced them.

Among the clinical mammary symptoms, that which
appears the most constant, and an immediate proof of
progesterone deficiency, is bilateral mastodynia, with
a disagreeable sensation of swelling of the breasts
appearing more than three days before menstruation and
disappearing within the first 2 to 3 days of the cycle.

Several arguments suggest a causal relationship
between progesterone deficiency and evolution of adenomatous or fibrocystic disease :
- A treatment with progesterone or a progestative
in sufficient doses relieves mastodynia, reduces the
irregular nodular consistency of the breasts during the
premenstrual phase and stops the evolution of benign
tumors (Mauvais-Jarvis et al., 1978).
- The thermographical anomalies disappear within
a few weeks under the influence of a purely local treatment with percutaneous progesterone (Lafaye and Aubert,
1978). This is a direct effect of progesterone since the
progesterone concentration in the mammary tissue increases
due to the percutaneous treatment without any notable
modification of plasma levels, therefore without dis-
turbing other hormonal balances (de Boever et al., 1980).
- A progestative treatment improves the mammographic
appearances of benign breast diseases within 4 to 6
months (Duperray and Sitruk-Ware, 1979). The frequency
of benign breast tumors is higher in those using estrogen
alone, compared to those using an association of estro-
progestatives (Nomura and Comstock, 1976).
- With the estro-progestative association, containing
an identical dose of the same estrogen (ethinyl estradiol
50 µg/day), the occurrence of benign breast disease is
even lower when the dose of the same progestative is
higher (norethisterone acetate). With 4 mg/day of this
progestative, the incidence of new cases of benign mastopathy falls to 3.5 for 1 000 years/women, whereas it
is 10.6 per 1 000 years/women in the control population
not receiving any hormonal treatment.

ESTRO-PROGESTATIVE BALANCE AND VASCULAR PHENOMENA

It is easy to understand how a progesterone deficiency may increase the effect of estrogens on certain

tissues. Estrogens increase vascular permeability, inducing an extra-vascular plasma leakage and tissular
hydric retention in the uterus of the rat and mouse
(Cecil et al., 1966) and in the mammary gland of the
rabbit (Zeppa,1969). But this effect is progressively
reduced, or even suspended, if at the same time as
estrogen, increasing doses of progesterone or progestatives are injected (Dasgupta et al., 1970). It is also
produced in the human species : vascular permeability
is abnormally high in women during premenstrual tension
syndrome (Morton, 1950 ; Wong et al., 1972), which
corresponds to a plasmatic increase in the estrogen/
progesterone ratio (Backstrom and Carstensen, 1974). The
hydric retention induced by the increase in capillary
permeability is particularly sensitive in the breasts
as mastodynia (Morton, 1950 ; Wong et al., 1972), accom-
pagnied by a measurable modification of mammary volume
(Milligan et al., 1975) and thermographical anomalies
(Gros et al., 1969 ; Nassar and Smith, 1975 ; Lafaye
and Aubert, 1978). The administration of progesterone
or progestatives to these women normalizes capillary
permeability (Morton, 1950) and relieves mastodynia
(Mauvais-Jarvis, 1978) and thermographical anomalies
(Lafaye and Aubert, 1978). It has also been possible to
reproduce mastodynia experimentally in post-menopausal
women, by modifying the estro-progestative ratio. In
105 women, post-menopausal for over 6 months, with
plasma estradiol levels less than 50 pg/ml, none presented mastodynia (bilateral painful swelling of the
breasts). When these women received estrogen treatment,
their estradiol level increased in varying proportions
according to each individual and the dose of estradiol
administered : out of 5 women whose plasma estradiol
did not rise above 50 pg/ml, none had mastodynia ; out
of 42 whose plasma estradiol rose to between 50 and
150 pg/ml, 12 (30 %) had mastodynia ; out of 58 women
whose plasma estradiol rose above 150 pg/ml, 9 were
treated with estradiol alone and 7 (80 %) of them had
mastodynia ; the other 49 were treated with the same
estradiol dose plus a progestative for 10 days/month and
only 7 (15 %) had mastodynia. These results confirm that,
on the one hand, mastodynia is more frequent when plasma
estradiol is high (Fig. 3), but, on the other hand, at
equivalent plasma estradiol levels, progestatives considerably decrease the frequency of mastodynia (Fig. 4).
It is in fact the ratio between active estrogens and
progestatives, rather than plasma estradiol levels alone,
that controls vascular phenomena in the breast and their
various (clinical, radiological, thermographical) con-
sequences.

Before treatment   During treatment

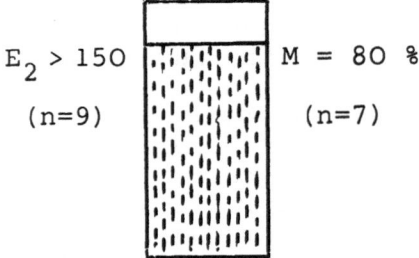

$E_2 > 150$ M = 80 %

(n=9)   (n=7)

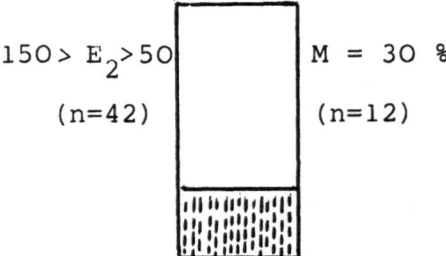

$150 > E_2 > 50$ M = 30 %

(n=42)   (n=12)

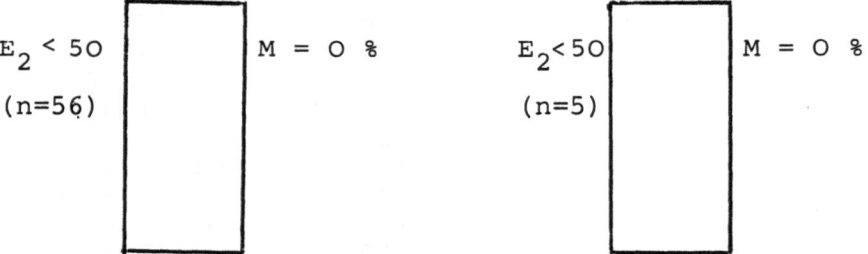

$E_2 < 50$ M = 0 % $E_2 < 50$ M = 0 %

(n=56)   (n=5)

Fig. 3.   Mastodynias before and during estradiol
          treatment in post-menopausal women.
          Relation to Estradiol plasma level.

          E_2 : plasma estradiol (pg/ml)
          M   : frequency of mastodynia (%)
          n   : number of subjects.

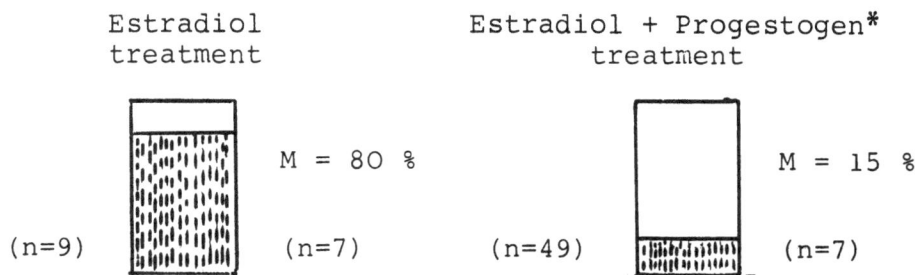

Fig. 4. Mastodynia during estradiol treatment with or without progestogen in post-menopausal women. (All women with plasma estradiol > 150 pg/ml) *P : Lynestrenol or ac. chlormadinone 5 mg/d x 10 d/month.

ESTRO-PROGESTATIVE BALANCE AND MITOTIC ACTIVITY OF SEXUAL EPITHELIUM

It is well established that the level of estro-progestative balance controls the mitotic activity of certain sexual epithelia. The human endometrium is an excellent model for this : estrogenic stimulation may induce epithelial hyperplasia of the endometrium and, at length, favor carcinogenesis (Antunes et al., 1979). Progesterone and progestatives, however, reduce epithelial hyperplasia (Thom et al., 1979), particularly when used at sufficient doses and associated with estrogens, prevent the appearance of hyperplastic zones (Sturdee et al., 1978), and obviate the estrogen-dependent cancer risk (Gambrell, 1978 ; Hammond et al., 1979). If progesterone controls the effect of estrogens on the epithelial cells of the endometrium, it is principally by decreasing specific estradiol receptor synthesis (Tseng and Gurpide, 1975). Estrogens also induce hyperplasia of the human galactophores (Huseby and Thomas, 1954), and the same type of estrogenic receptor has been identified in hyperplastic galactophores of the human breast (May-Levin et al., 1977 ; Martin et al., 1978). The concentration of these receptors is equally diminished by progesterone (Fournier and Kuttenn, 1980). In the case of hyperestrogenesis, or progesterone deficiency, one may expect the appearance of hyperplastic zones in the galactophores and, as with the endometrium, an increase in cancer risk.

Such benign mastopathies, whether spontaneous or iatrogenous, increase the risk of breast cancer.

BENIGN BREAST DISEASE AND RISK OF BREAST CANCER

The first prospective study, carried out by Warren
in 1940, showed an increase by 4 in the frequency of
breast cancer in women with benign breast disease. In
1973, Mc Mahon, for the "Breast Cancer Task Force" concluded with an increase of cancer risk to the same order
(Mc Mahon et al., 1973). In 1975, the prospective study
over 14 years from the Mayo Clinic showed a mean increase
by 3 of the risk of breast cancer but by 10 with benign
breast disease appearing after the age of 30 (Donnelly
et al., 1975). In 1976, a prospective study over 30 years
showed a 250 % increase in breast cancer mortality in
a group of 733 women with benign breast disease (Monson
et al., 1976).

In Haagensen's study (1977), the control of 5 000
fibrocystic diseases with macrocysts, between 1928
and 1971, shows a 4 fold increase in the incidence of
breast cancer.

In 1972, then in 1977, in a prospective study covering 7 years and 2 900 cases of benign breast disease,
the cancer risk appears multiplied by 2.5 to 16 according
to the histological aspect of the galactophores, atypical
hyperplasia representing the maximal risk (Black et al.,
1972 ; Kodlin et al., 1977).

IATROGENOUS BENIGN BREAST DISEASE AND CANCER RISK

Hoover et al. (1976) showed in a prospective study
over 10 years, that the risk of breast cancer is 7 fold
greater in menopausal women treated with estrogens if
benign breast disease appears or persists under treatment. In 1977, a retrospective study demonstrated that
if prolonged utilization of oral contraceptives does not
generally increase the risk of breast cancer, it may
increase this risk 11 fold in a particular group of
women with benign breast disease (Paffenbarger et al.,
1977). The prospective study of Lees et al. (1978) confirms that only the association of benign breast disease
together with the pill increases the risk of breast cancer
whereas the pill without benign breast disease does not
increase this risk.

Oral contraceptives induce a great variety of relationships between estrogenic and progestative activity,
on the one hand because of their chemical composition
and on the other hand because of the great diversity of

metabolism of the steroids from one woman to another (Weems-Chihal et al., 1975). The drugs with predominating estrogenic activity increase the frequency of benign breast disease (Nomura and Comstock, 1976), whereas those which have a strong progestative activity decrease the frequency of benign breast diseases (Royal College, 1977). Actually only women who find good estro-progestative balance with the pill accept its prolonged use. The others rapidly abandon their contraceptives because of minimal disagreeable symptoms, the most frequent of which are premenstrual tension, mastodynia and appearance of mammary nodules (de Lignières, 1976).

Thus, in the population using the pill for more than 4 years, there is an overall decrease in the frequency of benign breast disease and only very few groups of women prolong their consumption of estrogens for several years, despite the persistance of benign breast disease (Hoover et al., 1976 ; Paffenbarger et al., 1977). The utilization of the pill thus contributes, in practice, to the general decrease in the incidence of benign breast disease.

However, one cannot count on observing a corresponding decrease in the incidence of breast cancer given the current conditions of oral contraceptive use. In the vast majority of cases, the pill is used for far less than the 10 years necessary to influence carcinogenesis (Mc Cornack et al., 1977 ; Keifer and Scott, 1975). Moreover, the use of the pill by women over 35 years old is now exceptional (Ford, 1978), although this is the age at which the risk of breast cancer starts and estro-progestative balance should be controlled (Donnelly et al., 1975).

It thus appears that the situations of epithelium of the endometrium and of the galactophores are very similar in the human species. Estrogens also induce hyperplasia of galactophores (Huseby and Thomas, 1954). They increase the concentration of their own receptors which progesterone, on the contrary, decreases (Fournier and Kuttenn, 1980), exactly as has been described for the human endometrium. Durable hyperplasia of the galactophoric epithelium favors the action of carcinogenic agents and increases the incidence of breast cancer (Kodlin et al., 1977). Studies are necessary to determine whether progestative treatment reduces epithelial hyperplasia of the galactophores, as it does in the endometrium, and whether it also decreases the incidence of breast cancer (Sherman and Korenman, 1974 ; Mauvais-

Jarvis et al., 1975). Recently, it has been shown that progesterone deficiency is correlated to other risk factors of breast cancer, particularly late first pregnancy (Bulbrook et al., 1978). In addition, the hypothesis that the breast is more sensitive to estro-progestative imbalance than the endometrium should be verified. The level of estradiol accumulated by connective and adipose tissue is indeed higher in galactophoric epithelium surroundings than in the endometrium (Cortes-Gallegos et al., 1975). Thus, plasma progesterone levels to the order of 3 ng/ml in the luteal phase are generally sufficient to relieve all gross anomalies of the endometrium, whereas double or triple plasma progesterone levels are necessary for relief of the clinical, thermographical or radiological symptoms in the breast (de Lignières, 1976). Estro-progestative imbalance is relatively easy to check by endometrium biopsy, but it rarely induces local clinical symptoms (Whitehead et al., 1978). In the breasts, however, if biopsies cannot easily be carried out, the clinical symptomatology is often suggestive due to the vascular effects of the estro-progestative imbalance on the abundant connective tissue. As already described, the principal symptom is mastodynia. This symptom coincides exactly with an increase in the estradiol/progesterone ratio and its incidence may indicate the induction risk of a benign breast pathology (fibroadenoma in the young woman, fibrocystic disease around the age of 40), and finally of a malignant pathology. However, until now, this symptom, considered over-subjective and often confused with unilateral non-cyclic mastodynia (Tietze's syndrome, intercostal nevralgia, etc.), has never been taken into account in the statistical enquiries on breast cancer risk factors. For some women it has become so habitual and frequent in their families that it is not spontaneously declared to the practitioner as it is not considered a motive for consultation.

HORMONE DEPENDENCE OF CANCERS

Cancer cells may conserve a certain degree of hormone dependence long after the clinical appearance of the tumor. 70 % of the cancerous cells retain specific estradiol receptors. Their concentration is greater in post-menopausal women (Saez et al., 1978), in histologically differentiated tumors (Antoniades and Spector, 1979) and then indicate a better prognosis (Bishop et al., 1979).

The mitotic activity in some human breast cancers may, in vitro, remain stimulated by estradiol (Lippman et al., 1977) and inhibited by progesterone (Plata et al., 1973).

The presence of great concentrations of estrogenic receptors allows the post-menopausal tumors to conserve mitotic activity in spite of a decrease by 10 of estrogen production (Lippman et al., 1977). The main estrogen source is, at this time, the mammary adipose tissue (Nimrod and Ryan, 1975) or the malignant tumor itself (Varela and Dao, 1978).

Only 30 % of macroscopic breast cancers remain influenced by hormonal surroundings. Those which remain dependent on estrogen most often conserve specific estradiol receptors and also specific progesterone receptors, the latter appearing as soon as conventional estrogenic stimulation occurs (Mc Guire et al., 1978). The systematic determination of these estradiol and progesterone receptors should not only enable one more patient to be cured, but also avoid the profoundly mutilating surgery (surrenalectomy plus oophorectomy or hypophysectomy) in women who would not benefit from it. The administration of anti-estrogen substances is of great theoretical interest and should be capable of replacing major endocrinological surgery. Practically speaking, two difficulties have to be overcome : the utilization of anti-estrogens in the pre-menopausal phase and the risk of blocking the negative feed-back effect of estrogens on the pituitary-hypothalamus, thus inducing intense ovarian stimulation with compensatory production of estradiol. These drugs should only be used in pre-menopause in association with drugs blocking the pituitary secretion of gonadotrophins (progestatives for example). Also, until now, tamoxifen itself retains a certain estrogenic activity. In low doses its anti-estrogenic effect predominates and its estrogenic effect is negligible. However, when the dose has to be increased, the estrogenic effect becomes considerable and its therapeutic benefit disappears.

CONCLUSION

The recent results of epidemiological enquiries into plasmatic and tissular hormonal controls give human endocrinology a new coherance and a fresh therapeutic impulse. Far more than the possibility of intervening in cases of late stage cancer, endocrinology can be expected

to be applied in recognition of the hormonal situation
which otherwise might favor mammary carcinogenesis
(Wellings et al., 1975). Although in rodents the inter-
vention of prolactin is fundamental, in the human species
it is a lapse in the estradiol and progesterone balance
which appears capable, as in the endometrium, of faci-
litating the growth of the first cancer cells. The hormonal treatment of benign breast disease is thus necessary not only because it reduces the disconfort of the
patient (mastodynia) but above all because it constitutes
probably the only present possibility of attempting
to control the increasing incidence of breast cancer.

REFERENCES

Antoniades, K., and Spector, H., 1979, Correlation of
        estrogen receptor levels with histology and cyto-
        morphology in human mammary cancer. Am. J. Clin.
        Path., 71, 497-503.
Antunes, C.M.F., Stolley, P.D., Rosenshein, N.B., Davies,
        J.L., Tonascia, J.A., Brown, C., Burnett, L.,
        Rutledge, A., Pokempner, M., and Garcia, R., 1979,
        Endometrial cancer and estrogen use. N. Engl. J.
        Med., 300, 9-13.
Backstrom, T., and Carstensen, H., 1974, Estrogen and
        progesterone in plasma in relation to premenstrual
        tension. J. Steroid Biochem., 5, 257-260.
Baldwin, R.L., and Plucinski, T., 1977, Mammary gland
        development and lactation. In "Reproduction in
        domestic animals". H.M. Cole and P.T. Cupps, Eds.,
        Academic Press, New York, p 369.
Bishop, H.M., Blamey, R.W., Elston, C.W., and Haybittle,
        J.L., 1979, Relationship of oestrogen receptor
        status to survival in breast cancer. Lancet, 1,
        283-284.
Black, M.M., Barclay, T.H.C., Cutler, S.J., Hankey, B.F.,
        and Asire, A.J., Association of typical charac-
        teristics of benign breast lesions with subsequent
        risk of breast cancer. Cancer, 29, 338-343.
De Boever, J., Desmet, B., and Vandekerckhove, D., 1980,
        Variation of progesterone, 20α-dihydroprogeste-
        rone and estradiol concentration in human mammary
        tissue and blood after topical administration of
        progesterone in "Percutaneous administration of
        steroids". Mauvais-Jarvis P., Vichers C.F.H.,
        Wepierre J., Eds., Academic Press, New York, in
        Press.
Bulbrook, R.D., Moore, J.W., Clark, G.M.G., Wang, D.Y.,
        Tong, D., and Hayward, J.L., 1978, Plasma

oestradiol and progesterone levels in women with varying degrees of risk of breast cancer. Europ. J. Cancer, 14, 1369-1375.

Cardiff, R.D., Wellings, S.R., and Faulkin, L.J., 1977, Biology of breast preneoplasia. Cancer, 39, 2734-2746.

Cecil, H.C., Hannum, J.A., and Bitman, J., 1966, Quantitative characterization of uterine vascular permeability changes with estrogen. Am. J. Physiol., 211, 1099-1102.

Colin, C., Gaspard, U., and Lambotte, R., 1978, Relationship of mastodynia with its endocrine environment and treatment in a double blind trial with Lynestrenol. Arch. Gynäk., 225, 7-13.

Mac Cornack, F.A., Nathan, J.K., Covey, L.S., and Wynder, E.L., 1977, Oral contraceptive use. Epidemiology. New York State. J. Med., 77, 200-202.

Cortes-Gallegos, V., Gallegos, A.J., Sanchez Basurto, C., and Rivadeneyra, J., 1975, Estrogen peripheral levels vs estrogen tissue concentration in the human female reproductive tract. J. Steroid. Biochem., 6, 15-20.

Corvol, P., Mahoudeau, J.A., Valcke, J.C., Menard, J., and Bricaire, H., 1976, Effets sexuels secondaires des spironolactones. Mécanismes possibles de l'action anti-androgène. Nouv. Presse Med., 5, 691-696.

Dargent, D., Rivier, A., and Lasne, R., 1977, La fonction ovarienne des femmes atteintes de mastopathie non cancéreuse. Sénologia, 2, 11-17.

Dasgupta, P.R., Ghosh, M., Pande, J.K., and Kar, A.B., 1970, Antiestrogenicity of norgestrel. Curr. Science, 39, 467-468.

Desphande, N., Jensen, E.V., and Bulbrook, R.D., 1967, Accumulation of tritiated oestradiol by human breast tissue. Steroids, 10, 219-232.

Diamond, E.J., and Hollander, V.P., 1979, Progesterone and breast cancer. Mount Sinai J. Med., 46, 225-235.

Donnelly, P.K., Baker, K.W., Carney, J.A., and O'Fallow, W.M., 1975, Benign breast lesions and subsequent breast carcinoma in Rochester, Minnesota. Mayo. Clin. Proc., 50, 650-656.

Duperray, B., and Sitruk-Ware, R., 1979, Mammographie dynamique. Intérêt du traitement progestatif préalable. Nouv. Presse Méd., 8, 3058-3059.

Editorial, 1979, What does prolactin do in man ? Lancet, 1, 234-235.

Ford, K., 1978, Contraceptive use in the United States, 1973 - 1976. Family Planning Perspectives,

10, 264-269.

Fournier, S., and Kuttenn, F., 1980, Estradiol and Pro-
     gesterone receptors in breast fibroadenomas in
     women, in Press.

Franks, S., and Brook, C.G.D., 1976, Basal and stimulated
     prolactin levels in childhood. Horm. Res., 7,
     65-76.

Frantz, A.G., Kleinberg, D.L., and Noel, G.L., 1972,
     Studies on prolactin in man. Recent Prog. Horm.
     Res., 28, 527-573.

Gairard, B., 1979, Profil hormonal dans les mastodynies.
     Rev. Med., 20, 477-480.

Gambrell, R.D., 1978, The prevention of endometrial car-
     cinoma in postmenopausal women with progestagens.
     Maturitas, 1, 107-112.

Gräf, K.J., and El Etreby, M.P., 1979, Endocrinology of
     reproduction in the female beagle dog and its
     significance in mammary gland tumorigenesis.
     Acta Endocrinol. Suppl 222, p 1 - 33.

Gros, C., Gautherie, M., Bourjat, P., and Vrousos, C.,
     1969, Thermographie des affections mammaires.
     Radiol., 5, 68-81.

Mc Guire, W.L., Zava, D.T., Horwitz, K.B., Garola, R.E.,
     and Chamness, G.C., 1978, Receptors and breast
     cancer : do we know it all ? J. Steroid Biochem.,
     9, 461-466.

Haagensen, C.D., 1971, Diseases of the breast. Saunders
     Co Edit. Philadelphia, p 159.

Haagensen, C.D., 1977, The relationship of gross cystic
     disease of the breast and carcinoma. Ann. Surg.,
     185, 375-376.

Hammond, C.B., Jelovsek, F.R., Lee, K.L., Creasman, W.T.,
     and Parker, R.T., 1979, Effects of long term
     estrogen replacement therapy. II. Neoplasia. Am.
     J. Obstet. Gynecol., 133, 537-547.

Hoover, R., Gray, L.A., Cole, P., and Mac Mahon, B.,
     1976, Menopausal estrogens and breast cancer.
     New Engl. J. Med., 295, 401-405.

Huseby, R.A., and Thomas, L.B., 1954, Histological and
     histochemical alterations in the normal breast
     tissues of patients with advanced breast cancer
     being treated with estrogenic hormones. Cancer,
     7, 54-74.

Keifer, W.S., and Scott, J.C., 1975, A clinical appraisal
     of patients following long term contraception.
     Am. J. Obstet. Gynecol., 122, 446-458.

Kodlin, D., Winger, E.E., Morgenstern, N.L., and Chen,
     U., 1977, Chronic mastopathy on breast cancer.
     A follow-up study. Cancer, 39, 2603-2607.

Lafaye, C., and Aubert, B., 1978, Action de la progestérone locale dans les mastopathies bénignes. J. Gyn. Obst. Biol. Repr., 7, 1123-1139.

Large, D.M., and Anderson, D.C., 1979, Twenty-four hour profiles of circulating androgens and oestrogens in male puberty with and without gynecomastia. Clin. Endocrinol., 11, 505-521.

Lee, P.A., 1975, The relationship of concentrations of serum hormones to pubertal gynecomastia. J. Pediatr., 86, 212-215.

Lee, P.A., Xenakis, T., Winer, J., and Matsenbaugh, S., 1976, Puberty in girls : correlation of serum levels of gonadotrophins, prolactin, androgens, estrogens and progestins with physical changes. J. Clin. Endocrinol., 43, 775-784.

Lees, A.W., Burns, P.E., and Grace, M., 1978, Oral contraceptives and breast disease in premenopausal nothern Albertan women. Int. J. Cancer, 22, 700-707.

Leung, B.S., and Sasaki, G.H., 1973, Prolactin and progesterone effect on specific estradiol binding in uterine and mammary tissues in vitro. Biochem. Biophys. Res. Comm., 55, 1180-1187.

Lignières, B. de, 1976, Cybernétique hormonale du sein : II pathologie. Senologia, 1, 53-62.

Lippman, M.E., Osborne, C.K., Knazek, R., and Young, N., 1977, In vitro model systems for the study of hormone dependent human breast cancer. New Engl. J. Med., 296, 154-159.

Mac Mahon, B., Cole, P.C., and Brown, J., 1973, Etiology of human breast cancer : a review. J. Nat. Cancer Inst., 50, 21-42.

Martin, P.M., Kuttenn, F., Serment, H., and Mauvais-Jarvis, P., 1978, Studies on clinical, hormonal and pathological correlations in breast fibroadenoma. J. Steroid. Biochem., 9, 1251-1255.

Mauvais-Jarvis, P., and Kuttenn, F., 1975, L'insuffisance en progestérone est-elle cancérigène ? Nouv. Presse Med., 4, 323-326.

Mauvais-Jarvis, P., Sterkers, N., Kuttenn, F., and Beauvais, J., 1978, Traitement des mastopathies bénignes par la progestérone et les progestatifs. Résultats en fonction du type de mastopathie. J. Gyn. Obst. Biol. Repr., 7, 477-484.

Mauvais-Jarvis, P., Tamborini, A., Sterkers, N., Ohlgiesser, G., and Mowszowicz, I., 1975, La fonction hormonale du corps jaune ovarien au cours des affections mammaires bénignes. J. Gyn. Obst. Reprod., 4, 965-970.

May-Levin, F., Contesso, G., Guerinot, F., Delarue, J.C., and Bohuon, C., 1977, Rëcepteurs des estrogènes et de la progestérone dans les affections non carcinomateuses du sein. Path. Biol., 25, 233-239.

Milligan, D., Drife, J.O., and Short, R.V., 1975, Changes in breast volume during normal menstrual cycle and after oral contraceptives. Brit. Med. J., 4, 494-496.

Monson, P.M., Yen, S., Mac Mahon, B., and Warren, S., 1976, Chronic mastitis and carcinoma of the breast. Lancet, 1, 224.

Morton, J.H., 1950, Premenstrual tension. Am. J. Obst. Gynec., 60, 343.

Nagasawa, H., and Yanai, R., 1970, Effects of prolactin or growth hormone on growth of carcinogen-induced mammary tumors of adreno-ovariectomized rats. Int. J. Cancer, 6, 488-495.

Nagel, T.C., Freinkel, N., Bell, R.M., Friesen, H., Wilber, J.F., and Metzger, B.E., 1973, Gynecomastia, prolactin and other peptide hormones in patients undergoing chronic hemodialysis. J. Clin. Endocrinol. Metab., 36, 428.

Nassar, A.M., and Smith, R.E., 1975, Menstrual variations in thermal properties of the human breast. J. Appl. Physiol., 39, 806-811.

Newsome, J.F., Timmons, R.L., Van Wyck, J., and Dugger, G.S., 1971, Pituitary stalk section for metastatic carcinoma of the breast. Ann. Surg., 174, 769-773.

Nimrod, A., and Ryan, K.J., 1975, Aromatization of androgens by human abdominal and breast fat tissue. J. Clin. Endocrinol. Metab., 40, 367-372.

Nomura, A., and Comstock, G.W., 1976, Benign breast tumor and estrogen hormones : a population based retrospective study. Am. J. Epidemiol., 103, 439-444.

Paffenbarger, R.S., Fasal, E., Simmons, M.E., and Kampert, J.B., 1977, Cancer risk as related to use of oral contraceptives during fertile years. Cancer, 39, 1887-1891.

Pearson, O.H., and Manni, A., 1978, Hormonal control of breast growth in women and rats. Curr. Top. Exper. Endocrinol., 3, 75-92.

Peck, D.R., and Lowman, R.M., 1978, Estrogen and the postmenopausal breast. J.A.M.A., 420, 1733-1735. 1733-1735.

Plata, E.J., Aoki, T., Robertson, D.D., Chu, E.W., and Gerwin, B.I., 1973, An established cultured cell line (HBT-39) from human breast carcinoma. J. Natl. Cancer Inst., 50, 849-862.

Rajendran, K.G., Shah, P.N., Bagli, N.P., Mistry, S.S., and Ghosh, S.N., 1975, Steroid biosynthetic potential of gynaecomastic tissue in man. Horm. Res., 6, 329-335.

Royal College of General Practitioners, 1977, Effect on hypertension and benign breast disease of progestagen component in combined oral contraceptives. Lancet, 1, 624.

Saez, S., Martin, P.M., and Chouvet, C.D., 1978, Estradiol and progesterone receptor levels in human breast adenocarcinoma in relation to plasma estrogen and progesterone levels. Cancer Res., 38, 3468-3473.

Sherman, B.M., and Korenman, S.G., 1974, Inadequate corpus luteum function : a pathophysiological interpretation of human breast cancer epidemiology. Cancer, 33, 1306-1312.

Sitruk-Ware, R., Seradour, B., and Lafaye, C., 1980, Treatment of benign breast diseases by progesterone topically applied. In "Percutaneous absorption of steroids". Mauvais-Jarvis P., Vichers C.F.H., Wepierre J. Eds., Academic Press, New York, in Press.

Sitruk-Ware, L.P., Sterkers, N., Mowszowicz I., and Mauvais-Jarvis, P., 1977, Inadequate corpus luteal function in women with benign breast diseases. J. Clin. Endocrinol. Metab., 44, 771-774.

Sturder, D.W., Wade-Evans, T., Paterson, M.E.L., Thom, M., and Studd, J.W.W., 1978, Relations between bleeding pattern, endometrial histology, and estrogen treatment in menopausal women. Brit. Med. J., 1, 1575-1577.

Thibault, C., and Levasseur, M.C., 1979, in "La fonction ovarienne chez les mammifères". I.N.R.A. and Masson, Paris, p 57.

Thom, M.H., White, P.J., Williams, R.M., Sturdee, D.W., Paterson, M.E.L., Wade-Evans, T., and Studd, J.W.W., 1979, Prevention and treatment of endometrial disease in climacteric women receiving estrogen therapy. Lancet, 1, 455-457.

Thorner, M.O., Round, J., Jones, A., Fahmy, D., Groom, G.V., Butcher, S., and Thomson, K., 1977, Serum prolactin and estradiol levels at different stages of puberty. Clin. Endocr., 7, 463-468.

Tseng, L., and Gurpide, E., 1975, Effects of progestins on estradiol receptor levels in human endometrium. J. Clin. Endocrinol. Metab., 41, 402-404.

Turkington, R.W., Underwood, L.E., and Van Wyk, J., 1971, Elevated serum prolactin after pituitary stalk section in man. New Engl. J. Med., 285, 707-710.

Vandaele, W., 1977, Progrès récents dans la connaissance du cycle sexuel des chiennes. Précautions à prendre lors de l'emploi de progestogènes. Ann. Med. Vet., 121, 369-381.

Varela, R.M., and Dao, T.L., 1978, Estrogen synthesis and estradiol binding by human mammary tumors. Cancer Res., 38, 2429-2433.

Vignon, F., and Rochefort, H., 1974, Régulation des récepteurs des estrogènes dans les tumeurs mammaires : effet de la prolactine in vivo. C.R. Acad. Sc. Paris, 278, 103-106.

Warren, S., 1940, The relation of "chronic mastitis" to carcinoma of the breast. Surg. Gynecol. Obstet., 71, 257-273.

Watson, G.H., Korach, K.S., and Muldoon, T., 1977, Obstruction of estrogen-receptor complex formation. Further analysis of the nature and steroidal specificity of the effect. Endocrinology, 101, 1733-1743.

Weems-Chihal, H.J., Peppler, R.D., and Dickey, R.P., 1975, Estrogen potency of oral contraceptive pills. Am. J. Obstet. Gynecol., 121, 75-81.

Wellings, S.R., Jensen, H.M., and Marcum, R.G., 1975, An atlas of subgross pathology of the human breast with special reference to precancerous lesions. J. Nat. Cancer Inst., 55, 231-273.

Whitehead, M.I., Mc Queen, J., Minardi, J., and Campbell, S., 1978, Clinical considerations in the management of the menopause : the endometrium. Postgrad. Med. J., 54, suppl.2, 69-73.

Widholm, O., Kantero, R.L., Ascelson, E., Johansson, E.D.B., and Wide, L., 1974, Endocrine changes before and after the menarche. Urinary excretion of estrogen, FSH and LH, and serum levels of progesterone FSH and LH. Acta Obstet. Gynec., 53, 197-208.

Winters, J.S., and Faiman, C., 1973, The development of cyclic pituitary gonadal function in adolescent females. J. Clin. Endocrinol. Metab., 37, 714-718.

Winters, S.J., Banks, J.L., and Loriaux, D.L., 1979, The histamine H2-antagonist cimetidine is an anti-androgen. Gastroenterology, 76, 504-508.

Wong, W.H., Freedman, R.I., Levan, N.E., Hyman, C., and Quilligan, E.J., 1972, Changes in the capillary filtration coefficient of cutaneous vessels in women with premenstrual tension. Am. J. Obstet. Gynecol., 114, 950-953.

Zeppa, R., 1969, Vascular response of the breast to estrogen. J. Clin. Endocr., 29, 695-700.

LIST OF INVITED SPEAKERS

Adnet J.J., Laboratoire Pol Bouin, Centre Hospitalier
     Universitaire, 51100 Reims, France.

Baldwin R.W., Cancer Research Campaign Laboratories,
     University of Nottingham, Nottingham, England.

Brux J. de, Institut de Pathologie, 53 rue des Belles
     feuilles, 75116 Paris, France.

Cabanne F., Centre Georges-François Leclerc, 1 rue
     du Professeur Marion, 21034 Dijon Cedex, France.

Franchimont P., Institute of Medicine, Radioimmunoassay
     Laboratory, University of Liège, Belgium.

Heuson J.C., Institut J. Bordet, Centre des tumeurs
     de l'université libre de Bruxelles,
     1000 Bruxelles, Belgium.

Hollmann K.H., Hopital Marie-Lannelongue, 133 avenue
     de la Résistance, 92350 Le Plessis Robinson,
     France.

Lasfargues E.Y., Tumor Cell Biology Laboratory,
     Institute for Medical Research, Camden, N.J. 08103.

Lignières B. de, C.H.U. Necker-Enfants-Malades, 149-161
     rue de Sèvres, 75730 Paris Cédex 15, France.

Ozzello L., Department of Pathology, University of
     Lausanne, School of Medicine, Lausanne,
     Switzerland.

Robert L., Laboratoire de Biochimie du Tissu Conjonctif,
     94010 Créteil, France.

Tubiana M., Institut Gustave Roussy, 94800 Villejuif,
        France.

Verley J.M., Hopital Marie-Lannelongue, 133 avenue de la
        Résistance, 92350 Le Plessis Robinson, France.

Wellings S.R., Department of Pathology, School of Medicine.
        University of California, Davis, California, 95616.

Zajdela A., Department of Cytopathology, Institut Curie,
        26 rue d'Ulm, 75005 Paris, France.

INDEX